THE BALANCED BODY

A Guide to Deep Tissue and Neuromuscular Therapy

Second Edition

THE BALANCED BODY

A Guide to Deep Tissue
and Neuromuscular Therapy

Second Edition

Donald W. Scheumann

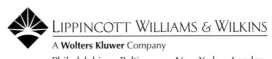

LIPPINCOTT WILLIAMS & WILKINS
A **Wolters Kluwer** Company

Philadelphia · Baltimore · New York · London
Buenos Aires · Hong Kong · Sydney · Tokyo

Editor: Peter Darcy
Managing Editor: Eric Branger
Marketing Manager: Christen DeMarco
Project Editor: Jennifer D. Weir
Indexer: Barbara DeGennaro
Designer: Armen Kojoyian
Compositor: Maryland Composition
Printer: Quebecor World, Dubuque
Art Direction: Jonathan Dimes
Artwork: David Rini, MFA, The Fine Art of Illustration

530 Walnut Street
Philadelphia, Pennsylvania 19106

351 West Camden Street
Baltimore, Maryland 21201

Library of Congress Cataloging-in-Publication Data

Scheumann, Donald W.
    The balanced body : a holistic approach to deep tissue and neuromuscular therapy / Donald W. Scheumann.—2nd ed.
      p. cm.
    Includes bibliographical references and index.
    ISBN 0-7817-3575-0
      1. Massage therapy. I. Title.

RM721 .S326 2002
615.8′22—dc21

2002066129

The publishers have made every effort to trace the copyright holders for borrowed material. If they have inadvertently overlooked any, they will be pleased to make the necessary arrangements at the first opportunity.

To purchase additional copies of this book, call our customer service department at **(800) 638-3030** or fax orders to **(301) 824-7390**. For other book services, including chapter reprints and large quantity sales, ask for the Special Sales department.

For all other calls originating outside of the United States, please call **(301)714-2324.**

Visit *Lippincott Williams & Wilkins on the Internet*: http://www.lww.com. Lippincott Williams & Wilkins customer service representatives are available from 8:30 am to 6:00 pm, EST, Monday through Friday, for telephone access.

04 05 06
4 5 6 7 8 9 10

TO JEANNE ALAND, WHO ALWAYS BELIEVED IN ME.

—DS

Preface

No man is an island, entire of itself; every man is a piece of the continent, a part of the main
—John Donne

As members of the human race, we do not exist in isolation from each other, but within webs of complex, interwoven relationships. We are all linked to each other through the dynamic interactions of families, friends, co-workers, communities, and nations. The repercussions of each person's acts resonate through those around him or her, often extending far outside the range of the immediate environment. It is becoming increasingly apparent that the manner in which we conduct our lives creates an imprint that has far-reaching impact.

Perhaps the most significant relationship we have is with our own body. The body's sensory apparatus provides the medium for contact with the world around us. We communicate to others through speech and touch. Our bodily movements and facial expressions reveal inner thoughts and feelings, often more deeply and honestly than our words. Unfortunately, for many of us this relationship is the one to which we devote the least amount of attention. We are often out of touch with our own physicality, which diminishes our capacity to establish meaningful relationships with other people. To be truly effective in our dealings with the world around us, it is imperative that we not only have an acquaintance with but some measure of mastery over the world within us as expressed through the body.

The physical body itself has an immediate, on-going relationship with the earth through its interaction with the earth's gravitational field. When the body is aligned and harmoniously balanced within the force of gravity, movement flows easily, stress is minimized, pain is reduced, and vitality is increased. Under these conditions, our feelings are more accessible and our thoughts more clearly delineated. We are more effective in our interactions with others and our impact on the world around us is powerful. A body that is distorted through poor posture and tense muscles is straining against the effects of gravity, creating potential conflict that can interfere with our ability to recognize and act on authentic, internal motivations.

Physical hands-on methods of manipulating soft tissues to improve the health and function of the body have existed for millennia. However, it is only within the past century, in Western cultures at least, that body therapies have been developed whose primary goal is to organize the body along a gravitational orientation to reduce internal stress and thus improve the relationship between body and mind. A major forum for this approach to body therapy has been the Esalen Institute in Big Sur, California. Many of the pioneers of holistic, integrative styles of massage therapy have introduced their work at Esalen, from where it has proliferated throughout the United States.

The system of massage therapy described in this book draws inspiration from this holistic perspective. The holistic view of health care has served as the foundation and philosophy of the Atlanta School of Massage, where I received my initial education in massage and was introduced to deep tissue therapy. The education I received there taught me the value of combining various massage modalities to affect a person on many levels. Generally, any single method of massage therapy emphasizes improvement in one or two of the body's systems. Systematically blending several massage approaches in an intelligent manner creates a synergistic effect that can greatly enhance the results of body therapy.

My intention in creating this textbook was to make available a comprehensive course in integrative soft tissue manipulation presented in an easy-to-learn format of experiential lessons. The chapters are laid out so that the student progresses through the body logically and systematically to gain a thorough understanding of the design and functions of the various body segments as well as their relationship to each other. Students are always encouraged to view the effects of their interventions on the body as a whole, no matter how small the area of focus may be. A key concept in following a holistic perspective to massage therapy is that change effected anywhere in the body affects the entire body.

The crux of this integrated system is a type of massage known as deep tissue therapy. Deep tissue massage therapy acts as a bridge between the structural realignment approaches to body therapy and relaxation-oriented styles of massage. It combines the benefits of both of these modalities by effectively reducing or eliminating the many layers of tension the body has accumulated since childhood. By extracting this tension from the soft tissues, structural integrity is promoted and the body's natural state of fluid ease can be re-established. Deep tissue therapy, as presented in this course, is supplemented with other styles of body work that address the neurologic, circulatory, respiratory, and energetic systems as well as the body's connective tissues.

Due to the comprehensive scope of this integrated deep tissue therapy approach, it has broad appeal to a wide range of clients' needs. The primary goal of this work is to minimize stress to the body by reducing muscular imbalances that distort its relationship to the gravitational field. In so doing, the body will naturally be less subject to pain and wear-and-tear. Injuries are less likely to occur, and an overall sense of well-being is encouraged. Within this overall context of establishing optimal physical functioning, the ability to perform specific rehabilitative work and perform general relaxation and stress reduction massage are among the skills of a well-trained deep tissue therapist.

This textbook provides the necessary tools to train a fully qualified deep tissue therapist. The philosophical and theoretical underpinnings of the integrated deep tissue therapy system are laid out at the beginning of the book. The rationales for including each of the massage modalities that are incorporated in the system are fully explained. The intent behind and approach to performing the techniques selected from these modalities are described as well. All the deep tissue and neuromuscular therapy techniques used are fully explained and illustrated. Concise, essential guidelines for practicing proper body mechanics while performing the techniques are also provided.

One of the major challenges in designing a training manual for deep tissue therapy is to try to convey the quality of touch and intent necessary to make the deep tissue strokes effective and safe. To help meet this challenge, explanations of the effects of deep tissue and neuromuscular therapy techniques on the myofascial and nervous systems are included. The characteristics and functions of different types of skeletal muscle are described as well as the kinesthetic feeling of various kinds of tense, aberrant tissues, as part of learning the palpatory skills necessary to be a competent therapist.

A unique feature of this book is the inclusion of 10 guidelines for developing a conscious, caring, and sensitive approach to performing deep tissue therapy. These guidelines summarize the qualities and principles necessary to perform deep tissue therapy properly. They elucidate the foundation on which the integrated deep tissue therapy system rests.

It would be counter-productive to try to describe step-by-step deep tissue therapy sessions that can be applied by rote to every client. Every person's body is different. Everyone's patterns of tension, areas of pain, and movement habits are unique. A skilled deep tissue therapist knows how to assess and work with each individual's myofascial patterns of distortion by designing therapy sessions specifically targeted to that client's requirements. The necessary information and guidance to implement individualized sessions of deep tissue therapy is provided throughout the book. Postural evaluation outlines accompany each lesson along with range of motion charts of the major joints. The origins, insertions, and actions as well as common trigger points of every muscle that appears in the deep tissue routines are listed.

The deep tissue routines are sequenced according to a structural realignment model. This approach was taken to help students better understand functional relationships between the various body segments and to reinforce the overlying concept of this system, which is to always consider the body as a unified entity. The first part of each deep tissue lesson contains practical information about the musculoskeletal system and kinesiologic concepts relating to the areas of the body being studied, a component that is often missing in massage texts. Acquiring a thorough understanding of how the body moves is essential to understanding postural distortions and muscular tension patterns and, therefore, to being able to design effective therapy sessions.

As explained within the body of the text, the deep tissue routines described in this book are meant to be learning tools and act as broad outlines for deep tissue therapy sessions on a particular area of the body. The overall sequence and pattern of a deep tissue session is delineated, along with descriptions and illustrations for performing deep tissue and neuromuscular therapy techniques on every major muscle within the designated section of the body. These sessions are to be practiced in their totality when learning the work so that the student can become expert in all the necessary techniques. However, within the context of an actual session with a client, these session outlines are to be used more for reference purposes. They may be adapted to suit each client's unique patterns and needs. When all the lessons have been learned and assimilated, the therapist may feel free to combine material from several sessions when it serves the best interest of the client.

It is my desire that students studying this textbook will acquire the knowledge, skill, and confidence to think creatively and allow the foundation of this integrated deep tissue therapy system to grow within them as they approach a level of mastery. No two people ever perform massage therapy in exactly the same way. There are certainly principles and precautions that should never be ignored or transgressed when it comes to the health, safety, and integrity of both client and therapist. However, there is always room for adaptation and exploration. For example, if a therapist finds that performing a particular stroke the way it is described in the text is awkward or causing discomfort, that therapist should feel free to find an alternative way to execute it.

This approach to massage therapy is meant to be, at its best, transformational. It is hoped that clients receiving integrated deep tissue therapy acquire the means to improve their relationship with their body and find greater ease within their life. It is my desire that as interest in massage therapy continues to grow and its benefits are experienced by more people, the possibility of living in harmonious relationship with our self and with others does not remain a hopeful platitude but becomes a vital reality.

Acknowledgments

To the editorial staff at Lippincott Williams & Wilkins, who provided strong support and guidance: Pete Darcy, Eric Branger, and Kathleen Scogna.

To the artists who did such a phenomenal job drawing the illustrations.

To all of my colleagues, past and present, at the Atlanta School of Massage.

To the many teachers along the way who have contributed to my quest to understand the body, movement, and life.

To James Fryzel, who gave so generously of his time to pose for many of the illustrations.

To Chris MacHarg, who helps me in so many ways and is always there to listen.

To Leslie Stevens, for giving her perspective on the first three chapters.

To all the reviewers, who offered many helpful suggestions for improving the manuscript.

D. Scheumann

Contents

Introduction to the Integrated Deep Tissue Therapy System

1

Overview of the Integrated Deep Tissue System

INTRODUCTION

This is a training manual for learning an integrated approach to massage therapy, emphasizing deep tissue and neuromuscular therapy. It is designed for students who have completed an introductory program of basic massage procedures. This course will incorporate and expand on techniques used in Swedish and other forms of circulatory massage, while introducing many other methods of addressing soft tissue dysfunction.

Integrated deep tissue therapy is a highly effective method of soft tissue treatment in that it combines several modalities that emphasize different aspects and qualities of the myofascial system. When combined, these techniques provide a comprehensive protocol for reducing or eliminating many different manifestations of restriction in muscles and fascia and provide the means to return the body to a healthy, strong, and vital condition.

The integrated deep tissue approach to massage therapy aligns with the Wellness Model proposed by Dr. John Travis in the 1970s.[1] This model has served as a prototype for many complementary health-care treatment protocols and holistic health centers that have been created since that time.

Travis and his co-author, Regina Sara Ryan, viewed wellness as an on-going dynamic process of self-activated participation in the health and welfare of one's being. According to this perspective, humans are composed of a series of integrated systems that all work synergistically toward optimal health and well-being. This means that our physical, mental, emotional, and spiritual states are vital factors in determining the condition of our bodies and our outlooks on life.

According to Ilya Prigogene's Nobel Prize winning theory of dissipative structures,[2] human beings, as well as all living organisms, are examples of an organizing principle known as the open system. An open system operates by taking in energy, metabolizing or converting it for use, and then releasing or dissipating energy back into the environment. All our vital processes depend on the

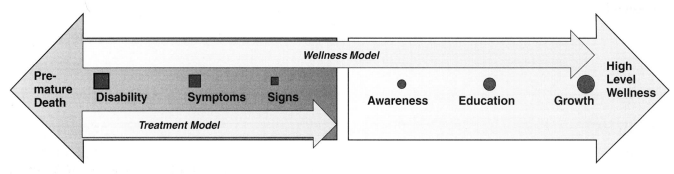

FIGURE I-I The Wellness Model. (Reprinted with permission from Travis JW, Ryan RS. Wellness workbook. Berkeley, CA: Ten Speed Press, 1981.)

smooth and efficient transformation of energy for the health and integrity of the human system to remain intact.

The three primary ways that we receive energy are through the air we breathe, the food we eat, and the sensory input received by the nervous system and sense organs. In a state of health, the physiologic pathways provided for conduction and transformation of energy throughout the body operate effectively and efficiently. When our biologic conduits falter, the stage is set for disease and breakdown to occur.

Massage therapy provides excellent assistance in the maintenance of high-level wellness as it directly or indirectly affects many of the systems that transport and transform energy within the body. The circulatory, respiratory, muscular, endocrine, and nervous system functions can all be improved through the application of manual massage techniques.

As the flow of energy through the body is improved, psychological and physiologic activities are affected. When the body is performing at peak levels, our ability to interact with our environment is vastly improved. This can have a direct effect on the quality of our relationships and our mental and emotional outlooks in general.

Dr. Travis' Wellness Model depicts the process of achieving wellness as a journey along a continuum (Fig. 1-1). The midpoint of the scale, labeled neutral, represents a condition of moderate well-being where the individual is capable of functioning in everyday life without too much difficulty. For many, this average state of health has been

accepted as the norm, and maintaining it is considered the best-case scenario.

The left side of the scale depicts gradual decline from the neutral state of wellness through a series of signs and symptoms of degenerating health that can eventually lead to disability or even premature death. It is hoped that a person experiencing this slide into dysfunction will seek adequate care and return to the neutral point of wellness. The halting of physical and/or psychological breakdown and the rebuilding of health is called the Treatment Model. Most traditionally recognized physical and psychological therapies are based on this goal.

The right side of the scale depicted in the Wellness Model represents what Travis calls high level wellness. This half of the continuum describes movement toward expanding states of greater well-being beyond the neutral stage of adequate functioning. These states of more complete fulfillment and happiness are motivated by increased awareness, pursuit of education, and personal growth. Achievement of these states is largely self-motivated as a person seeks out ways to explore opportunities for expansion of consciousness, creative expression, and productivity.

The Wellness Model describes a potential for personal excellence that we are all capable of achieving. Any method of treatment or intervention that leads a person back along the road to health can potentially provide the momentum to motivate that individual to seek the knowledge that will guide him or her to the highest level of wellness that person is capable of manifesting.

INTEGRATED DEEP TISSUE SYSTEM

The integrated deep tissue therapy method of bodywork encompasses the spectrum of the illness/wellness scale in that it can be used to provide assistance and education at almost any point along the continuum. It must be stated that this approach to massage therapy does not attempt

to replace any form of medical treatment, physical or psychological. Massage therapists are not trained to diagnose, treat, or give prescriptions for any kind of medical condition, nor are they qualified to provide psychological evaluations or counseling.

Massage therapists are trained to work with the body's soft tissues to reduce tension and alleviate restrictions in the myofascial system and to increase fluid circulation within the body. Massage therapy education includes instruction in manual techniques applied to the body's myofascial tissues to improve their function as well as instruction in stretching and joint mobilization techniques.

Massage therapists need to be familiar with the factors that lead to soft tissue dysfunction, including postural abnormalities and movement habits that can result in misuse, abuse, and injury to the body. They must also understand the role of the mind and emotions in creating heightened activity of the sympathetic nervous system that can lead to muscular tension and pain.

A person who practices integrated deep tissue therapy may be viewed primarily as an educator. Through manipulation and realignment of the body's soft tissues, the therapist teaches the client to experience the benefits of becoming more relaxed, balanced, and pain free. The client may then be motivated to gain the necessary information to make lifestyle improvements that will assist in sustaining this higher state of well-being. These adjustments may include receiving regular massage therapy, instituting a fitness program, improving nutrition, and learning meditation or other forms of stress reduction.

Integrated deep tissue therapy incorporates viewpoints and methodologies from both Western and Eastern approaches to health. Many of the soft tissue techniques used were developed within the context of the Western rehabilitative therapy model. A primary goal of these techniques is to improve muscle function by enhancing oxygen and nutritive levels within muscle fibers, reducing the effects of scar tissue and other adhering factors in the myofascia, and decreasing pain by minimizing irritation to nerve endings due to trapped waste products.

The techniques of energy balance and enhancement utilized are mostly drawn from Eastern bodywork modalities. The perspective on health provided by the Wellness Model and advocated by the integrated deep tissue therapy system is decidedly holistic, as are many of the traditional Asian health-care practices. (For a good introduction to the holistic perspective offered by Chinese medicine, the reader is referred to Beinfield and Korngold[3].) The holistic perspective views all aspects of a person—including the body, mind, lifestyle, and relationships—as important contributing factors to the overall state of health.

ORIGINS

In embracing both the rehabilitative and holistic perspectives on health care, the integrated deep tissue therapy system follows in the tradition of many bodywork

approaches that have been developed or promoted since the 1960s. A variety of sources have contributed to weave the tapestry that makes up this comprehensive style of body therapy. The techniques incorporated are shown in Figure 1-2.

The overriding goal of integrated deep tissue therapy is to establish an internal environment whereby energy may be taken into the body, utilized, and dissipated back into the environment in a fluid, efficient manner. This is largely accomplished through assessing and removing restrictions in the myofascial system, which manifest as shortened or adhered areas within the muscles and fascia resulting in limited function and possibly pain. As the physical body is restored to a condition of optimal performance capability, many signs and symptoms of malfunction often dissipate. A better self-image and a more positive outlook toward life in general may accompany this improvement in physical well-being.

One of the first people to develop a method of bodywork based on this concept of comprehensive, overall body assessment and realignment was Dr. Ida Rolf. Her style of therapy is called Structural Integration, commonly known as Rolfing. Dr. Rolf was a biochemist who began to formulate the principles and techniques of Structural Integration in the 1940s. She developed a 10-session series of bodywork in which the fascial network is manipulated to realign the vertical axis of the body to the earth's gravitational field. Many of the newer styles of deep tissue therapy and myofascial work are at least partially derived from Dr. Rolf's pioneering concepts.

Neuromuscular therapy, or trigger point release work, rests on a foundation laid by Dr. Janet Travell. Dr. Travell was a cardiologist who served two presidents as White House physician. She did much research in the area of muscular involvement in pain causation and relief. Her

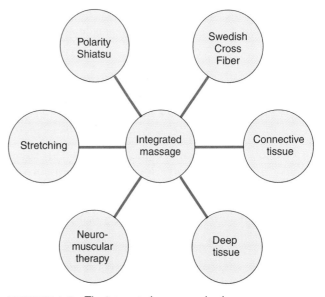

FIGURE 1-2 The integrated massage wheel.

two-volume work, *Myofascial Pain and Dysfunction, The Trigger Point Manual,* co-authored with David Simmons, MD, serves as the seminal guide in this field.

The pioneering psychologist, Dr. Wilhelm Reich, developed many of the concepts of mind and body interaction that are incorporated in various styles of bodywork as well as several forms of somatic psychotherapy. Among other thought-provoking concepts, Dr. Reich proposed theories about how the shape and tone of the body are greatly influenced by the inner psychic structure.

He also discovered that patterns of chronic tension based on restricted feelings become lodged in the neuromuscular system, contributing to conditions of neurosis. By confronting these holding patterns in the soft tissues through physical manipulation, various exercises designed to amplify the tension, and conscious breathing, Dr. Reich found that the unconscious tension blocks could be released and the underlying feelings expressed.

Polarity therapy is a comprehensive holistic health-care practice that includes physical manipulations performed while the patient is on a massage table. It was developed by Dr. Randolph Stone and was based on his many years of study of traditional healing systems worldwide. The basic premise of polarity therapy is that health is built on freeing blockages in the underlying energetic pathways that provide organizational templates for the physical and psychological structures. Dr. Stone's writings and work have a broad interface with many styles of bodywork, including structural integration, acupressure, craniosacral therapy, myofascial release, and energetic forms of healing, like therapeutic touch.

The above list of pioneers in the art of healing whose works have illuminated the integrated deep tissue therapy system described in this manual is only a partial one. Many other talented individuals have also participated in the design and refinement of techniques that are incorporated in this fluidly adaptable synthesis of massage modalities. Their contributions are acknowledged and appreciated.

COMPONENTS OF THE INTEGRATED DEEP TISSUE SYSTEM

The techniques incorporated in the integrated deep tissue method are depicted on a wheel (Fig. 1-2) rather than in a list. This is done to illustrate that they need not always be applied in a predetermined sequence but can be blended and mixed as required by the specific situation.

In each lesson in this text, the techniques are described in a prescribed order that is suggested as a general protocol for approaching the body. This sequence opens the body progressively, beginning with preparatory contact between therapist and client, then warm-up of the tissues,

and then work on the deeper layers. Within this basic structure there is much room for adaptability by moving through the techniques on the wheel according to the unique needs of the individual.

DEEP TISSUE THERAPY

The heart of the integrated deep tissue system is, naturally, deep tissue therapy. Many varying styles of deep tissue therapy have been developed over the years, but there are characteristics common to all of them. The primary function of deep tissue therapy is to reduce the level of stress imposed on the body by chronically shortened muscles. This is accomplished by applying a combination of slow compressive and lengthening procedures to the involved musculature.

The effects of chronically shortened, tense muscles are many. Circulation of blood and lymph is inhibited. Constricted muscles act as dams, blocking fluids from flowing freely throughout the body. It must be remembered that in an open system, energy exchange must be efficient for the system to function properly.

Muscles rely on a steady intake of oxygen and nutrients to provide the necessary energy for muscular contraction and relaxation to occur. The waste products of muscle metabolism are released into the venous blood supply to be transported out of the muscles and processed for removal from the body. If this cycle is disrupted, the muscles become toxic from lack of nutrition and build-up of waste products and can no longer perform their job effectively.

Toxicity within the muscle tissue irritates nerve endings, resulting in weakness and possible sensations of pain. This internal toxicity taxes the immune system and creates an environment in which disease can more easily take hold.

The primary function of muscles is to provide movement for the body. This is accomplished by paired groups of muscles alternately contracting and lengthening to move the bones to which they are attached. Muscles must be free to respond to stimuli from the nervous system, which sends the impulses that direct them to contract.

The fine motor skills the body is capable of performing rely on this precise balancing act of muscular contraction and relaxation. Stated in a simplified manner, as one set of muscles contracts, it pulls a bone in a particular direction, causing the opposing muscles to lengthen and yield for the movement to occur. To move the bone in the opposite direction, the sequence of events is reversed, with the lengthened muscles receiving the stimulus from the nervous system to shorten, thus moving the bone in the other direction. The currently contracted muscles then relax and lengthen to allow the bone to move.

Muscles that are chronically contracted disrupt the symmetry of balanced forces acting on the skeleton. They hold bones out of position, causing postural distortions that result in structural stress. Soft tissue integrity is compromised when the body is not in balance with the field of gravity. Fascial tissue builds up around points of stress to reinforce those areas from being pulled further out of alignment. Ligaments are also put under strain to brace misaligned joints.

Chronic uneven muscular pulls on the skeleton cause some muscles to remain contracted while opposing muscles are stretched beyond their resting length and are weakened. This results in lack of adaptability in movement, which makes the body more prone to injury. Muscle fibers that cannot lengthen are more likely to be torn during a rapid, forceful movement. Injury is most likely to occur at the musculotendinous junction or where the tendon blends with the periosteum of the bone. Unless the factors creating these stresses on the soft tissues and skeleton are relieved, the body will continue to degenerate into states of greater dysfunction and pain.

Deep tissue therapy is designed to return the body to a state of ease and balance by eliminating the uneven pulls on the skeleton caused by contracted muscles and constricted fascia. Muscular strain in the body may be assessed by watching how a person stands and moves. Manual testing of the degree of movement available at the joints also aids in determining which muscles are short, or contracted. After recognizing the patterns of muscular distortion, the deep tissue therapist systematically releases the shortened muscles and stretches the constricted fascia to re-establish freedom of movement of the bones.

Slow compressive strokes applied along the length of a muscle recalibrate the nerve receptors that determine muscle length, allowing contracted muscles to relax. These receptors are called **muscle spindles** and are located within the muscle belly parallel to the contractile fibers. Slow stretching of the muscle after the deep tissue strokes are applied also activates the **Golgi tendon organs**, which are the nerve receptors within the tendons that also help to determine the degree of tone in the muscle.

If a muscle is stretched quickly, causing the muscle spindles to lengthen rapidly, an impulse is sent through the nervous system directing the muscle to contract. This mechanism is known as the **stretch reflex**. It is a protective device that prevents muscles and tendons from being damaged from overstretching. If, however, a muscle is stretched slowly, causing the muscle spindles to lengthen slowly, the stretch reflex is overridden. A message is sent from the nervous system to allow the muscle to relax and lengthen further.

Deep tissue strokes are also performed along the borders of adjacent muscles to release fascial adhering and reduce build-up of scar tissue that may be preventing the muscles from moving independently of each other. In deep tissue therapy, muscle groups are also freed in layers, from superficial to deep, to allow each muscle to perform its appropriate actions without restriction. Removing these glitches from the musculature frees obstructions that are binding the muscles and not allowing full movement capability.

The benefits of deep tissue therapy are many. As the soft tissues of the body are realigned and balance is returned to the skeleton, there is much less strain imposed on the nervous system. This results in better posture and freer movement, which greatly reduce the risk of injury. Coordination is improved. Minimizing strain around joints reduces the incidence of osteoarthritis and the possibility of ligament tears. Reducing the amount of energy used in holding chronically contracted muscles increases the overall level of vitality and promotes clearer thinking. All the body's systems benefit from having more metabolic energy available to fuel them.

NEUROMUSCULAR THERAPY

Neuromuscular therapy is a specialized form of deep tissue work that treats a specific manifestation of muscular dysfunction known as trigger points. Trigger points are tiny areas of irritation that form within strained bands of muscle tissue. They refer sensations of pain, weakness, or numbness to either surrounding or distant areas of muscle tissue.

Trigger points are present in the majority of cases of chronic muscular pain. They are formed as a result of muscular strain. This can be the result of some kind of trauma, including an accident, exposure to cold or infection, or overuse of a particular set of muscles. Areas of strain also form in misaligned areas of the body where muscles have to work constantly to maintain distorted positions of the bones. Trigger points always manifest in areas of musculature that are shortened. It is common to locate trigger points in contracted muscles that are being treated by deep tissue therapy.

The exact mechanism of trigger point activation is unknown. Dr. Travell postulated that the constant presence of waste products within a damaged group of muscle **fibrils**, apparently produced by unrelenting cellular metabolism in that section of the muscle, stimulates nerve endings in the area to send amplified input into the spinal cord.[4] This stimulus is then thrown back into the peripheral nervous system through weakened or **facilitated nerve pathways**. The impulses traveling along these nerve routes activate pain sensations in a specific portion of the muscles stimulated by those particular nerves. The areas affected by trigger points are called **referred pain zones**.

Trigger points are self-perpetuating. They accompany a phenomenon known as the stress-tension-pain cycle. Stress can be generated by a number of factors, including physical trauma, as discussed above. Emotional trauma produces many of the same symptoms as physical stress, including muscular tension.

The body attempts to isolate areas of trauma through a process known as **muscle splinting**. This is a protective mechanism whereby muscles around the injured area contract to isolate the trauma and prevent movement that could lead to further damage. Scar tissue tends to build up in this area as well as taut bands of muscle fibers that are unyielding. The lack of circulation that occurs within these frozen bands of tissue, in addition to the cellular damage brought about as a result of the trauma, fosters the formation of trigger points.

The activation of trigger points produces discomfort and pain in the musculature. Sensations of pain in the body invariably raise a person's stress level. This leads to heightened tension, which fosters the conditions that increase pain, and thus the cycle is perpetuated.

Neuromuscular therapy attempts to disrupt the stress-tension-pain cycle by locating trigger points and deactivating them. Manual pressure applied directly to the trigger point for 8 to 12 seconds disrupts the flow of nerve impulses activating the referred pain zone, diminishing the sensations of pain felt there.

There are several hypotheses as to why compression of a trigger point disrupts the pain cycle. Oxygen levels at the location of a deactivated trigger point have been found to be measurably less, leading to the conclusion that diminished oxygen reduces the rate of unbridled cellular metabolism that perpetuates trigger point firing. Pressure on the trigger point may also instigate the release of endorphins and enkephalin, two of the body's natural pain fighters.

To prevent the trigger point from becoming reactivated, it is important to keep the muscle fibers around it lengthened. The therapist should stretch the affected muscle after treating it and instruct the client to continue to stretch that area on a regular basis.

The tissue breakdown that led to the formation of trigger points is not necessarily repaired by pressure point treatment. The goal of neuromuscular therapy is to reduce the active firing of trigger points to manage pain and stress levels in the body. This form of therapy works best when accompanied by other massage modalities that keep the muscles lengthened and relaxed, thus reducing the likelihood of future trigger point formation and activation.

SWEDISH MASSAGE

Swedish massage is classified as a circulatory style of massage. Its broad, sweeping strokes promote increased blood flow through muscle tissue which facilitates metabolic efficiency. The Swedish style is also quite effective at inducing relaxation in the body by enhancing parasympathetic nervous system activity. It is often performed as a full-body massage, which helps to bring a sense of wholeness, continuity, and integration to the recipient.

Within the integrated deep tissue approach, Swedish techniques are used to warm up the tissues in preparation for deeper, more specific work. Swedish strokes are also incorporated to initiate the process of re-establishing the proper directions for the myofascial tissues to follow to eliminate stress-producing misalignment. The massage therapist can utilize these strokes almost like a sculptor, shaping and remolding the body into a better-organized configuration of muscle and bone.

Integrated deep tissue therapy is primarily a nonverbal form of communication with the body's nervous system and soft tissue components, designed to re-educate the reflex arcs to produce more effective movement patterns. The relaxing, pleasurable, lengthening sensations generated by Swedish massage strokes are the perfect vehicle for introducing sensations of ease and comfort.

CROSS FIBER

Cross fiber techniques are incorporated along with the Swedish strokes to further relax the muscle groups and assist in the elimination of myofascial restrictions. The application of strokes perpendicular to the direction of muscle fibers rather than parallel to them is the distinguishing characteristic of all styles of cross fiber manipulation.

The cross fiber strokes used in the integrated deep tissue system are performed bilaterally. This means that they are applied across the muscle fibers in both directions, forward and back, rather than in one direction only. The procedure consists of rolling bundles of muscle fibers over each other using either the fingers or broad side of the thumb to release adhesions. Adhered muscle fibers diminish circulation of blood and lymph and inhibit the ability of the muscle to fully contract and lengthen.

CONNECTIVE TISSUE TECHNIQUES

Connective tissue manipulations are designed to stretch the fascial membranes that surround and penetrate the musculature. The fascial component of muscles is both strong and flexible and is responsible for providing support to all the body's structures. The degree of fascial mobility is an important factor in determining the shape of the body. As inhibiting factors in the fascia are released through slow stretching and low-force compressive movements, a renewed quality of expansiveness and freedom can be introduced to the body.

Many varieties of connective tissue release work have been formulated. The maneuvers presented here have been chosen for their effectiveness in spreading fascial membranes in conjunction with deep tissue therapy. Freeing the surrounding fascia is necessary to accommodate muscle lengthening that occurs due to the release of contracted fibers brought about by the deep tissue strokes.

STRETCHING

Lengthening the soft tissues through stretching movements serves several important functions. The therapist stretches the recipient's muscles during a massage treatment for them to better assimilate the neuromuscular changes that have occurred during the session. Stretching on one's own after receiving a deep tissue therapy treatment is highly encouraged. Maintaining muscle length through stretching reduces the overall level of stress in the body and helps eliminate many of the muscular imbalances that can result in pain and injury.

Massage is essentially a passive process for the recipient in that during the session the client's body is manipulated and moved primarily by the therapist. For the changes brought about by deep tissue bodywork to become permanent, the client must activate the recalibrated reflex arcs achieved in the session through volitional movement based on the body's new alignment. Otherwise, the previous aberrant muscle patterns will soon return and progress toward greater body function will be halted.

ENERGY WORK

Techniques of energy balancing are based on the premise that the body is formed and nourished by patterns of energy currents that determine the state of health and vitality of the individual. When these energy pathways are flowing freely, all the body's systems are fortified and continued growth and development are assured. Weakening or blockage of the energy currents eventually leads to breakdown within the body.

The two methods of energy balancing that are included in this course are polarity and Shiatsu. They are both complete systems of bodywork and health care that require extensive specialized training to learn in their entirety. Practitioners of this style of deep tissue therapy are not to be considered experts in either of these modalities unless they have acquired the education to meet the necessary requirements. A few techniques from both of these healing systems have been included to enhance the effects of the deep tissue therapy.

Polarity therapy likens the body's energy currents to the flow of magnetic forces, with positive and negative poles (Fig. 1-3). Balance between these two poles is mediated by a third, or neutral, pole. Blockage through any of

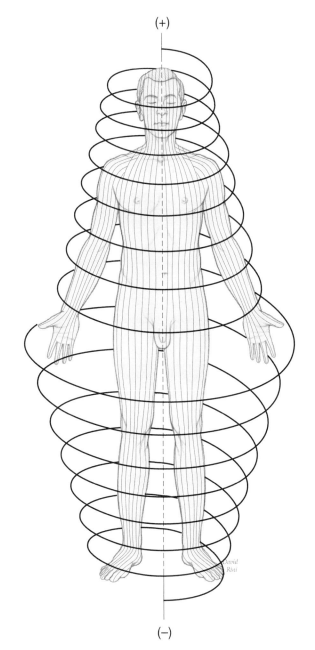

(+)

(−)

FIGURE 1-3   Polarity energy currents.

these three poles weakens the natural flow of energy. This inhibition of energy flow manifests physically as myofascial restriction.[5] Most of the polarity procedures described in these lessons consist of contacts where the therapist places his or her two hands on the client's body corresponding to this flow of energy to enhance the body's natural healing abilities.

Polarity procedures are applied at the beginning of the session to help induce relaxation and a state of readiness on the part of the client. The simple polarity holds described are very effective at reducing sympathetic nervous system stimulation, allowing the client's body to

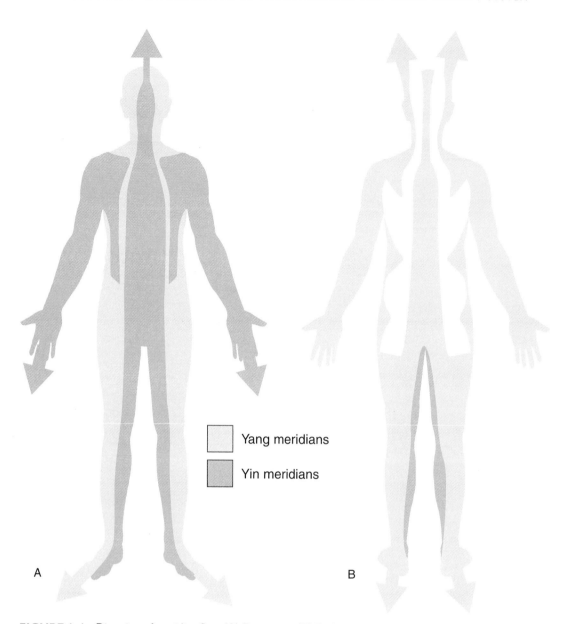

Yang meridians

Yin meridians

FIGURE I-4   Direction of meridian flow. (**A**) Front view. (**B**) Back view.

assimilate the effects of the massage treatment more effectively. The sustained contact characteristic of the opening polarity maneuvers, along with their innately nurturing quality, assists in building a bond of confidence and trust between the therapist and client.

Shiatsu is a Japanese style of bodywork that encourages the flow of the life energy, or **qi**, through a series of energy channels known as **meridians** (Fig. 1-4A and B). It is administered through a combination of compressive strokes and stretching of the body along these pathways. The Shiatsu procedures described in this course were chosen to bolster the effects of the accompanying deep tissue release work. By improving the flow of the vital life energies of the body, the release of soft tissue restrictions usually occurs more easily and is sustained for a longer period.

Methods of bodywork exploring the combination of Eastern and Western modalities are becoming increasingly popular. The reader is referred to two books, *Informed Touch* by Finando and Finando[6] and *Acupuncture, Trigger Points and Musculoskeletal Pain* by Baldry,[7] for more information on this topic.

REFERENCES

1. Travis JW, Ryan RS. Wellness workbook. 2nd ed. Berkeley, CA: Ten Speed Press, 1988.
2. Travis JW, Ryan RS. Wellness workbook. 2nd ed. Berkeley, CA: Ten Speed Press, 1988: xxii.
3. Beinfield H, Korngold E. Between heaven and earth: a guide to Chinese medicine. New York, NY: Ballantine, 1992.

4. Travell JG, Simons DG. Myofascial pain and dysfunction: the trigger point manual. Baltimore, MD: Williams & Wilkins, 1983: 35.

5. Stone R. The wireless anatomy of man and its function. In: Polarity therapy: the complete collected works. Sebastopol, CA: CRCS Publications, 1999; ZS1: charts 15 and 16.

6. Finando D, Finando L. Informed touch: a clinician's guide to the evaluation and treatment of myofascial disorders. Rochester, VT: Healing Arts Press, 1999.

7. Baldry PE. Acupuncture, trigger points and musculoskeletal pain. 2nd ed. London: Churchill Livingstone, 1993.

SUGGESTED READINGS

General

Tappan FM, Benjamin P. Tappan's handbook of healing massage techniques: classic, holistic, and emerging methods. Upper Saddle River, NJ: Prentice Hall, 1998.

Shiatsu

Lundberg P. The book of Shiatsu. New York, NY: Simon & Schuster, 1992.

Polarity

Burger B. Esoteric anatomy: the body as consciousness. Berkeley, CA: North Atlantic Books, 1998.

Stone R. Polarity therapy: the complete collected works. Sebastopol, CA: CRCS Publications, 1999; ZS1, 2.

Swedish and Connective Tissue

Fritz S. Mosby's fundamentals of therapeutic massage. 2nd ed. St. Louis, MO: Mosby-Year Book, 1999.

Neuromuscular Therapy

Chaitow L. Modern neuromuscular techniques. London: Churchill Livingstone, 1996.

Learning the Work

INTRODUCTION

The latter portion of this book consists of the integrated deep tissue therapy lessons. Each lesson contains essential information for learning and understanding this system of deep tissue therapy. The book is not to be considered a self-teaching guide. It is best used as a supplement to instruction by an experienced instructor who has mastered the system and can give the student the necessary guidance and feedback. While learning the work, the lessons should be read and practiced in the order presented in the book. They have been organized to teach the student a logical, sequential approach to mastering the concepts of integrated deep tissue therapy.

The routines given in the lessons do not represent exact reproductions of specific bodywork sessions that would actually be performed on a client. Rather, they outline a general sequence of possible moves for an area of the body. Each routine describes techniques for releasing most of the muscles associated with that particular part of the body. Although the therapist needs to know all these techniques, he or she would not use every procedure described on any one client.

The student will practice all the techniques in each lesson on a partner in class; this is done so that both students can learn the material effectively. There is no way to determine which techniques would be most beneficial for any individual without assessing that person according to his or her own particular needs.

FORMAT OF THE LESSONS

Each lesson is divided into two parts. The first portion presents information and assessment tools that provide the foundation for acquiring the skills of a deep tissue therapist. The second part of the lesson describes the techniques that are used in the integrated deep tissue system, based on its six components.

The first part of each lesson is divided into the following sections.

INTRODUCTION

This section presents general concepts and information pertaining to the area of the body under discussion. It acquaints the student with the overall design of this body segment and describes the relationships between the muscles and bones.

MUSCULOSKELETAL ANATOMY AND FUNCTION

This portion of the lesson expands on the information mentioned in the introduction. The material discussed here focuses on the related muscles' anatomy and movement capabilities as they pertain to integrated deep tissue therapy.

CONDITIONS

These are common problems, diseases, indications, and contraindications that the deep tissue therapist may encounter. It is not an inclusive list; it is designed to point out highlights. The student is encouraged to do further research in this area as needed. (*Taber's Cyclopedic Medical Dictionary*[1] is an excellent reference for medical conditions and terms.)

MIND/BODY CONNECTION

The holistic scope of the work is discussed in this section. Students are introduced to concepts about the relationship between thoughts, beliefs, and emotions and the physical state.

POSTURAL EVALUATION

An outline for a full analysis of the segments of the body being studied is included here. Postural evaluation is one of the major assessment tools of the deep tissue therapist. It provides the necessary information to outline a plan of bodywork for an individual client. It also serves as a guide to assess changes in the client's body due to the application of integrated deep tissue therapy.

EXERCISES AND SELF-TREATMENT

Included here are exercises the client can do on his or her own that will stretch and strengthen the muscles that have been treated in the sessions. These exercises can be taught to the client so that they can be performed between massage sessions and will enhance the results of the deep tissue therapy.

QUICK REFERENCE CHARTS

1. *Indications/Contraindications.* This chart gives a brief synopsis of common reasons to perform massage treatments and conditions that could make receiving treatments inadvisable.
2. *Essential Anatomy.* This chart lists the muscles, bones, and bony landmarks that will be referred to and/or worked on in the lesson.
3. *Conditions/Muscles Involved.* This chart outlines the most common muscles involved in certain postural deviations.
4. *Range of Motion.* Most of the possible movements for each major joint are listed, along with the muscles that perform those actions. Testing range of motion lets the therapist know if the client is restricted in normal movement and requires additional work on the involved muscles.

LESSON SEQUENCE

The order of presentation of the integrated deep tissue lessons has been planned to maximize the learning process by giving the student a clear understanding of the organization of the body according to structure and function. The author is indebted to the pioneering work of Dr. Ida Rolf, who conceived a unique vision of the body's design and created a logical, effective plan to reorganize the soft tissues within the field of gravity.[1]

Integrated deep tissue therapy is not considered a form of structural integration in the Rolfing tradition, in that it does not follow the progressive 10-session series plan that is characteristic of that style of bodywork. (See Suggested Readings for information about the theory and principles of Rolfing.) The overall layout of the lesson plans in this book does follow, in a very general way, the sequence of treatment that Rolf advocated. This sequence is suggested as an effective order in which to perform a series of deep tissue therapy sessions done with a client over a period of time. It exemplifies the eighth guideline in *The Principles of Conscious Bodywork* (see Chapter 3, page 23).

The sequence of the lessons is as follows:

1. Trunk
   a. *Chest*. Opening the chest helps to establish better breathing habits. One of the first manifestations of inhibited feelings and bodily sensations is restricted breathing. Releasing the breathing mechanism is crucial for the rest of the deep tissue work to be fully effective. The increased oxygen intake acquired by full, deep breathing is necessary to fuel the metabolic changes that are brought about by deep tissue therapy.
   b. *Spine and Back Muscles*. The spine supports the weight segments of the upper half of the body. It must be aligned properly to perform this function properly. When the vertebrae are aligned, the nerves passing through the spinal column are unimpeded. Lengthening the spine helps to organize the soft tissues and bones of the trunk. Freeing the back muscles helps to further balance the chest area in the front of the trunk.
2. The Upper Extremity
   a. *Scapula*. This is the root of the upper extremity. Many of the muscles that attach the arm to the body are anchored on the scapula. Freeing the scapulae extends the range of motion of the arms and takes pressure off the ribcage.
   b. *Shoulder and Upper Arm*. Treatment proceeds progressively from the proximal portion of the arm to the distal portion. Release of the rotator cuff muscles and other muscles of the shoulder helps to reposition the arm and improve alignment of the upper body.
   c. *Forearm and Hand*. The muscles that control the hand are the smallest of the upper extremity. Reestablishing refined movement of the hand helps strengthen its connection to the brain and contributes to the reduction of tension throughout the body.
3. The Lower Limb
   a. *Foot, Leg, and Knee*. Reflexively, this body segment mirrors the hand and forearm. Massage work on both the feet and hands helps to tonify all the body's systems and contributes to an overall sense of well-being. The foot forms the foundation for vertical support of the entire body. This area needs to be realigned to accommodate the shifts that have occurred by opening the upper body.
4. Thigh, Abdomen, and Pelvis

   Work on the thigh muscles accompanies release of the core muscles of the trunk. Many of the thigh muscles attach on the pelvis, and they greatly affect pelvic positioning and overall body alignment. The progression of the sequence on the lower extremity is upward, from the foot to the pelvis.
   a. *Posterior Thigh and Hip*. The posterior thigh muscles draw the base of the pelvis downward and flex the knees. They counterbalance the actions of the quadriceps muscles on the anterior thigh. The hip muscles control the movements of the femur and tend to accumulate tension.

   The pelvis forms the body's center of gravity. Muscles attached to it tie the upper and lower portions of the body together. Increasing sensory awareness in the pelvic region facilitates well-coordinated full-body movement.

   The abdominal muscles provide support for the lower spine and assist in holding the viscera in place. The abdominal cavity is the seat of the **hara**, or vital life force. The body's ability to evolve to its full potential is greatly enhanced once the core has been freed.
   b. *Abdominal Muscles*. The abdominal muscles connect the chest to the pelvis and control motions of the trunk. The rectus abdominus muscle assists the hamstrings of the posterior thigh in pulling the base of the pelvis anteriorly. The quadratus lumborum, which is the deepest abdominal muscle, forms the back wall of the abdominal cavity. It counterbalances the rectus abdominus by elevating the iliac crests and moving the base of the pelvis posteriorly.

c. *Lateral Thigh, Adductors, and Intestines.* Balancing the lateral and medial thigh muscles helps to reduce lateral shifting of the pelvis and realigns the knee joint. The outer portion of the thigh is a reflex zone to the large intestine, so working on it during the same session as the intestinal region encourages better results.[2] The intestines are treated after the abdominal muscles have been relaxed.

When the body is toxic due to sluggish elimination of intestinal waste, it adversely affects the muscles' ability to metabolize the waste products that are squeezed out during deep tissue therapy. Proper function of the intestines aids in maintaining a more healthful internal environment in the body, which helps sustain the chemical changes brought about by deep tissue therapy.

d. *Anterior Thigh and Iliopsoas.* The abdominal muscles and thigh muscles should be released before work on the iliopsoas complex is attempted. Both the rectus femoris and psoas muscles tilt the iliac crests of the pelvis anteriorly, in opposition to the hamstrings and rectus abdominus, which tilt the iliac crests posteriorly. The psoas is the deepest core muscle. Its release can have profound effects on the entire body.

5. Upper Pole—Head and Neck

Work on the upper pole commences after balance of the pelvis has been achieved. The head and pelvis are the two weight segments positioned on either end of the spine. They serve to counterbalance each other. The head and pelvis have a direct relationship to each other both structurally and reflexively.

a. *Neck and Head Extensors.* These muscles prevent the head from tipping forward. They are called into use often and tend to accumulate tension. It is difficult to maintain tension release in the rest of the body until the neck has been freed. It is recommended that some relaxation work on the neck area be done at the beginning of each massage session.

b. *Neck and Head Flexors.* The front portion of the neck seldom gets addressed in standard massage sessions, but it is extremely important that it receive the same attention as the rest of the body. These muscles counterbalance the often overused extensor muscles at the back of the neck and are subject to damage from neck-related injuries.

c. *Head, Face, and Jaw.* Release of the cranial, facial, and, particularly, the jaw muscles completes the balance of the upper pole and integrates the head to the neck. Relaxation of this area promotes increased parasympathetic activity, reducing mental agitation and diminishing stress levels. The realignment of the head on the neck completes the process of total body re-education, allowing the client the opportunity to fully embrace the changes the experience of integrated deep tissue bodywork has produced.

DESIGNING A SESSION

The lesson plans give the full scope of the integrated deep tissue system, but they do not provide the step-by-step details of actual massage sessions. The plan for each bodywork treatment is constructed by the therapist with input from the client.

There are four parts to putting together an integrated massage session. They are as follows:

■ The interview.
■ Assessment of the client.
■ The session.
■ Homework and follow-up.

THE INTERVIEW

1. *Talk to the Client.* Before beginning to work on a client, a massage therapist needs to get to know him or her somewhat. Find out why this person has come to receive bodywork. What are the expectations? Take a brief history of the client's previous experience with massage.

2. *Ask Questions.* Ask about previous injuries, surgeries, medical conditions, current medications, etc. Elicit as much as possible about the client's state of health and any factors that will affect receiving massage.

3. *Talk about how the Client is Feeling.* What is the client's emotional state? What factors are affecting it? Remember that people are not bringing just their bodies to the massage table—they are bringing their total selves. Factors affecting their well-being are important for the massage therapist to know.

Feelings are a major component of how we experience ourselves through our bodies. The client's emotional state will play a part in the design of the sessions and may color the therapist's approach. For instance, if a person is expressing sadness, it may be determined that a nurturing style of touch would be more beneficial at this time than a more forceful, penetrating approach.

4. *Establish Goals with the Client.* It is a good idea for the therapist to discuss what he or she would like to accomplish in the session, based on what the client has expressed. Then the client has the opportunity to align with the goals, modify them, or add to them.

ASSESSMENT OF THE CLIENT

1. *Observe the Client.* The most important assessment tool the integrated deep tissue therapist uses is postural analysis. Through observing a client's posture and movement, it can be determined what the body's major tension patterns are and how to guide the client to a more effective use of the body to reduce the likelihood of future problems and discomfort.

    Postural evaluation is used to monitor changes occurring during massage sessions. Take time to observe the client both before and after the session to assess the effects of the work. The body may respond differently than anticipated, and some modifications made need to be made.

2. *Use the Charts.* Range of motion and conditions charts provided in the lessons should be used to assist in determining which muscles are contracted, based on the information gathered from the body reading. For example, if it is observed that the client rolls his left shoulder forward, the therapist would check the range of motion chart for the shoulder joint and find which muscles medially rotate the shoulder. The client could also perform the same movements with his left and right arms to check if there is restriction in range of motion of both shoulder joints.

3. *Assess Other Factors.* Facial expressions, vocal tone, and gestures can all be indicators of a person's general state of being and can help in assessing the person's reaction to the bodywork, both while receiving it and afterward.

THE SESSION

There are two levels of organization within the integrated deep tissue therapy method presented in the lessons. The first level deals with the order of application of the six components of the integrated system within a massage session.

To open the body effectively, a suggested sequence of treatment is to:

1. *Open* the energy pathways to relax the body and prepare the soft tissues for the work that is to follow. The two techniques used to accomplish this are polarity and Shiatsu.

2. *Warm up* the myofascia and enhance metabolic functioning by increasing blood flow through the body. Swedish and cross fiber techniques serve this purpose.

3. *Eliminate* restrictions within the fascial component of the soft tissues so that the muscles have room to lengthen. The connective tissue techniques are designed for this purpose.

4. *Relax* tension held in chronically shortened muscles. Deep tissue strokes achieve this result.

5. *Break up* cycles of pain generated by trigger point formation in the muscles. Neuromuscular therapy targets this phenomenon.

6. *Teach* the muscles and the mind to incorporate the newfound freedom that the application of all these techniques has created. Stretching serves this purpose.

Outlined above are the six stages of the integrated massage system. In a deep tissue session, this is a highly effective sequence to follow to achieve maximum results. After the initial sequence has been applied to an area, the techniques may be interwoven into the massage as dictated by the response of the client's tissues. This intermingling of the massage components gives a richer dynamic to the sessions and allows the therapist to tailor the approach to be maximally effective.

The second level of organization of the integrated deep tissue therapy method deals with the order in which the body is processed over a series of sessions. The recommended protocol is to process the body in the following sequence:

1. *The trunk*—chest and back.
2. *The upper extremity*—shoulder, arm, and hand.
3. *The lower limb*—foot, leg, and thigh.
4. *The core*—abdomen and pelvis.
5. *The upper pole*—neck and head.

The above list refers to the order in which each body segment is emphasized over a progressive series of bodywork sessions. Following this sequence will assist in reorganizing the body effectively through reinforcing the counterbalancing relationships of the segments. The number of sessions required to bring satisfactory full-body integration varies. The therapist may choose to focus on any one segment for several sessions in a row and may return to that area again in future sessions.

The deliberate omission of a detailed, nonflexible treatment plan is in recognition of the inherent organic nature of this style of bodywork. The therapist is encouraged to monitor the rate of the client's progress and work within his or her individual pattern of unfolding.

Although one specific body segment is emphasized in a single session, other areas of the body should also be addressed. The principle of working with counterbalancing relationships applies not only over a series of bodywork sessions, but also within each session. This means that a degree of full-body balance and integration is sought with each treatment. There are many ways that this can be accomplished.

Below are some suggestions for achieving balance within each deep tissue session:

- Follow the suggestions listed in the lessons under the category "Accessory Work." They present useful ideas for creating complete bodywork sessions.
- Include some work on the neck and the feet in each session to more fully facilitate the experience of release and integration throughout the body.
- The suggested order in which to process the body over a series of treatments can also be applied within an individual session. In other words, in a 60- or 90-minute time span, the therapist may progress through the 5 segments of the body, selecting the appropriate type of work and amount of time to spend on each one.

HOMEWORK AND FOLLOW-UP

After the massage session, the therapist may choose to show the client some exercises and self-care treatments he or she can do to further facilitate the release that took place in the session. The exercises described in the lessons were chosen specifically for this purpose. It is helpful to first demonstrate the exercise for clients and then watch them perform it, offering guidance on proper form and execution.

Always encourage clients to take time to relax and reflect on their feelings and sensations after receiving bodywork. Strongly urge clients to allow time to rest after a deep tissue therapy session. It takes time for all the changes brought about by massage to take effect. A period of rest helps the body greatly during this period of assimilation. Suggesting that the client write about the experience in a personal journal can also enhance the effects of the massage by providing a means for the client to acknowledge consciously any internal differences they feel due to the deep tissue work.

The therapist should let the client know that he or she is available if any questions or concerns arise in the days following the massage. The therapist may also want to call the client a few days after the session to check up on him or her and to allow discussion of the reactions to the work. Setting some mutually agreed-on, long-term goals for the time the client will receive therapy can also be a useful endeavor.

REFERENCES

1. Thomas CL, Venes D, eds. Taber's cyclopedic medical dictionary. Philadelphia, PA: FA Davis, 2001.
2. Sills F. The polarity process: energy as a healing art. Dorset, UK: Element Books, 1988: 122, Figure 6.16.

SUGGESTED READINGS

Rolf IP. Rolfing and physical reality. Rochester, VT: Healing Arts Press, 1990.
Rolf IP. Rolfing: the integration of human structures. New York, NY: Harper and Row, 1997.

Guidelines for the Deep Tissue Therapist

CARING FOR THE CLIENT

Choosing to receive massage therapy can be a challenging proposition for some people. They may feel threatened by the thought of removing clothing and putting themselves in a vulnerable situation with someone they do not know well. Establishing a safe, nurturing environment for the client should be a primary concern of the massage therapist.

There are many ways in which a therapeutic climate can be fostered. The massage office should have a pleasing appearance and be well equipped with accessories that aid in increasing the client's comfort level. Various-sized pillows, towels, and bolsters help in positioning a person's body for maximum ease and effectiveness of soft tissue release during massage. The capability to regulate temperature level with heaters, blankets, and fans is essential. Attending to a client's physical needs sets a caring tone that helps facilitate openness and trust.

The therapist should make it clear to the client that their relationship is in the form of a partnership. The client works with the therapist in determining goals for the bodywork. The client also sets parameters for the work by determining how much he or she is willing or able to let go at any particular time. For example, if during a session the client wishes to stop, for any reason, the therapist should quit working immediately and check with the client. Knowing that boundaries are being completely honored by the therapist often gives the client a sense of security that allows him or her to explore feelings and reactions more fully and experience the opportunities offered for a more complete healing.

The attitude of the therapist also contributes greatly to the therapeutic value of the bodywork. An effective therapist exhibits compassion and concern without becoming overly absorbed in the client's problems or feelings. An appropriate attitude of detachment is necessary to be able to make decisions and offer guidance that is helpful to the client's well-being.

INCORPORATING THE MIND/BODY ASPECT OF INTEGRATED DEEP TISSUE MASSAGE

THE NATURE OF TENSION

One of massage therapy's primary values is its effectiveness at relieving tension in the body. Tension manifests physically as chronically contracted muscles. It contributes to many problems, including pain, irritability, and diminished function. The manifestations of tension are often what prompt a person to seek massage therapy.

The mechanical techniques of massage therapy confront tension directly, through lengthening and relaxing contracted muscle fibers with a combination of pressure and movement. However, these results can be short-lived because when the client is again confronted with stress-producing experiences, the tension and its ensuing problems often return. It may be necessary to explore the nature and sources of tension more fully with clients so that they are capable of neutralizing its effects when it invades the body.

Tension itself is a form of resistance. It is the body's attempt to defend itself against a perceived threat. Mild short-term tension, which accompanies low-level stress reactions, can be a useful response. The increased muscular tone and heightened activity of the sympathetic nervous system that accompany mild stress can actually improve a person's ability to respond to a threatening situation. For example, the tension we feel when driving in traffic, although not necessarily making us feel very good, does tend to improve our reflexes and mobilize our senses so that we can react to potentially dangerous events more quickly and effectively. Stress becomes a problem when it is overbearing and unyielding. Exposure to long-term stressful conditions produces chronic tension.

EMOTIONS AND TENSION

Psychological sources of stress can be as devastating as physical ones. Very often people are unaware that the condition of their mind forges a direct link to their body. When worry, fear, anger, and other highly charged emotional states are unrelenting, they can have a devastating effect on the body through their tension-producing nature. As long as these emotional irritants are present, the body cannot maintain an environment of relaxation.

To complicate matters, areas of chronic physical tension lodged in the body may have been triggered by emotional stimuli that occurred years before. If a perceived threat is strong enough, is of a sustained duration, or is both, it can create an area of muscular tension that becomes locked in the body and is no longer responsive to

a conscious directive by the mind to release. This type of unrelenting muscular tension was labeled "armoring" by psychologist Wilhem Reich.[1,2] Armoring refers to the protective nature of the muscle block. It manifested to prevent the person from experiencing an unwanted or unacceptable feeling. There are many sources for these blocks, but the result is always the same—an area of deadened feeling due to muscular restriction.

Deep tissue therapy offers an effective means to uncover places of frozen tension in the body. We all contain an invisible matrix of memories and emotions that hold our muscles in distorted positions. In some cases, these distortions may be necessary as they allowed us to survive life experiences that would otherwise have been overwhelming to our fragile psyche. Much armoring occurs in childhood, before a person has acquired the necessary inner mechanisms that allow humans to effectively absorb or counter an intense emotional barrage.

As muscular tension softens during deep tissue therapy sessions, the underlying feelings sometimes resurface. In some instances, the client may choose to explore these feelings and their source. If this is the case, the therapist should recommend that the client talk to a qualified psychological counselor.

WORKING WITH EMOTIONAL RELEASE

Muscles that have become tense are painful. The lack of movement within the tense muscle belly prevents fresh blood, which is loaded with oxygen and nutrients, from reaching starving cells. Waste products that irritate nerve endings and dull the muscle fibers' responsiveness are trapped within the muscle, creating a swamp-like stagnation.

Over time, the uncomfortable feelings generated by the contracted muscles are repressed by the conscious mind, leaving only a vague blanket of numbness over the area. Any underlying feelings that may have triggered the initial tension are buried within deadened muscle tissue. The physical and emotional pain has not gone away, it is merely held suspended within steadily degenerating tissues and is still acting on the person at an unconscious level. Many people lack vitality or feel trapped in unproductive patterns of behavior because of the pervasive influence of these tension patterns.

As the muscle tissues are freed from their chronic gripping and the associated feelings surface, the client may experience a loosening of blocked emotions along with the muscular release. Depending on the source of the original inhibition, an emotional outpouring can manifest in a number of ways, including crying, laughing, a feeling of great relief, and/or insight into the nature of the physical-emotional blockage. Muscular and emotional release are similar in many ways. Both represent a yielding of a restrictive pattern involving the mind, musculature, and nervous system.

The signs of an impending emotional release are many and varied. Therapists need to be aware of them so that they will know how to act appropriately should an emotional outpouring take place.

One of the first indications that inner feelings are surfacing is a change in the client's breathing pattern. He or she may begin to hold the breath or take deeper or more rapid breaths. Blood flow to the skin may change. The client may become more flushed or the skin may become paler. The therapist may feel a change in the temperature level on the surface of the client's body.

The degree of tension in the musculature, particularly in the jaw, chest, and abdomen, may suddenly increase. The client may begin to fidget or become unusually subdued. If the eyes are closed, the therapist can look for rapid movement under the eyelids. The client may suddenly open the eyes and begin to look around or stare off into space.

The therapist should make note of changes in the level of communication offered by the client. A person who has been talkative and becomes uncharacteristically quiet, or one who was quiet and unexpectedly begins to converse, may be experiencing the surfacing of feelings. There are many other signals of a possible emotional outpouring as well. Therapists should be attentive and note any changes in clients' demeanors that might indicate that strong feelings are rising.

What is the proper course of action on the therapist's part if a client should experience an emotional release? First of all, the therapist needs to check with the client to make sure his or her needs are being met. Every massage office should be equipped with tissues, extra blankets, and water in case the client requires them. Beyond making sure that the client feels safe and comfortable, the therapist does not need to do anything except to be present and nonjudgmental.

It is not the therapist's responsibility to facilitate the client's feelings. The therapist should not try to push the client to express feelings, nor should the therapist discourage an honest outpouring of emotion if it should spontaneously occur. It is important that the therapist stay calm and centered while the client is experiencing emotional release. Any attempt by the therapist to actively suppress emotional expression on the part of the client can heighten the feelings of shame and embarrassment that many people experience when revealing withheld feelings.

The deep tissue therapist should deal with an emotional release in very much the same manner as a muscular release. The therapist should acknowledge the opening, give the client space to fully experience and absorb it, and be available to offer any assistance or support that may be required. It is often not necessary to verbally discuss the nature of the release or the reasons behind the emotions, unless the client wishes to do so. Most of the time, providing a compassionate and nurturing presence is all that the client requires from the therapist to process the feelings.

There is component of fear accompanying much emotional release. Feelings are often suppressed due to fear of expressing them, for whatever reason. That fear will resurface as the client lets go of the restricted emotions. With reassurance and support provided by the therapist, most clients feel a great relief once the feelings are expressed. It is as if a huge burden has been lifted off the person. If the client requires additional guidance in assimilating the feelings uncovered in the deep tissue session, the therapist may suggest that he or she seek the services of a professional counselor or psychologist.

ETHICAL CONSIDERATIONS

The role of the massage therapist is as an educator and facilitator for the body's natural healing processes. Massage therapy does not itself create healing or wholeness. It serves as a form of input that may assist persons in recovering their own innate capacities for health. Therefore, one should not fall into the trap of taking responsibility for the healing that may occur on the client's part. Nor should one blame oneself if the best effort has been given and all the desired results have not been achieved. One's full trust must be placed in the process itself, hoping that the client will extract the maximum benefit possible from the massage experience.

As stated previously, a massage therapist is principally a teacher. He or she offers valuable lessons to clients by guiding them through maneuvers that encourage the body to reorganize itself into a state of optimal functioning and well-being. Another aspect of this learning is derived from the massage therapist's attempt to embody the principles of growth within his or her own actions. One of these principles, honesty, is a quality that is highly valued in a professional bodyworker. Living by this creed helps to assure that the therapist will maintain a massage practice based on personal integrity and ethical behavior. In a therapeutic setting, honest assessment and acceptance of one's present condition is also the first step in making the changes that lead to increased happiness and fulfillment. Observing this level of integrity exemplified in the therapist greatly assists the client in having the perseverance to cultivate more productive and healthful habits.

PRINCIPLES OF CONSCIOUS BODYWORK

The following principles provide guidelines for the most beneficial application of the deep tissue therapy techniques. They encapsulate many of the concepts discussed in this book and serve as important reminders to the deep tissue therapist in the endeavor to maintain the highest standard of excellence when performing integrated deep tissue therapy. The therapist should commit these principles to memory and strive to embody them in the deep tissue work.

1. *Respect the Client.* When a client chooses to receive bodywork, that person is entrusting the body to the therapist and also expressing vulnerability to the therapist. Your responsibility is to honor and care for that person to the best of your ability. Every opportunity given to you to work on someone in this manner should be viewed as a privilege. Honor your clients for their desire to grow and for allowing you to grow with them. Each individual is unique and precious. The gift that conscious bodywork offers is the reminder that we are all unfolding into our own perfection.

2. *Be Attentive.* The therapist needs to stay present and focused to attune to the process of opening that is occurring within the session. Communication is being exchanged continually between the therapist and client. This interchange happens in many ways. As much as possible, the therapist needs to be able to track the client's experience of the work through touch, observation, and communication. Through the hands, the therapist receives messages about the response of the client's tissues to the work being done. It is crucial that these messages are interpreted correctly for the therapist to make the appropriate choices about how to interact effectively with the client's body. The client will be much more open to change if he or she feels that the therapist is attentive and responsive.

3. *Move Slowly.* Within a massage session many different dynamics may be experienced in terms of pressure, speed, and flow. When working to change the state of the myofascial structures, the pace must be slow to be effective. Connective tissue, deep tissue, neuromuscular, and stretching techniques are all performed at a slow rate. Time is required for the tissues to respond to the stimulus being applied. When deep pressure is administered quickly, there is not adequate time to respond to the client's reaction to the force in order to make appropriate adjustments. This is how injuries occur. If the therapist is moving slowly, there is enough time to ease up pressure or remove the hands from delicate tissues before damage results. A slow pace is also more conducive to the quality of self-awareness that fosters transformational growth on the client's part.

The massage experience establishes a relationship between the therapist and client whereby the client is often led into the same frame of mind as the therapist. Messages are received through the therapist's touch, quality of breathing, and inner attitude. A slow, fluid quality transfers more of a feeling of integration and deep relaxation to the massage recipient. This encourages the state of healing that people seek from deep tissue massage.

4. *Never Force the Tissues.* There is an old saying that states that a blossom will open on its own when it is ready. Any attempt to pry the flower open from its bud will only result in ruining the flower. The same is true with the body. An effective massage therapist learns how to interact with the soft tissues in such a way that they are encouraged to give up their holding patterns willingly. When the body is opening up freely, the therapist experiences a melting sensation under the fingers as they sink into the tissues. It is as if the hands were a boat being carried along by moving waters.

When resistance is encountered, the best tactic is to wait patiently for the internal conflict to be resolved before moving further. Pushing against resistant tissues sets up a tug-of-war situation between the therapist and recipient. In this kind of struggle, both the therapist and recipient lose. The therapist may plow through the blockage with assertive force and maybe even succeed in creating an opening, but all the effort and pain produced in the attempt has probably lodged somewhere else in the client's body. Resistance in the muscles is a natural defense against invasion. It is the body's way of protecting itself against what it perceives as intrusion, whether physical or emotional. Matching force with force is never very fruitful if the goal is to bring someone around to your point of view. Kindness, patience, and understanding are much more effective means to melt resistance.

5. *Work on "The Edge."* This guideline is closely related to the previous one. Working on the edge describes an approach to soft tissue manipulation that creates the most productive environment for change to occur. Working in this realm means that the therapist has found the pace, pressure, and rhythm that provide the ideal stimulus for the client's tissues to release tension patterns and move into

dynamic equilibrium. In other words, transformation is happening. When the qualities of pace, pressure, and rhythm are not in cadence with the client's tissues, the massage is not being very productive, and the results will be disappointing. Using the dynamic of pressure as an example, if the force of the stroke is too light, the client will not feel the muscles and fascia lengthening and consequently will not feel tension in the tissues melting. If the pressure is too deep, the sensations of pain become overwhelming and block any other stimulus to the nervous system, inhibiting the positive benefits of the work. When the pressure is just right, the client's experience is that the body is becoming freer, and the person is able to experience the pleasure of profound release.

6. *Move the Body Toward Greater Ease.* Massage should be an educational process. Through the medium of touch, the therapist is teaching the client what the body could feel like if it were in a better balance. When easy, pleasurable movement is presented to the mind and nervous system, they will tend to embrace and incorporate it, if given the opportunity. Throughout any bodywork session, the therapist is monitoring the state of tension in the client's muscles and through stroking and positioning of the body, creating the greatest degree of comfort. Often, changing the position or angle of a body part on the table will relax the muscles around it and increase the effectiveness of any techniques applied to those muscles. Pads and bolsters can be used to change the alignment of the body on the table for more effective muscle release. Teaching the body proper positioning creates efficient pathways of movement for the muscles and fascia to follow as they start to move back to their natural positions.

7. *Elongate Shortened Tissues, Strengthen Stretched Tissues.* Most deep tissue massage techniques are designed to bring balance to the body by lengthening shortened muscle fibers and the fascial sheaths that surround them. Muscles act in pairs. When a muscle contracts, its opposing muscle is stretched. If the muscle stays contracted, the antagonistic muscle will remain in an overly lengthened position, which usually has the effect of weakening it. Therefore, once the shortened muscles have been released, the stretched muscles should be strengthened with specifically targeted exercises.

Muscles need to be free to contract and lengthen at the slightest instigation for the body to maintain its ability to respond and adapt to stimulus. To bring harmony to muscular relationships, the massage therapist evaluates where tissues are shortened through observation and palpation and elongates them through a combination of compression and stretching techniques. When the shortened muscles

regain their proper length, the pull on the opposing muscles is reduced and they also return to a resting state. This allows the reflex arcs to once again do their jobs, and the body's full capacity for adjustment returns.

8. *Seek to Re-establish Balance.* As stated above, muscles operate in counterbalancing relationships. The body as a whole operates the same way. When part of the body shifts in one direction, the rest of the body makes compensating adjustments to maintain some sort of functional integrity. Anyone who has tried to balance a stack of blocks knows that when one block is moved out of position, the whole stack has to be readjusted to prevent the blocks from falling into a pile. In organizing the body efficiently, the bodyworker is conscious of the body's counterbalancing nature and works accordingly. This means that massage sessions are structured so that the body's oppositional relationships are taken into account. When focusing on the top of the body, do some work to align the bottom half of the body with it. Juxtapose work on the back of the body with work on the front. Integrate the right side of the body with the left side. Balance the deep, inner muscles with the more surface muscles, and so forth. Approaching the body in this manner within each session will give longer-lasting and much more profound results.

9. *Release Blockages so the Energy Can Flow.* An open body is analogous to a flowing river. The water in a river is constantly moving, finding its way along the path of the riverbed. The surface of the water may at times appear still, and yet underneath there are always deep currents flowing. The river exhibits a quality of fluidity and ever-changing dynamics amidst a backdrop of timeless constancy. When the body is unified in harmonious balance, it exhibits the same ease of flow and adaptability as the rushing river. There is an ease of movement within an aura of tranquillity that appears almost liquid in nature. The tissues seem to ripple with a sense of aliveness.

When the body is viewed with this image in mind, blocks to the flow of the life force become readily apparent. The breath may appear uneven or shallow, and muscles seem knotted in stiffness and immobility. The body structure is out of alignment. There is a feeling of strain emanating from it. The massage therapist develops an awareness of the areas of blockage and seeks to remove them in much the same way one would remove a log that is damming the flow of water in a stream.

10. *Approach the Body from the Perspective of Wholeness.* The words "heal" and "whole" are derived from the same root.[3] Therefore, "to heal" means "to make whole." The ultimate goal of inte-

grated bodywork is to help guide a person to a state of completeness or wholeness. The body is the vehicle used for this healing to take place.

In the process of learning various massage techniques, the body is broken down into parts to be labeled and analyzed. The student learns how atoms make up molecules, which combine to create cells, which build all the physiologic systems. Muscles are delineated in the same manner. Bundles of muscle tissues are given special names and described as performing specific actions. When massaging the body, the therapist may also compartmentalize his or her work by addressing individual systems with techniques designed to facilitate their specific functioning. However, a person is not just the sum of all these systems. We do not experience ourselves internally as a conglomeration of parts with strange Latin names.

A human being is a locus of consciousness that transcends all the individual facets. It is this expansive quality that allows us to go beyond our limitations and fulfill our capabilities. Conscious bodywork offers the potential to tap into this experience of finding and expressing our unique qualities and individual natures.

REFERENCES

1. Lowen A. Bioenergetics. New York: Penguin, 1975.
2. Lowen A. The language of the body. New York: MacMillan, 1958.
3. Neufeldt V, ed. Webster's New World Dictionary of American English. 3rd College edition. New York: Simon & Schuster. 1986: 621.

The Lessons

4

Integrated Deep Tissue Therapy System Techniques

INTRODUCTION

The integrated deep tissue therapy system, while incorporating many facets of stress-reducing relaxation styles of massage, embraces a broader vision of high-level wellness. It teaches a precise methodology for normalizing the muscular system, thereby reducing unbalanced pulls on the skeleton which lead to loss of structural integrity and eventual physical breakdown. Circulation of fluids is improved, resulting in better metabolic functioning. Pain-producing elements within the myofascial tissues may be eliminated, diminishing excessive activity of the sympathetic nervous system, which is characteristic of high-stress states.

An important by-product of a relaxed, stress-free body is a calm and powerful mind. Excessive firing of nerves brought about by the strain of holding muscles in distorted positions disturbs mental equilibrium. It stimulates random mental chatter in the brain, which leads to unclear and unproductive thought patterns. As the body is brought to a state of dynamic equilibrium and poise through the deep tissue therapy techniques, the nervous system is able to return to its optimal, efficient state of low-level firing. This reduces the production of static within the central nervous system that creates disturbance in the mind.

THREE LEVELS OF ASSESSMENT USED IN DEEP TISSUE THERAPY (BOX 4-1)

The systematic approach to processing the soft tissues presented here requires three levels of client assessment. The first level of assessment the deep tissue therapist must master is the ability to recognize the unique patterns of muscular compensation brought about by distortions in the myofascial system in each client. An individual's posture and movement characteristics are largely determined by the limitations imposed by restricted soft tissues. After the therapist has evaluated these patterns, he or she must then determine which ones are most detrimental (i.e., causing pain, producing wear and tear on joints, straining ligaments and muscle tissue, or leading to fascial build-up and bracing).

Deep tissue therapy sessions are built around minimizing these dysfunctional patterns of distortion. Because every person's muscular relationships are unique and ever-changing, no two deep tissue therapy sessions are exactly the same. Each treatment is designed to neutralize the counterproductive soft tissue patterns that are generating problems.

The second level of assessment involves the ability to envision the body's progression to a balanced state over time by organizing a logical, effective plan of treatment. It takes time and patience to undo the effects of years of trauma and lack of proper movement education. The therapist's job is to guide the client to a condition of pain-free, unrestricted movement capability through a combination of progressive deep tissue therapy treatments and supplemental stretching and strengthening exercises.

In Chapter 2 an effective protocol for efficiently reorganizing the body was introduced. To summarize, the spinal unit and upper extremity are approached first, followed by the lower extremity. Work on the lower extremity begins with the feet, because they form the structural foundation for the vertical body. The deep tissue therapy sessions then progress upward to the body's core, which consists of the abdominal cavity and pelvis. The pelvis, being the lower pole of the spinal column, is the body's movement and instinct control center.

After the core is freed up, work progresses to the upper pole of the spine, the neck and head region, which is the intellectual control center. Structural integrity between the two poles needs to be reestablished for whole-body dynamic alignment to be realized fully. This sequence of learning and applying deep tissue therapy provides students with practical knowledge of how the natural counterbalancing relationships in the body manifest.

The third level of assessment involves evaluating the state of the muscular system through observation and palpation. It takes place primarily as the therapist is working on the client's body. The deep tissue therapy techniques are designed to manipulate and stretch myofascial tissue. Just as an assortment of specialized tools are used by a mechanic to perform specific tasks, a variety of deep tissue strokes are incorporated by the therapist to address the full range of muscular qualities and conditions.

Part of the skill of mastering deep tissue therapy is acquiring the ability to recognize the manifestations of myofascial aberrations and the knowledge of proper application of the appropriate techniques to correct them. It must be remembered that the primary goal of deep tissue therapy is to reestablish the proper balance of muscular forces around the skeleton. This is accomplished by lengthening chronically contracted muscles and treating other restrictive conditions that are inhibiting the function of muscle fibers, like scar tissue and trigger points.

To release contracted muscles, slow compressive strokes are applied along their length, from origin to insertion, covering the tendons and muscle bellies. Shorter, focused strokes are then used to treat smaller sections of the muscle that may be aberrant. These strokes may be applied parallel to the muscle fibers or across them, depending on the nature of the restriction. They are also used on the tendinous attachments to the bones to aid in minimizing scar tissue formation and to stimulate the Golgi tendon organs to send messages through the nervous system to direct the muscle to lengthen and relax.

BOX 4-1

Three Levels of Assessment

1. Determining the client's patterns of muscular tension and compensation
2. Planning the sequence and number of sessions required to minimize compensatory patterns
3. Evaluating the condition of the myofascial tissues and correcting imbalances with deep tissue therapy

The muscular system is worked in layers, from superficial to deep. It is crucial that the deep tissue therapist have a thorough knowledge of muscle anatomy to be able to distinguish the various layers of muscles that are being affected. None of the layers should be neglected in a deep tissue treatment. Each has unique characteristics and tends to store different manifestations of tension.

The superficial layer of muscle is the level most affected by the environment. It, along with the skin and adipose tissue, forms a barrier between the external world and the internal body. Invasions from the environment are often trapped in the superficial layer of muscles. These invasive elements include exposure to extreme temperatures and trauma resulting from accidents or falls. Tension tends to migrate from the surface of the body to deeper levels. If the deeper layers of muscle are overemphasized in a deep tissue therapy treatment, the origin of many tension patterns in the surface muscles may be easily overlooked.

The deeper layers of muscle, which are often called on for maintaining postural positions, store stress patterns that result from trauma, faulty movement habits, and psychological conditioning. The ropy, knotted fibers characteristic of tense muscles, along with trigger points, usually manifest at this level. Releasing these muscular conditions while reorganizing the superficial layer of muscles brings longer-lasting results. Imbalances between the layers of soft tissue distort the body with tension-producing compensations. By freeing all the soft tissue layers, the body becomes functionally integrated throughout.

USING THE LESSON MATERIAL

Incorporating all three levels of assessment allows the therapist to perceive the continuum of myofascial influences acting on the client's body. In assessing a client and planning a course of action for treatment, the therapist moves from level 1 to level 3. The information presented in the lessons and the deep tissue routines provides the necessary foundation to plan and execute a series of sessions effectively. Chapter 2 describes how the lessons and routines are organized and gives an overview of the information they contain. The therapist's job is to adapt each routine to fit the specific requirements of the client based on the three levels of assessment.

To determine the client's patterns of muscular tension and compensation, the therapist makes use of the postural evaluation outline, along with the range of motion and conditions charts. The sequence of the routines presented in this book provides an effective map for planning a course of treatment. It is a good idea to discuss with the client the approximate number of sessions that will be required to bring the body to a state of better functioning, so that a level of commitment to deep tissue therapy is agreed to at the beginning. Most people experience a significant improvement in their state of health and well-being within 5 to 10 sessions.

A deep tissue therapy session is generally scheduled in a 60- or 90-minute format, depending on the preference of the therapist and the needs of the client. The session is structured as follows:

- Opening: polarity and Shiatsu.
- Warm-up: Swedish and cross fiber techniques.
- Connective tissue release.
- Deep tissue and neuromuscular therapy.
- Stretch.
- Accessory work.
- Closing: foot reflexology move or polarity.

Table 4-1 provides an approximation of the amount of time spent on each section.

This timeline is very flexible. It is only meant as a

TABLE 4–1	Timing a Deep Tissue Session	
Sequence	**60-Minute Format**	**90-Minute Format**
Opening	3 minutes	3 minutes
Warm-up	5 minutes	7 minutes
Connective tissue release	5 minutes	5 minutes
Deep tissue and neuromuscular therapy	38 minutes	65 minutes
Stretch	2 minutes	2 minutes
Accessory work	5 minutes	6 minutes
Closing	2 minutes	2 minutes

general guideline to help the therapist use the session time efficiently. The large block of time given to the deep tissue and neuromuscular therapy techniques allows the therapist to intersperse techniques from the other sections as needed. In addition to the time given to the work on the massage table, the therapist must factor in the time spent with the client before and after the session, which could add up to an additional 30 minutes to the appointment time.

Each routine contains instructions for deep tissue release on all the muscles in that particular body region. It is not necessary to perform deep tissue therapy on all of the muscles listed in a routine. Contracted muscles are chosen for focus based on the therapist's observation of the client's unique patterns of distortion. The client's history of traumas and reported areas of pain are also taken into account when deciding which muscles should be targeted for deep tissue release and neuromuscular therapy treatment.

The illustrations accompanying the descriptions of the strokes demonstrate the technique performed fully on a willing recipient. In this way, the student can see the completed stroke. When working with clients, their level of comfort in receiving massage must be taken into account. For some clients, draping may need to be adjusted so that less of the body is exposed. Some strokes may need to be stopped before the therapist reaches the muscle attachment, particularly in the pelvic region. The therapist and client should discuss these issues beforehand so that the client is assured that his or her boundaries are respected.

POSTURAL AND MOVEMENT MUSCLES

Understanding the characteristics of skeletal muscles helps the therapist to anticipate the types of problems that are likely to be encountered in specific muscles. Skeletal muscle serves two important functions: movement and support. The skeletal muscles move the human structure through space. They exhibit an extraordinary dynamic range, capable of producing large bursts of motion that propel the body against the force of gravity or controlling tiny subtle movements that allow the fingertips to trace the contours of a single strand of hair. The skeletal muscles also support the position of the bones in relation to each other against the force of gravity to maintain postural integrity.

To carry out these functions, two distinct types of skeletal muscle have evolved. The muscles that are mostly responsible for movement are called *phasic*, whereas the support, or postural, muscles are known as *tonic*. As the roles of the muscles become defined, their biochemical properties diverge. A muscle's role as phasic or tonic is not strictly determined at birth. It can change depending on the types of movement activities in which a person engages.[1] For instance, a long-distance runner will not have exactly the same distribution of movement and postural muscles as that of a computer operator, because they use their muscles in vastly different ways.

CHARACTERISTICS OF POSTURAL MUSCLES

Postural, or tonic, muscles support the body against the force of gravity. They are referred to as the workhorse muscles because they have to be able to perform for long periods, sustaining a semi-contracted state (Box 4-2.) They are made up of a large percentage of slow-twitch

BOX 4-2

Major Postural Muscles

Adductor longus	Pectoralis major
Adductor magnus	Piriformis
Erector spinae muscles	Quadratus lumborum
Gastrocnemius	Rectus femoris
Hamstrings	Soleus
Iliopsoas	Sternocleidomastoid
Levator scapulae	Upper trapezius

red fibers, which have a plentiful blood supply so they do not produce a large amount of fatiguing waste products.

Additionally, these muscles maintain a high level of endurance because their fibers do not all contract in unison, but rather segmentally. The motor units in the fibers fire irregularly, like blinking holiday lights. As one section of the muscle contracts, other portions of it are able to relax. It is like long-distance runners passing the baton to each other at intervals to distribute the workload among several athletes. Because the fibers contract in relay fashion, these muscles do not tire easily and therefore can offer long-term support to the body. Not enough fibers contract at one time to produce movement of the bones, but they are able to maintain a continuously toned state that braces the structure against the force of gravity.

Tonic muscles are slow to respond to reflex stimulus. They cannot contract and relax quickly, like phasic muscles. Their movement capabilities are limited, as is their ability to sustain heavy loads. They tend to cramp easily if called on to move quickly or exhibit great strength.

When a person's posture is distorted, the postural muscles have to work very hard to brace misaligned joints and tend to become hypertonic. This permanent highly contracted state of muscles fosters the formation of trigger points. The body also produces additional connective tissue in these muscles to bolster their bracing capability.

The overabundance of connective tissue confines the muscle in its contracted state, preventing it from being able to lengthen. Thus, the body becomes congealed into a distorted shape. Because of the unyielding nature of built-up connective tissue, the person cannot willfully move the body into the proper position. Slow, focused stretching exercises must be performed by the person on a regular basis to release bonding within the fascial tissues, in addition to receiving connective tissue release work to release the muscles from their confinement and return the body to its natural, lengthened state.

CHARACTERISTICS OF MOVEMENT MUSCLES

As stated previously the movement, or phasic, muscles are responsible for moving the body through space. They are made up predominantly of fast-twitch red fibers, which contract and release rapidly in response to stimulus. The movement muscles are linked to the body's many reflex arcs. They can move the body quickly to adapt to unanticipated events, like stepping off an unseen curb. The fast-twitch fibers have a relatively low blood supply available to them, causing them to fatigue quickly and produce large amounts of lactic acid that are not quickly flushed out of the muscles. Although the movement muscles have more short-term strength than the postural muscles, they tire much faster and need more recovery time.

When there is muscular imbalance, movement muscles tend to weaken in response to postural muscles shortening. Because the deep tissue compressive manipulations are designed to lengthen contracted muscles, the postural muscles are often the focus of deep tissue sessions. As postural muscles are released, allowing the musculoskeletal relationships to become more integrated, the movement muscles naturally become stronger. If particular movement muscles remain weak even after treatment, additional strengthening exercises may be recommended to improve their function.

Because the phasic muscles often have to make quick adjustments, their fibers are prone to micro-tearing. This tearing often occurs at the musculotendinous junction. The constant pull of the muscles against the attached bones can lead to inflammation of the tendon, known as tendinitis. Movement muscles can also become hypertonic, like postural muscles. Repetitive use of certain muscle groups for a specific activity, such as hammering nails, can lead to chronic contraction of those muscles. The quick changes in length that are sometimes required of movement muscles to stabilize the body's equilibrium can lead to spasms and permanently contracted states.

PALPATION

Palpation is the art of sensing or feeling changes in the tissues. It is incorporated along with the massage strokes to generate an instantaneous feedback loop. In other words, to gauge the effect of a stroke, a massage therapist is sensitive to the reaction of the client's tissues, as perceived by the therapist's hands, as various techniques are performed. If necessary, the therapist can make adjustments to the stroke in pace, pressure, or intention to yield the desired outcome, which is the resolution of aberrations in the myofascia.

The hands are extremely sensitive instruments for performing massage, particularly the fingertips, as they contain a high percentage of nerve receptors. These nerve receptors are capable of perceiving temperature differences, textural qualities and variations, degrees of hardness or softness, moisture, degrees of depth, and minute movements. The ability to register all of these characteristics allows the therapist to tune into the client's tissues at a very subtle level.

Skill in palpation is developed through practice. Over time, the brain develops the capacity to absorb more and more input coming from the nerve receptors, increasing the capacity of the therapist to distinguish and assimilate all the signals coming through the hands. Although the fingers and palms contain a higher number of nerve receptors than other parts of the body used to perform massage strokes, palpatory proficiency can also be acquired with the elbow, knuckles, and forearm through regular, concentrated practice. Chaitow and Freyman[2] provide a large selection of palpatory exercises.

Accurate palpatory assessment requires the ability to visualize clearly the soft tissues that are being targeted. Therefore, a thorough knowledge of anatomy is necessary to train the hands to move through the layers of the body accurately and safely. The therapist must be able to palpate the condition of the skin and the underlying layers of adipose and fascia. Sensing the qualities of the skin can yield much information about the underlying tissues. An abnormally warm area on the skin may indicate inflammation in the soft tissues beneath it. Skin that feels tight and cannot slide easily over the underlying tissues may indicate binding in the superficial fascial membranes.

To palpate the muscles accurately, the therapist needs to be familiar with their shape, the directions of their fibers, and their points of attachment on the bones. The therapist must also be able to distinguish the differences between normal and abnormal muscle tissue. A normal muscle that is free of tension and restrictions has a springy, resilient quality. It yields to pressure and maintains even tone. Healthy muscles have a translucent quality when palpated, meaning that other tissues can easily be felt through them. They do not feel painful to the touch, even when deep pressure is applied.

Abnormal muscle tissue embodies the effects of strain and imbalance. Unhealthy muscles can be weak and flaccid or dense and tough. Their fibers are more pronounced than those of healthy muscles. They may feel stringy or ropy and crunch when rolled across. Highly contracted muscles feel thick and hard. They are not resilient when pressed, but rather resistive. Muscles that are under tension, being held in a stretched position, can feel like taut cable wires. Unhealthy muscle tissue usually feels painful to the touch, but it can also feel numb or deadened, particularly if the abnormal condition is long standing. With experience, the various states of muscle health can be palpated accurately and appropriate techniques applied to them to counteract the effects of strain and improper usage.

Knowledge of the shape and function of the skeleton is equally as important as the ability to visualize muscles when palpating the body. All muscles are anchored to bones, which they pull on to move them. Much of the damage done to muscles through trauma and stress occurs at their attachments to the bones. Tracing the contours of the bones is an extremely important aspect of deep tissue therapy. Repairing damage at the tendinoperiosteal junction helps to reduce much of the pain experienced due to pulled muscles.

GUIDELINES FOR PERFORMING THE MODALITIES

ENERGY WORK

Polarity and Shiatsu moves are used at the beginning of the deep tissue therapy sessions to prepare the client for the massage work that is to follow. The initial contact between client and therapist establishes the quality of their interaction. It allows the client time to relax and become accustomed to the therapist's touch. The therapist uses this time to establish rapport with the client and build an environment of trust and safety.

The goal of energetic styles of bodywork is to allow the body to open up so that energy can flow more effectively. Whether one wishes to think of energy as life force or merely conscious awareness of the body's internal activities, the opening moves establish a bond between the therapist and client that enhances the level of receptivity in both parties.

POLARITY

The polarity contacts introduce each deep tissue session. Polarity techniques are described at the beginning of each routine for the part of the body being emphasized in that lesson. The polarity touch is very soft. It is usually administered with full, open hands. The therapist should place the hands on the client's body slowly and lightly. The palms and fingers touch the surface of the body with only enough pressure to make contact with the client's skin. The therapist's hands should have the quality of hovering on the surface of the client's body. A useful image is to try to imagine placing your hand on a leaf floating on the surface of a pond. Use only enough pressure to feel the leaf against your palm without submerging it in the water.

Dr. Randolph Stone, the developer of polarity therapy, used terminology from magnetism when describing the direction of energy flow through the body. The direction of outwardly flowing energy was described as the positive pole. The inwardly flowing direction was called the negative pole. Described in bodily terms, the upper portion of the body is the positive pole, whereas the lower portion is the negative pole. The right side and front of the body are considered positive, and the left side and back of the body are considered negative. To enhance the flow of energy between the therapist and client, opposite poles should be connected, whenever possible, just like connecting batteries in an electronic device. In other words, the therapist's right hand (positive pole) makes contact with the negative pole of the client's body, while the therapist's left hand (negative pole) makes contact with the client's positive pole. Directions for appropriate placement of the therapist's hands are given in the description of each polarity move in the lessons.

After the therapist establishes contact with the client's body, the polarity move is generally held for 1 to 2 minutes. During this time the therapist sits or stands upright in a relaxed, receptive stance, and his or her breathing pattern should be even and calm. There should be no strain on the body or distractions in the mind so that the therapist may be fully sensitive to the sensations in the hands. Feelings of warmth or mild vibration in the therapist's palms and fingers while contacting the client's body are common sensations, as is heightened attunement to the rhythms of the client's various pulses. The therapist may also become aware of subtle shifts and movements in the client's body. These movements emanate from the fascial layers of the body. Clients often report becoming deeply relaxed and more in tune with the feelings in their body as a result of the focused contact.

No analysis of the sensations is necessary for treatment to be effective. The therapist's focus is on being receptive to all the input that is being received from the client's body to become more in tune with the client. Receptivity and compassion are the qualities the therapist should cultivate while administering polarity therapy. To release the polarity hold, the therapist very slowly removes the hands from the client's body while maintaining focus on the client's comfort and welfare. It is helpful to time the release of the hands to the client's inhalation, as if the client was gently pushing the therapist's hands off the surface of the body as it expands to take in a breath.

SHIATSU

The Shiatsu moves are performed after the polarity hold is released. A few easy-to-perform techniques have been chosen from the vast repertoire of Shiatsu procedures. As explained in Chapter 1, the goal of Shiatsu is to enhance the flow of qi, or life force, through a complex series of channels, or meridians, that run through the body. This is accomplished by applying a series of compressive moves that trace the course of the channels. Whereas some Shiatsu techniques move very specifically along the path of a meridian, the techniques chosen for this course are more general, usually covering several channels at a time.

Many of the Shiatsu moves incorporated in the lessons involve compression moves done with the hands along the length of a limb, moving proximal to distal. To begin the sequence, the therapist faces the client's body and holds the limb with both hands. The thumbs are placed on the lateral side of the limb. The palms cover the center of the limb, while the fingers wrap around the medial side. A combination of compression, squeezing, and slight medial rolling of the limb is used in coordination with both therapist and client exhalations. The stroke begins by pressing the thumbs into the lateral side of the limb. The stroke is continued by pressing down on the top of the limb with the palms as the thumbs maintains contact; the therapist adds a squeezing action with the fingers to embrace the limb fully with the hands. The stroke is completed by rolling the limb slightly medial while maintaining the pressure on it with the hands.

Effective Shiatsu incorporates the therapist's whole body, not just the hands. The weight and motion of the body into the stroke supplies the necessary compressive force, not the contraction of arm or hand muscles. The correct body motion for the move described above begins with the stance. The therapist's feet are a little wider than hip distance apart and separated from each other lengthwise by the distance of a comfortable walking stride. Both knees are slightly flexed, with awareness focused on the pelvis as the initiator of movement. At the beginning of the stroke, about 70% of the body's weight is on the back foot. As the stroke continues, weight is shifted forward, timed with the pace of the stroke and with exhalation. At the completion of the stroke, about 70% of the therapist's weight is on the front foot. The spine stays long, and the shoulders, arms, and hands remain relaxed throughout the entire stroke. The therapist slides the hands a little further down the limb, shifts weight back to the back foot, and begins the compression sequence again. The therapist continues in this manner to the wrist or ankle.

SWEDISH MASSAGE

The Swedish strokes are introduced immediately following the polarity and Shiatsu maneuvers. Although Swedish massage is only mentioned in the routines after the energy techniques, it may be incorporated throughout the session at the therapist's discretion. The strokes should be applied with a sense of fluidity and continuity to promote a quality of integration throughout the soft tissues. More than any other technique, Swedish massage generates a sense of unity in the body. Its use enhances the benefits of every other modality.

Swedish massage contains a huge repertoire of strokes.

The three basic Swedish techniques—effleurage, pétrissage, and friction—are utilized in the integrated deep tissue therapy system to warm up the tissues, enhance fluid circulation, and create a unifying bridge between the other modalities used in this therapeutic approach.

Effleurage strokes are smooth gliding strokes executed over the surface of the skin. One or both hands may be used depending on the particular pattern of the stroke. Effleurage is used to warm up the tissues, soothe the nervous system, and relax tense muscles. Various degrees of pressure may be applied depending on the purpose of the stroke and the preference of the client. Lubricant is utilized to prevent friction or sticking to the client's skin. Although the palmar surfaces of the hands are the most commonly employed tools, other parts of the hand or arm may be used as well, including the knuckles, thumbs, and forearms.

Basic effleurage patterns should move from bone to bone whenever possible to stroke the entire length of the muscles. Effleurage strokes are used to delineate muscular arrangements to the client's nervous system, promoting relaxation-inducing sensations of length. An effleurage stroke that is stopped before it reaches a muscle's bony attachment tends to generate feelings of shortness and tightness that are counter-productive to the goal of massage.

The following are descriptions of effleurage style strokes used in this course that may not be familiar to all readers:

- *Shingles* is an effleurage variation in which one hand replaces the other by gliding under it every 2 or 3 inches throughout the length of the stroke. It creates a pattern reminiscent of overlapping roof shingles.
- *Swimming* is a forearm variation of effleurage, commonly performed on the back or thighs. The therapist places both forearms parallel to each other on the mid-back or mid-thigh. The therapist simultaneously shifts his or her weight forward and slides and rolls the forearms apart, allowing them to glide over the skin until they are should-width apart. At that point, the therapist draws the arms back together, without losing contact with the skin, to begin the stroke again. The motion is somewhat similar to the arm movement used by swimmers in the breaststroke.
- *Thumb gliding* is an effleurage stroke incorporating the full lengths of the thumbs. The thumbs alternately glide over the skin in an overlapping pattern similar to the path of windshield wipers. It is commonly used on smaller body parts such as the palm of the hand, the plantar surface of the foot, and around the knee.
- *Draining* is a two-handed effleurage stroke performed on either the arm or leg, moving from the distal to the proximal end. Both hands are wrapped around the extremity at either the ankle or wrist, with the fingers embracing the sides of the extremity while the thumbs cross each other over the mid-section. The webbing between the thumb and index fingers of both hands makes full contact with the central rounded contour of the limb. Light pressure is maintained as the hands glide up the limb toward the proximal end. Upon reaching the proximal end, the hands separate and slide down the medial and lateral sides of the limb to begin the stroke again. Contact with the skin is never broken.

Swedish pétrissage strokes are used to further relax muscles and pump fluids through them with grasping, squeezing motions of the hands. One- or two-handed variations are commonly employed. Knuckle kneading is a form of pétrissage using the knuckle side of an extended-finger fist position. The knuckles are rolled back and forth over a small section of the body at a comfortable pace and pressure.

Friction strokes are used to relax contracted muscle fibers and to realign scar tissue. The therapist presses into the client's tissues, pinning the skin directly under the fingers or palm to the underlying muscle and fascia. The skin and muscle are then moved as one unit to separate adhered muscle fibers. The pressure is firm so that the skin does not glide independently over the muscle tissue, which can cause irritation. Friction strokes are performed in circular motions or back-and-forth cross fiber patterns.

CROSS FIBER

Cross fiber techniques form a bridge between circulatory styles of massage therapy and deep tissue therapy. They are utilized to release adhesions in bundles of muscle fibers, which reduce fluid flow through the muscle and also hold it in a contracted state. The two primary strokes incorporated in the integrated deep tissue system are fingertip raking and a rolling technique using the full length of the thumb. These techniques are based on strokes developed by Therese Pfrimmer,[3] one of the originators of cross fiber style therapy. Both strokes require a generous application of lubricant to provide a smooth, back-and-forth gliding motion across the muscle fibers.

Fingertip raking is executed with a hand position formed from a cupped palm and curved fingers that are slightly spread apart. The fingertip pads roll across the muscle at a 90° angle to the direction the fibers are running in a continuous back-and-forward motion that progresses along the full length of the muscle between its two attachments.

The rolling stroke uses the broad side of the thumb all the way from its tip to the thenar eminence on the palm. To execute the stroke, the entire palmar surface of the hand is placed on the body with the thumb straight and comfortably extended from the hand in its natural position at approximately a 60° angle. The length of the thumb lies parallel to the direction the muscle fibers are running. As the hand glides back and forth across the muscle, the thumb rolls over the muscle fibers. This causes the bundles of fibers to slide against each other, spreading them and releasing fascial restrictions that may be keeping them bunched together. A helpful image in performing the stroke properly is to think of the thumb like a rolling pin being rolled back and forth across a ball of dough, flattening it out.

Both cross fiber strokes are performed at a moderate pace. The therapist should be able to cover the entire length of an average-sized muscle in five or six back-and-forth strokes. Because they roll across muscle fibers, cross fiber strokes allow the therapist to feel the condition of the fibers more effectively than strokes that run parallel to the fibers. Stringy or ropy fibers are signs of adhesion and should be focused on for several consecutive strokes.

Cross fiber strokes should not be performed over the same section of muscle for more than five or six passes in a row or they can lead to irritation of the skin. If the fibers still feel dry and stringy after several passes, the therapist should move on, perhaps returning to that section of fibers later to re-check it.

CONNECTIVE TISSUE

The goal of working on the body's fascia is twofold—to make the ground substance more fluid, and to release collagen bonds that are causing muscles to adhere. The techniques used to spread fascial membranes often incorporate slow stretching and pulling actions.

It has been found that steady, sustained stretching of fascial membranes helps to free restricting links that form within the collagen mesh. The key to successful fascial release is the ability to sense the limit of the tissue's ability to stretch and to hold the stretch until a yielding or lengthening sensation is felt. The tissues should never be forced with more pressure or stretch than they can comfortably accommodate.

Connective Tissue Strokes

1. *Fascial Lift and Roll.* This is a skin and muscle-rolling technique designed to release adhered areas in the superficial fascia. Both hands are used. The thumbs are placed end-to-end on one side of the tissue to be rolled. The fingers are positioned on the other side. The tissues are lifted and pressed toward the fingers with the thumbs. They are then rolled between the fingers and thumbs (Fig. 4-1). If the skin can be lifted easily off the underlying tissues it may be rolled independently. Otherwise, the skin, adipose, superficial fascia, and muscle tissue may all be lifted and rolled. Always move slowly and deliberately. Adhered areas may feel quite painful. Begin the rolling action on a

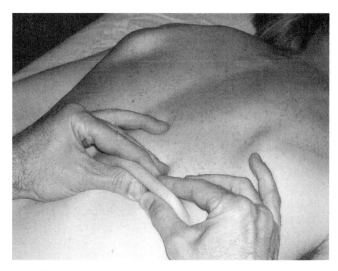

FIGURE 4-1   Fascial lift and roll technique.

section of tissue that is relatively easy to lift, gradually moving toward the more resistive areas. Never force the tissues.

2. *Myofascial Spread.* This stroke may be executed using fingers, knuckles, or the base of the palms. A very small amount of lubricant may be used. The therapist's hands should be able to pull the client's skin without slipping over it. Press into the midline of the section of tissue to be released until slight resistance is felt. Allow the hands to draw apart evenly until the client's tissue will not stretch any further. Hold at that point until the resistance yields and your hands can slide further apart (Fig. 4-2).

   This stroke is designed to release binding in the fascial membranes.

3. *Myofascial Mobilization.* The fingers, knuckles, palm, or forearm may be used for this stroke. The myofascial tissues are rolled against the underlying muscles and bones with a back-and-forth or circular movement (Fig. 4-3). This technique is used to free myofascial tissue that is adhering to itself. It re-establishes the ability of tissues to slide freely over each other.

DEEP TISSUE

The term *deep tissue therapy* has many connotations. It may be interpreted as the application of deep pressure to muscles, or as therapy to the deeper lying muscle groups in the body. Perhaps the most encompassing description of deep tissue therapy is that it is therapy that has a *deep* impact on the client. At its core, deep tissue therapy is transformative in nature. It has the capability to transform the dysfunctional characteristics of the body's soft tissues to minimize pain and stress as well as enhance function on many levels. To accomplish these goals, deeper pressure on the tissues may be

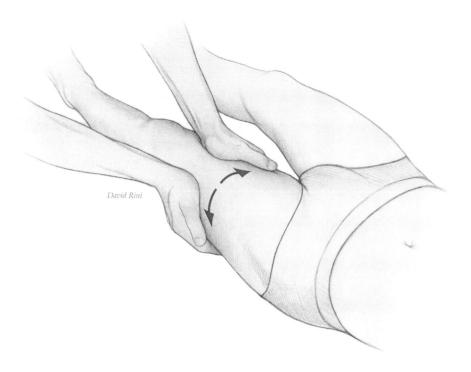

David Rini

FIGURE 4-2   Myofascial spread.

required at times. However, the pressure of strokes should never feel uncomfortably painful or at all intrusive to the client.

Pain is subjective. There is no constant, measurable amount of pressure to which every person will have the same response. The experience of touch as painful or pleasurable depends on many factors, including the degree of tension in the tissues, possible injurious conditions in the muscles, and the person's interpretation of the quality and intent of the touch. To be able to relax and willingly

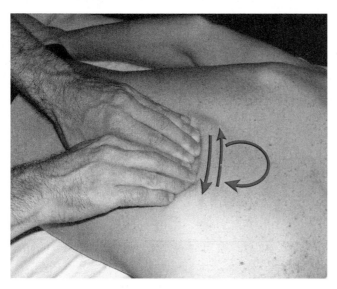

FIGURE 4-3   Myofascial mobilization.

accept deeper gradations of pressure, the client must be assured that the therapist is mindful of the effects of his or her touch on the client's body. The therapist must be capable of making the necessary adjustments to prevent touch from becoming painful, harmful, or intrusive. The organic, ever-changing nature of the interaction between the therapist and client during a deep tissue session requires constant vigilance to ensure that the quality of therapy remains productive.

After the warm-up phase of the session is completed, the deep tissue strokes are implemented. The lessons provide descriptions of the application of the strokes to specific muscles. They do not give details about the pace, depth, or number of repetitions of each stroke because, as stated above, those factors are variable, depending on the state of receptivity of the client's tissues and the client's attitude toward the work. Palpatory assessment and ongoing verbal communication with the client are necessary to determine the precise quality of the deep tissue techniques. The approach to deep tissue therapy will be different with every individual. Even the same client will require varying degrees of pressure on different muscle groups, depending on their condition.

The overall goal of the deep tissue strokes is to relax contracted muscles. This is accomplished by the application of slow, compressive force into the muscles accompanied by gradual movement of the stroke along the length of the muscle. This compressive force slowly lengthens the fibers in the muscle belly, similar to sustained stretching of a muscle.

Deep tissue strokes that are designed to lengthen shortened muscles are performed parallel to the muscle fibers. In this book, they are referred to as elongation strokes. They must be performed very slowly; otherwise, the stroke will activate the stretch reflex, causing the muscle to contract even more and defeating the purpose of deep tissue therapy.

When an elongation stroke is being performed at the appropriate pace, the tissues feel as if they are yielding, or melting, under the therapist's touch. If resistance is encountered as the therapist is stroking along the muscle, he or she should stop at that point and hold the stroke steady until the resistance melts. The therapist may need to lessen the degree of pressure being used to achieve the requisite softening of the muscle tissue before continuing the stroke.

Muscles are released in progression from the surface to the deeper layers. The therapist must be thoroughly familiar with the musculature and be able to picture the muscles' shapes and positions in relation to each other so that he or she knows when a particular muscle is being reached. Deeper muscles cannot be palpated directly. Their fibers are felt *through* the layers of muscle above them. If the surface muscles are contracted and tense, their fibers are not pliable enough for the therapist to feel through them to the deeper layers. Therefore, the surface layers must be released before the deeper layers are accessible.

As the therapist applies pressure, he or she sinks into the tissues only to the level of mild to moderate resistance. The feeling of resistance is a result of the muscle's contracting to defend itself against potentially harmful pressure. Deep tissue strokes may be applied with more force than connective tissue strokes, but never to the point at which the client has to tighten the muscles against the pressure. As soon as the soft tissues contract to defend themselves, tension is reintroduced into the body and deep tissue therapy is becoming counterproductive.

The client will sometimes experience sensations of pain during the work. Unhealthy conditions in muscle tissue are usually painful when touched. These include trigger points, scar tissue, bands of taut fibers, and spasms. When these conditions are encountered, the therapist should explain to the client the cause of the painful reaction. There is an element of fear associated with painful sensations. Educating the client about the nature of the painful response often calms the feelings of apprehension, lessening the subjective sensation of pain. The therapist always works with the client's input to ensure that the threshold of uncomfortable pain sensations is not crossed.

Signs of muscle relaxation are varied. As a muscle releases, it feels like it is able to spread more easily and has a softer tone as pressure is applied to it. Contracted fibers may fibrillate, or visibly jump, as they are relaxing. Sometimes a pulsation runs through the entire length of the muscle. Stringy, taut fibers become less pronounced as fluid circulation is enhanced.

Knots, or lumps, within a muscle belly are indications of deeply contracted fibers with accumulated waste products caused by fatigue, overuse, or trauma. These areas are usually painful to the touch and respond well to static compression maintained within the client's tolerance level for up to 30 seconds. Tiny lumps within the fibers that feel like crystals, or grains of sand, may be the result of waste product build-up or indications of scar tissue formation. They can also be found in tendinous fibers near the tendon's insertion on the bone. These small knots are usually tender when pressed and respond well to small, precise cross fiber strokes directly over them.

During the deep tissue session, the therapist should periodically pause to assess the progress of the work. Periodic pauses allow the client to relax and assimilate the experience more fully. Softly palpating the muscles worked with the palms of the hands allows the therapist to assess the degree of relaxation produced. The therapist may choose to ask the client for feedback about his or her feelings or reactions in response to the work done thus far. To enhance the assimilation process, a polarity contact may be administered to an area of the body after deep tissue therapy is completed.

Assessment of change may include range of motion stretches that use the muscles that have just been released to evaluate the degree of lengthening and relaxation that has occurred. Additional effleurage strokes performed from the muscles' origins to insertions reinforce the nervous system's reprogramming of the muscles resting lengths.

Deep Tissue Strokes

On Muscle Bellies

1. *Elongating/Lengthening* (Fig. 4-4A and B). This stroke is a slow gliding compression movement performed parallel to the muscle fibers, from origin to insertion. The fingers, knuckles, base of the palm, thumbs, elbow, or forearm may be used. It is the primary technique used to return a contracted muscle to its resting length.
2. *Spreading* (Fig. 4-5). These techniques are used to palpate aberrations in small sections of muscle fibers. They are incorporated within taut bands of fibers to locate trigger points precisely.

   The fingers, thumbs, knuckles, or elbow may be used. Although the thumb pads are the most sensitive part of the body used for delivering deep tissue strokes, it is best to perfect the use of these other body parts to save wear and tear on the thumbs.
   - *Up-and-Down.* Move parallel to the muscle fibers, covering 1-inch sections at a time.

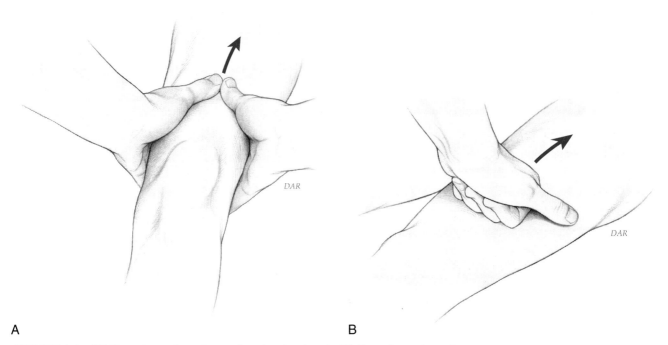

A

B

FIGURE 4-4 (**A**) Deep tissue elongation stroke using thumb pads. (**B**) Deep tissue elongation stroke using knuckles.

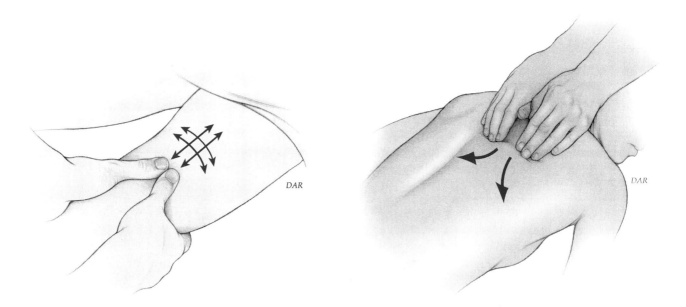

FIGURE 4-5 Position for spreading techniques.

FIGURE 4-6 Fanning stroke.

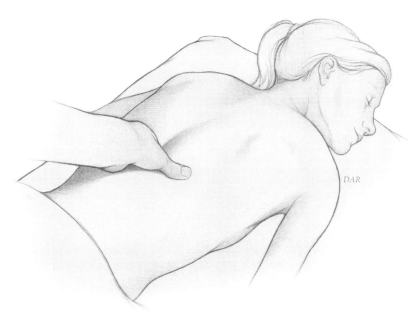

FIGURE 4-7   Static compression using the thumb.

- *Side-to-Side.* Move perpendicular to the muscle fibers in back-and-forth motions in 1-inch segments.
- *Combination.* Perform up-and-down and side-to-side strokes on the same section of muscle, creating a 1-inch square.
- *Fanning.* The hands spread apart from each other in an arc pattern 3 to 4 inches wide. This stroke stretches fascial membranes (Fig. 4-6).
3. *Static Compression* (Fig. 4-7). Lean directly into the muscle tissue at a 90° angle to the surface of the body. Thumbs, fingers, knuckles, or elbows may be used. This stroke is used on extremely contracted sections of

muscle fibers. It is also used to treat trigger points and acupressure points.
4. *Sifting* (Fig. 4-8). This is a cross fiber style stroke. Grasp a section of muscle tissue between your fingers and thumb. Roll the fibers to release adhering factors and to locate trigger points within taut bands of tissue.

TENDONS

The following procedures are used to treat tendons (thumbs, elbow, fingers, or knuckle may be used) (Fig. 4-9):

1. Stroke on the tendon toward the insertion point on the bone.

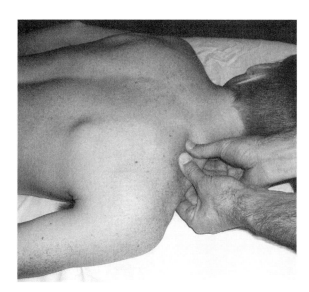

FIGURE 4-8   Sifting technique.

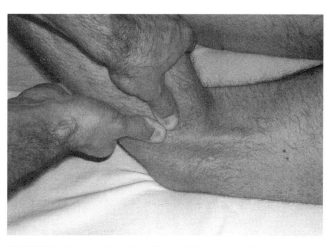

FIGURE 4-9   Hand position for working on a tendon.

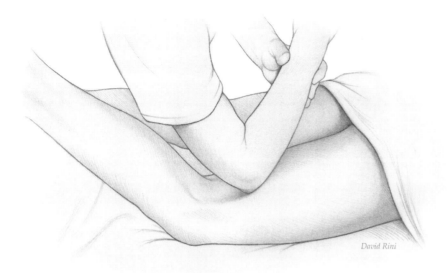

David Rini

FIGURE 4-10   Deep tissue elongation stroke between muscle bellies.

2. Do short cross fiber strokes across the tendon.
3. Hold static compression where the tendon attaches to the bone.

SEPARATING MUSCLES (FIG. 4-10)

Stroke along the borders of muscles to separate them from each other, using elongation strokes. The thumb, elbow, or knuckles may be used.

NEUROMUSCULAR THERAPY

The purpose of neuromuscular therapy is to seek out and treat trigger points, which may be causing pain or muscular weakness. A description of trigger points and their formation is provided in the introduction to neuromuscular therapy in Chapter 1.

Trigger points are located in one of two ways. The first way they may be encountered is while performing deep tissue strokes on a muscle. A trigger point is always found within a taut band of muscle fibers that are tender to the touch. An indication that a band of fibers houses a single trigger point or a group of points is that the fibers will twitch and elicit a pain response when the therapist's finger strums across them. Once the taut band of fibers is located, the therapist carefully seeks out the point within the fibers that delivers the most pronounced pain sensation when compressed.

If active, the trigger point will also produce painful feelings within a particular remote site, known as a referred pain zone. A trigger point found in a specific location will always refer sensations to the same distant site. Travell and others have spent much time mapping the referral patterns of trigger points. These maps are available in many books and in chart form (trigger point charts are available at medical bookstores and massage supply stores). The predictability of trigger point referral patterns provides the key to the second method of locating trigger points.

During the interview that takes place before the deep tissue session, the client may describe areas of soft tissue that commonly cause pain and discomfort. The pain may be active or most pronounced after certain physical activities, or when the person's stress level is high. The client is probably describing referred pain sites activated by trigger points. The therapist should try to pinpoint the exact location and dimension of the pain zone. A practical way to accomplish this is by the therapist tracing the perimeter of the pain zone on the client's body, with permission, while the client describes it. The therapist can also draw the area of pain on a piece of paper containing a blank figure of the human body. Once the location and size of the referred pain pattern is known, the associated trigger point can be found with the use of a trigger point chart.

The procedure for treating trigger points is simple. Once the location of the trigger point is pinpointed, the therapist presses on it directly using the thumb, finger, or elbow (Fig. 4-11). The degree of pressure applied should elicit a mild pain response at the site of the trigger point and at the referral zone. After explaining this to the client, the therapist may incorporate a simple pressure-determining scale graded from 1 to 3 (1 signifying too little pressure, 2 signifying appropriate pressure, and 3 signifying too much pressure). By using this scale with the client, the therapist can always gauge pressure perfectly to the client's reaction. This scale can also be used when per-

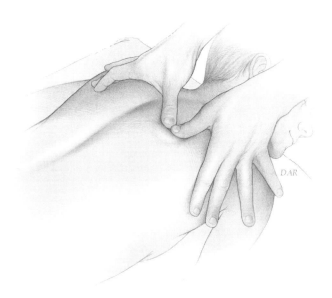

FIGURE 4-11   Hand position for neuromuscular therapy trigger point release.

forming deep tissue strokes to determine the proper amount of pressure.

Trigger points are always painful when pressed but are not usually noticeable otherwise. The pain produced by a trigger point is registered at the referral site, not at the location of the trigger point itself. Treatment performed solely at the referral pain site may offer temporary relief or comfort, but it will not relieve the pain permanently because the source of the irritation (which is the trigger point) has not been deactivated.

Trigger points are treated with static compression for approximately 8 to 12 seconds. That is usually enough time to interrupt the pain messages delivered by a trigger point to its corresponding referral zone. During the holding period the client should experience a significant drop in the level of pain sensation. The therapist needs to monitor the client's experience of the pain pattern to measure the effectiveness of the treatment. Again, a simple verbal device can be used to gain information about the level of pain sensation. Every few seconds, as the therapist continues to press, the client is asked if the degree of pain is more, the same, or less. If the treatment is successful, the client should report a continual lessening of the pain.

Immediately after deactivating the trigger point, the therapist should stretch the affected muscle to attain it natural resting length. Trigger points manifest within contracted bands of fibers. The more regularly a muscle is stretched, the less likely it is to harbor trigger points. The client should be taught exercises to perform between treatments to stretch the affected muscles.

Mapping and treating trigger points can become rather complex, especially if the trigger points have been active for a long time and the client has several areas of chronic pain. Stacks of trigger points can develop in muscles that overlay each other. Each trigger point in the stack needs to be treated in succession from the surface muscles to the deeper layers. Several trigger points can also be clustered around each other within the same muscle. They may have the same or different referral zones connected to them. Referral pain zones themselves can develop trigger points, known as satellite trigger points.

Satellite trigger points develop their own patterns of pain referral that extend into other areas of the body. If left untreated, trigger point activity can gradually spread throughout the body. The therapist must carefully map each pain zone and track down the trigger point or points that is causing it to fire. Maintaining a body map for each client which charts each pain zone and associated trigger points is very helpful in dealing with cases of chronic pain.

The length of time that pain relief from trigger point treatment lasts is variable. Among other factors, it depends on the activities and lifestyle of the client. Job-related repetitive movements that are aggravating trigger points may have to be relearned or curtailed. Stress management techniques should be incorporated to reduce excessive stimulation within the nervous system. Regular exercise, including slow, sustained stretching, should be practiced on a regular basis. If the necessary steps are taken, relief from trigger point pain may last anywhere from several days to forever.

At the client's next deep tissue therapy session, the therapist should ask about the duration of pain reduction in the referral zones. If necessary, trigger points can be re-treated. If no pain relief is reported, a consultation with a physician for possible causes of the pain other than musculoskeletal dysfunction should be suggested.

BODY MECHANICS

Of all the essential skills necessary to become a competent deep tissue therapist, one of the most important is learning to use proper body mechanics. Correct body alignment and movement support efficient execution of the strokes, minimizing wear and tear on the therapist both physically and mentally. Straining to perform the techniques is not only detrimental to the therapist's body, it interferes with the qualities of relaxation and openness that the therapist strives to transmit to the client through the strokes.

Almost all massage strokes require the transmission of weight from the therapist's body, moving from the feet and legs to the spine, then passing from the shoulder girdle through the arms and hands to the recipient. Leaning into the client's body is the means by which pressure for the strokes is generated. The study of body mechanics is largely based on learning how to transfer weight through the body structure without creating strain in the muscles.

Problems that occur due to a misaligned skeleton are compounded while performing massage. In addition to contending with the force of gravity, the body structure must distribute many extra pounds of pressure generated by the compressive movements of the strokes. When the body is not properly positioned, strain around unstable joints can become tremendous, leading to tissue breakdown and eventually disability.

The basic principles of alignment that apply when standing upright are also utilized in performing massage. The best way to understand correct alignment is to become familiar with the proper position of the skeleton to minimize structural stress. When correct placement of the bones is sensed or visualized, the nervous system directs the muscles to perform the necessary actions to maintain that position.

The complex, precise coordinating actions the muscles must perform to move the body are carried out almost entirely at an unconscious level. Any attempt to consciously control the muscles severely inhibits the nervous system's job of orchestrating smooth muscle function. Using this principle in mastering massage techniques requires learning the correct position of the body for delivering each stroke and developing the kinesthetic awareness to sense when the body is deviating from this position.

The major principles of good body mechanics have been divided into five questions the therapist can easily memorize and recall when performing massage to quickly assess if he or she is using the body properly (Box 4-3).

THE FIVE-QUESTION CHECKLIST

1. Are the centers of my joints aligned?
   - My thumb is comfortably extended, not flexed or hyperextended.
   - My spine is straight from the sacrum to the atlas.
   - When my knee is flexed, it lines up over the second toe of the foot.
   - When my leg is straight, the knee is not hyperextended.
   - The tips of my elbows are pointed outward, not rolled inward.
   - My scapulae are relaxed and dropped; the humerus is resting comfortably in the shoulder joint.
   - My wrists are in a neutral position.

2. Is my body facing the direction of my stroke?
   - My shoulders and hips are lined up in the same direction.
   - My hands are lined up to my center of gravity (a point at the midline of the body, 2 inches below the navel).
   - My legs and feet are moving in the same direction as my upper body.
   - My legs are approximating a parallel position, with my feet at least hip-width apart (imagine standing on skis).

3. Am I moving with my whole body?
   - At the beginning of the stroke, most of my weight is on my back foot.
   - My weight shifts forward as I apply pressure and/or the stroke travels forward.
   - The force needed to perform the stroke flows upward from my feet to my hands.
   - The more relaxed I am, the more easily the force can flow through my body.
   - Body movement is fluid and continuous; I am never *locked* in a position.

4. Am I lengthening as I apply pressure?
   - For every action, there is a reaction:
     - As I reach my back foot into the floor, my body lengthens upward.
     - As I reach forward, I lengthen backward.

BOX 4-3

Five Body Mechanics Questions

1. Are the centers of my joints aligned?
2. Is my body facing the direction of my stroke?
3. Am I moving with my whole body?
4. Am I lengthening as I apply pressure?
5. Am I breathing from my center?

- My joints feel properly aligned and not compressed.
- My body expands and softens as I apply pressure.
- My shoulders are relaxed and my shoulder girdle is wide; my spine is long.
- My muscles feel loose and long, not contracted and tense.

5. Am I breathing from my center?
   - The rhythm for each stroke comes from my breathing pattern.
   - I allow myself to relax and fall forward as I exhale into the stroke.
   - My lower body and upper body come into balance at my pelvis.
   - I breathe all tension out of my body as I work.
   - I yield rather than force.

THERAPIST SELF-CARE

Massage therapy is a demanding profession. It requires intense mental concentration and regular physical conditioning. As with any care-giving job, there is always the danger of burnout if the therapist does not provide adequate self-care. People who are constantly giving to others often neglect to take the necessary time to replenish themselves. A few simple practices done on a regular basis will assure that the therapist remains healthy and able to sustain a full-time massage practice.

1. *Exercise Daily*. Daily exercise is a requisite for taking care of the body adequately. Practicing proper body mechanics minimizes stress to the therapist's body, but it is not enough to counteract the compressive forces generated by performing massage therapy. The therapist's muscles and joints need to be lengthened and stretched regularly.

   Tai chi and yoga are both excellent practices that maintain flexibility and strength while reducing the build-up of stress. These systems also encourage deep breathing, which is extremely important for rejuvenating the body and mind. The self-awareness and mental control that tai chi and yoga foster help the massage therapist to increase the capacity to empathize with and stay focused on the client throughout the entire deep tissue therapy process.

2. *Take Time for Daily Reflection*. This helps the therapist to remain centered, enthusiastic, and committed while caring for others. There are many different ways to clear the internal clutter that accumulates from intense work involving constant interaction with other people. Activities like walking, gardening, reading, and meditating all have the capacity to provide an outlet for the therapist to unwind and relieve potentially toxic mental and emotional build-up.

3. *Eat Vitalized Food and Drink Water*. Massage therapy is intensive work. It involves constant physical activity, moment-to-moment decision-making, and unwavering vitality. In short, being a massage therapist calls on all of one's resources. Giving the body adequate reserves of energy through nutritious food and clean water is mandatory to sustain the level of activity required for the work. Maintaining a well-balanced diet is one of the cornerstones of healthy living.

4. *Receive Bodywork Yourself*. The experience of receiving regular massage therapy along with the activities mentioned above keeps the body operating at peak performance levels. It also reminds the therapist what the experience of being a massage recipient is like and what a profound impact he or she is having on clients by sharing deep tissue therapy skills.

REFERENCES

1. Chaitow L. Muscle energy techniques. New York, NY: Churchill Livingstone, 1996: 38–39.
2. Chaitow L, Freyman V. Palpation skills: assessment and diagnosis through touch. New York, NY: Churchill Livingstone, 1996.
3. Pfrimmer T. Muscles: your invisible bonds. Blyth, Ontario: Blyth Printing, 1983.

Connective Tissue

ROLE OF FASCIA

The connective tissues are the class of tissue that provides shape, support, strength, and continuity to all the structures contained within the human form. In a sense, it is the connective tissues that hold the body together. They include the bones, cartilage, ligaments, tendons, and fascia. Taken as a whole, the connective tissues are the most pervasive tissue in the body.

Fascia is a sheet-like membrane that wraps and interweaves all the muscles in the body (Fig. 5-1). (For an informative description of the composition and role of fascia, see Chapter 3 in *Job's Body: A Handbook for Bodywork*.[1]) It can be thought of as a multi-layered net that encases and connects all the soft tissue structures from just below the skin all the way down to the bones. Within the muscles (Fig. 5-2) it binds the muscle fibers together. Fascia even forms the walls of the individual muscle cells. Muscle is often referred to as myofascial tissue in acknowledgment of the inextricable relationship of muscle fibers and fascia.

To release constricted muscles fully, the distinct qualities and functions of muscle fibers and fascia must be considered. Muscle fibers actively shorten, or contract, to move the bones; they are passively lengthened by the shortening of other muscle fibers. Deep tissue massage techniques are designed to release chronically shortened muscle fibers through manual compression and slow stretching. However, a muscle cannot regain its resting length even when contracted fibers are relaxed if the surrounding fascial membranes are binding it. The constricted fascial casing will prevent the muscle fibers from expanding and thus maintain the restricted condition of the muscle. Techniques that address the unique characteristics of fascia must be applied to liberate contracted myofascial tissue fully.

Fascia is composed of three primary constituents: a fluid material called ground substance and two proteins (collagen and elastin). Each of these contributes a specialized property that gives fascia its diverse characteristics of

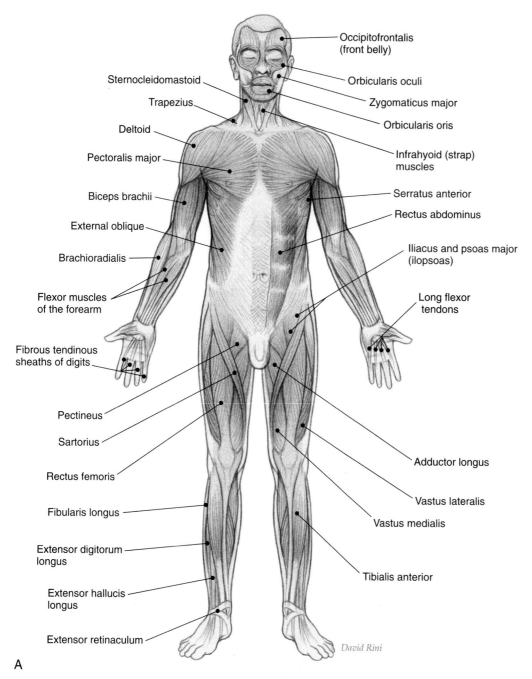

Occipitofrontalis
(front belly)

Sternocleidomastoid

Trapezius

Deltoid

Pectoralis major

Biceps brachii

External oblique

Brachioradialis

Flexor muscles
of the forearm

Fibrous tendinous
sheaths of digits

Pectineus

Sartorius

Rectus femoris

Fibularis longus

Extensor digitorum
longus

Extensor hallucis
longus

Extensor retinaculum

Orbicularis oculi

Zygomaticus major

Orbicularis oris

Infrahyoid (strap)
muscles

Serratus anterior

Rectus abdominus

Iliacus and psoas major
(ilopsoas)

Long flexor
tendons

Adductor longus

Vastus lateralis

Vastus medialis

Tibialis anterior

David Rini

A

FIGURE 5-1 **(A)** Superficial muscles—anterior. *(continued)*

fluidity, strength, and elasticity. Ground substance is the primary component of fascia. Chemically it is classified as a mucopolysaccharide. It is the same liquid that forms the interstitial fluid that bathes every cell of the body.

This ground substance is a gel, which means it has the capability of moving between a more fluid and a more solid state. The degree of viscosity of the ground substance is largely dependent on three factors—temperature, movement, and hydration. When the body is in motion, heat is generated which tends to promote a more fluid

state in the ground substance. Greater fluidity within the fascia promotes freer muscle tissue.

Exercise helps the body to remain supple partly due to this effect. Lack of movement causes the ground substance to thicken, which tends to inhibit muscular freedom. Because of this phenomenon the body feels stiffer when a person has been sitting or lying still for long periods. The elements of pressure and stretching used in fascial release techniques replicate natural muscle movements and help to return the ground substance to a fluid state.

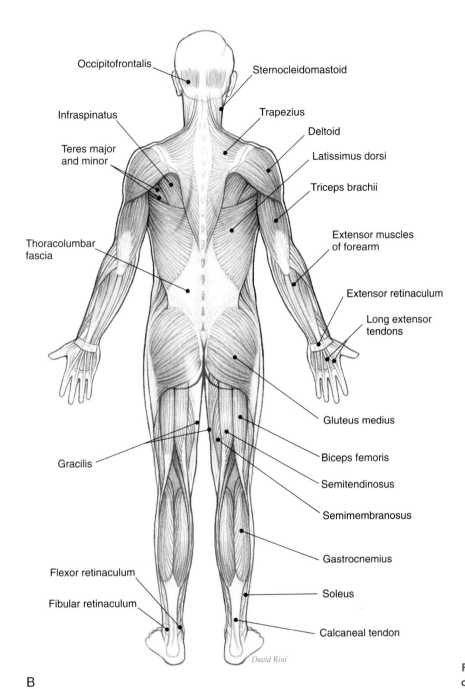

Occipitofrontalis

Sternocleidomastoid

Infraspinatus

Trapezius

Deltoid

Teres major
and minor

Latissimus dorsi

Triceps brachii

Thoracolumbar
fascia

Extensor muscles
of forearm

Extensor retinaculum

Long extensor
tendons

Gluteus medius

Gracilis

Biceps femoris

Semitendinosus

Semimembranosus

Gastrocnemius

Flexor retinaculum

Soleus

Fibular retinaculum

Calcaneal tendon

David Rini

B

FIGURE 5-1 *Continued.* (**B**) Superficial muscles—posterior.

Within the ground substance lie mesh-like layers of collagen, a protein composed of long ropy strands. Depending on the form of connective tissue, collagen can be configured in different patterns, but its basic role is to provide strength and support. Adjacent molecular chains of collagen readily link together due to the strong bonding capability of hydrogen, one of collagen's primary components. This creates an extremely durable webbing that can resist stretching better than steel wire. Ligaments and tendons contain a high concentration of collagen, making them very effective in holding the skeleton and muscles together.

Distributed within the collagen mesh of fascial membranes is another protein, called elastin, which has much greater flexibility than collagen. Elastin gives fascia more stretchiness than other forms of connective tissue, allowing it to change shape as muscles contract and expand. Fascia can be envisioned like the surface membrane of a jelly-filled balloon, with the ability to stretch and mold in response to internal changes but also with strong resistive force to contain and give shape to largely fluid contents.

In addition to giving it strength, collagen's affinity to bond causes fascial membranes to stick together like plas-

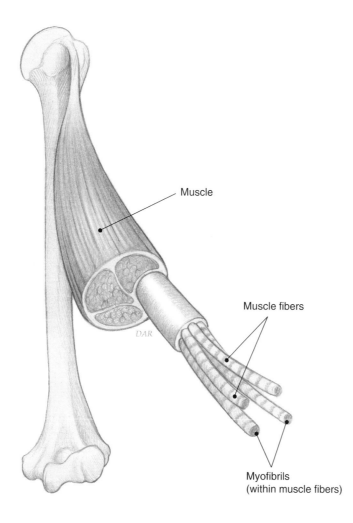

Muscle

Muscle fibers

DAR

Myofibrils
(within muscle fibers)

FIGURE 5-2   Every layer of a muscle is surrounded by fascia, from the surface down to the cellular level.

tic wrap. This can lead to muscular and postural problems. Under conditions of compression, which are aggravated by gravity's downward pull on the body, adjacent muscles tend to adhere to each other causing them to lose their differentiation. As muscles meld together, the body's movement capability is diminished and the structure begins to pull toward the ground.

The continuity of the fascial membranes throughout the body provides a medium to absorb and evenly distribute the impact arising from falls and from everyday movements like walking or jumping, much like the role of

shock absorbers in a car. Fascial planes thicken in areas of the body that are under stress due to postural misalignment, poor movement mechanics, or injury in order to provide additional bracing. These denser layers create a break in the flow of forces through the structure resulting in areas of weakness at the points of discontinuity. The weakened tissues are vulnerable to breakdown causing degeneration and injury. Realigning the lines of force that flow through the fascia adds immeasurably to the body's overall state of health and vitality by minimizing wear and tear on the muscles and skeleton.

WORKING WITH FASCIA

The goal of working on the body's fascia is twofold: to make the ground substance more fluid, and to release collagen bonds that are causing muscles to adhere. The techniques used to mobilize fascia often incorporate slow stretching and pulling actions. It has been found that steady, sustained stretching of fascial membranes helps to

free the restricting links that form within the collagen mesh. The key to successful fascial release is the ability to sense the limit of the tissue's ability to stretch and to hold the stretch until a yielding or lengthening sensation is felt. The tissues should never be forced with more pressure or stretch than they can accommodate comfortably.

Because contractile muscle fibers and fascial membranes are so intricately intertwined, it is physically impossible to touch one without affecting the other. The therapist's intention while manipulating tissues is the key to distinguishing which component of the myofascial unit is being emphasized. Helpful images for sensing tissue release when working on fascia can include visions of an ice cube slowly melting on a sidewalk or butter melting in a frying pan.

As the hands are placed on the body, pressure is applied only to the point at which resistance is first felt in the muscle tissue. This might be registered as a slight recoil or a feeling of the tissue thickening. The therapist then waits for a softening of the resistance, which allows the hands to continue to glide through the tissue until further resistance is encountered. This slow, methodical sensing of the tissue's reaction to the therapist's manipulation assures that the state of the fascia is being affected.

CONNECTIVE TISSUE ROUTINE

The description of the connective tissue procedures does not include the specific muscles being worked on because the goal of these strokes is to stretch the fascial membranes that wrap all of the muscles. The therapist's focus while performing these strokes is on sensing the softening and stretching of the tissues in response to the slow movements of the hands. The following chapters focus on lengthening and repatterning specific muscles.

NECK

POSITION

- The client is lying supine on the table.
- The therapist is sitting at the head of the table.

1. *Longitudinal Neck Release.* Place the fingers of both hands under the occipital ridge. Allow the fingers to sink into the tissues until a slight resistance is felt.

   Move the tissues of the neck with short up-and-down strokes without sliding over the skin (Fig. 5-3). Move the fingers down a couple of inches to the next section of the neck, about an inch below the first sec-

tion, and repeat the up-and-down stroke. Continue with this pattern to the base of the neck.

   Return to the occiput, placing the fingers further away from the midline than on the first pass. Repeat the sequence down the neck.

2. *Lateral Neck Release.* Place the fingers lengthwise on either side of the spinous processes of the neck, from underneath. Let them sink into the tissues. Slowly spread them laterally, away from the spine (Fig. 5-4). Slide farther down the neck and repeat. Continue, spreading in horizontal strips, to the base of the neck.

3. *Horizontal Neck Release.* Turn the client's head slightly to the side. Using your fingers, sink in along the anterior border of the sternocleidomastoid muscle. Slowly glide the fingers in a posterior direction as far as you can reach (Fig. 5-5). Repeat, in horizontal strips, throughout the length of the neck.

4. *Laterally Flex the Client's Neck.* Place your fingers into the front portion of the trapezius muscle on the flexed side, slightly behind the clavicle. Gradually sink in until mild resistance is felt and perform the short up-and-down movements with your fingers.

   Repeat moves 1 to 4 on the other side.

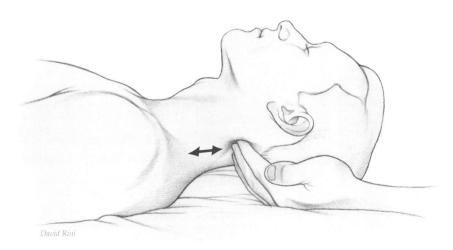

David Rini

FIGURE 5-3   Longitudinal neck release.

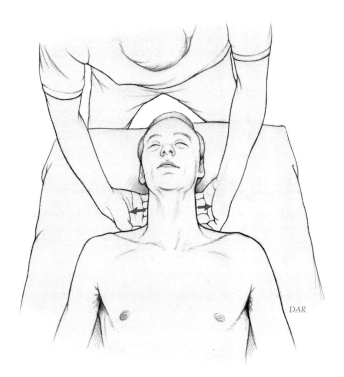

FIGURE 5-4 Lateral neck release.

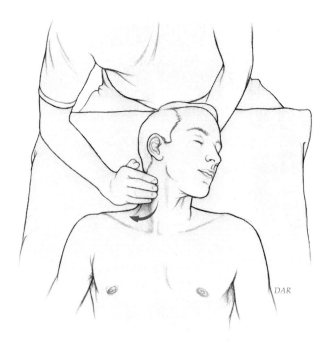

FIGURE 5-5 Horizontal neck release moving posteriorly.

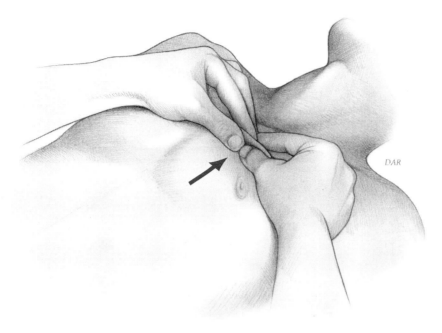

FIGURE 5-6 Lifting and rolling superficial fascia of the upper chest..

CHEST

POSITION

- The client is lying supine.
- The therapist is standing at the side of the table.

1. *Lift and Roll the Superficial Fascia of the Chest.* Grasp the skin of the upper chest lightly between your thumb and fingers. Roll it slowly superiorly toward the clavicle (Fig. 5-6). Cover as much of the chest as you can. When working with female clients, avoid the breast tissue.

2. *Fanning Strokes on the Upper Chest.* Place the fingers of both hands on the sternum. Sink into the tissues and spread slowly outward from the midline with a fanning stroke (Fig. 5-7). Repeat the stroke several times, moving in a superior direction toward the clavicles.

3. *Myofascial Mobilization of the Tissues over the Ribs.* Beginning at the lower portion of the ribcage, place

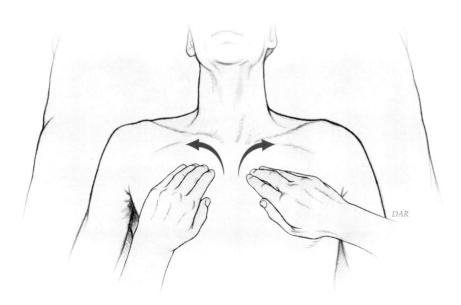

FIGURE 5-7 Fanning stroke on the chest.

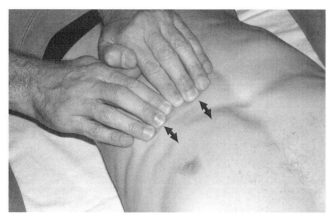

FIGURE 5-8 Myofascial mobilization of the tissues over the ribs.

your fingers on the lowest ribs and slide the tissues up and down over the rib (Fig. 5-8). Feel for areas where the tissue does not move or feels like it is sticking to the rib. Work to free all the tissue. Progress up the ribcage, working over each rib until you reach the clavicle. Repeat on the other side of the chest.

4. *Compress and Spread the Chest Tissues.* Holding the wrist, abduct the client's arm 90° and flex it at the elbow. Move the arm into various stretched positions while you compress and spread the stretched myofas-

cial tissues of the chest with the heel of your other hand (Fig. 5-9).

ABDOMEN

POSITION

- The client is lying supine with a bolster under the knees.
- The therapist is standing at the side of the table facing the client's abdomen.

1. *Lift and Roll the Abdominal Tissues.* Reach across the client's body, grasping the skin at the waistline between your thumb and fingers. Roll the skin, moving slowly toward the midline (Fig. 5-10). When you encounter tightness or resistance, slowly lift the skin away from the underlying muscle and hold until a softening is felt. Cover the entire side of the abdomen thoroughly, working in horizontal strips from the side of the trunk to the midline. Walk around to the other side of the table and repeat the procedure on the other half of the client's abdomen.

2. *Myofascial Stretch on the Abdomen.* Place the right palm on the abdomen, over the navel area. Place your left palm on top of your right hand. Begin to make a slow, clockwise spiraling motion, moving the skin over the underlying tissues (Fig. 5-11). Do not glide over the

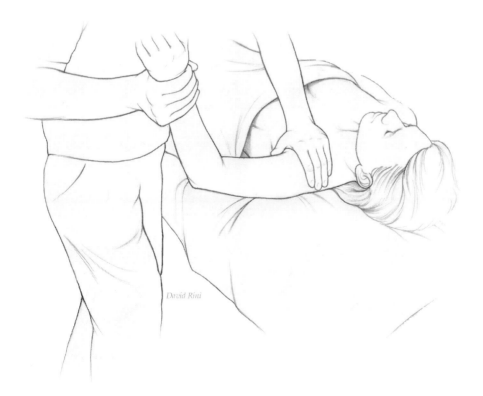

David Rini

FIGURE 5-9 Compress and spread the myofascial tissues of the chest.

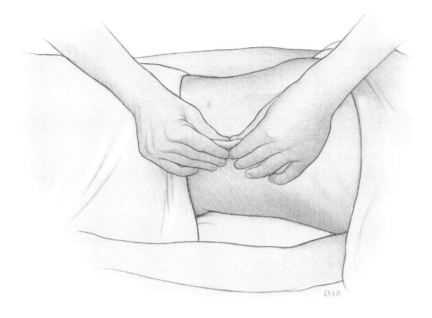

FIGURE 5-10 Lifting and rolling the abdominal tissue.

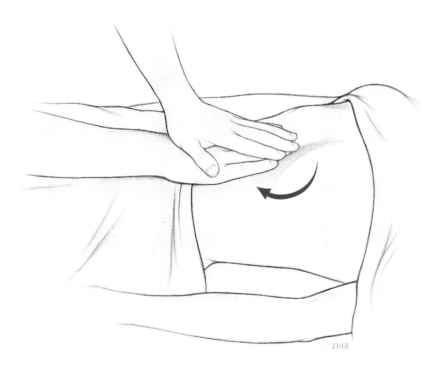

FIGURE 5-11 Myofascial stretch on the abdomen.

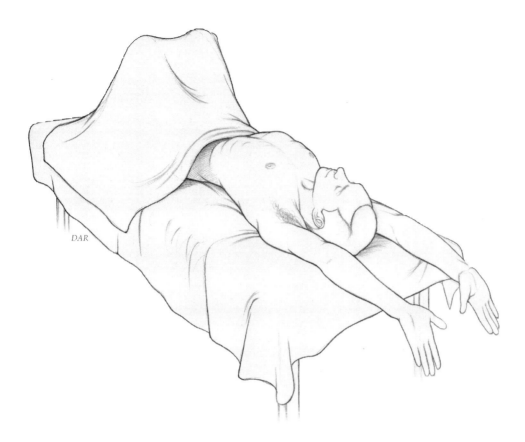

DAR

FIGURE 5-12 Abdominal stretch.

skin. Gradually increase the size of the spiral, stretching the skin and fascia to their maximm degree.

3. *Abdominal Stretch.* With the client's knees flexed, have him or her stretch both arms overhead and reach fully. Encourage the client to take a deep breath, lifting the chest and pulling the abdomen in while continuing to stretch the arms overhead, until a stretch is felt in the abdominal muscles (Fig. 5-12). A useful image to aid the stretch is to tell the client to imagine the navel touching the front of the spine as he or she reaches.

ARM

POSITION

- The client is lying supine.
- The therapist is standing at the side of the table, next to the client's hand.

1. *Myofascial Spread on the Palm.* The client's palm is facing away from the therapist. Using both hands, curve your fingers under the client's hand, pressing your fingertips into the palm. Slowly slide your hands apart, stretching the tissues of the palm (Fig. 5-13). Perform this move very slowly, pausing to allowing the fascia to stretch.

2. *Fascial Lift and Roll on the Forearm.* The client's arm is resting on the table. Place your hands in the skin rolling position, parallel to the muscle fibers, above the client's wrist. Roll and lift the tissues of the forearm, in horizontal strips, from wrist to elbow (Fig. 5-14).

3. *Myofascial Spread on the Forearm.* Flex the client's arm at the elbow. Place your hands around the forearm at the wrist, fingers sinking into the midline of the palmar side of the forearm with the same hand position as in no. 1 above. Slowly spread the fingers away from the midline, stretching the tissues (Fig. 5-15). Continue, in horizontal strips, to the elbow. Repeat the move on the other side of the forearm.

4. *Myofascial Spread on the Upper Arm.* The client's arm is lying on the table. Begin the stroke just above the elbow. Spread the tissues evenly from the midline out to the edges of the upper arm, using the heels of your hands or the broad side of your thumbs (Fig. 5-16).

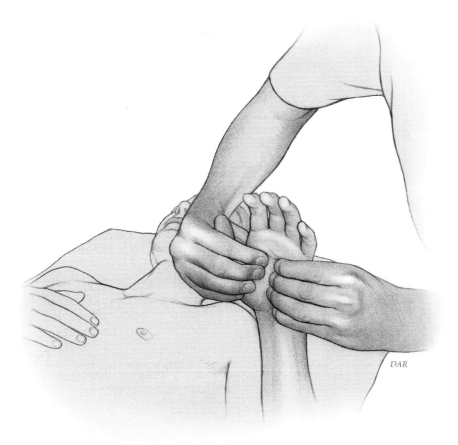

FIGURE 5-13   Spreading the fascia of the palm.

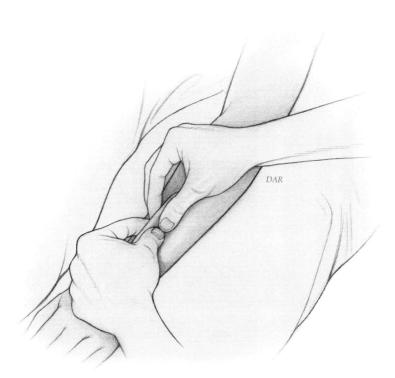

FIGURE 5-14   Lifting and rolling the forearm tissues.

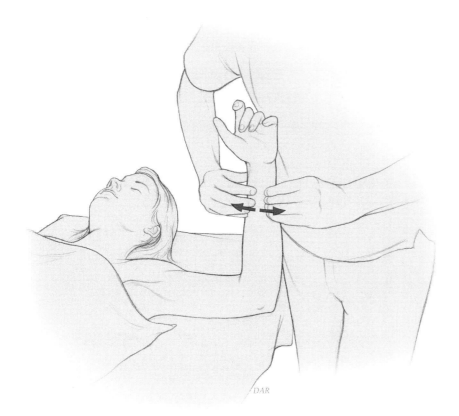

FIGURE 5-15 Myofascial spread on the forearm.

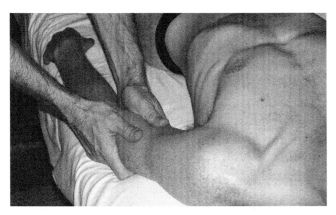

FIGURE 5-16 Myofascial spread on the upper arm.

BACK

POSITION

- The client is lying prone.
- The therapist is standing at the head of the table.

1. *Myofascial Mobilization of the Back*. With your fingertips or palms, sink into the tissues enough to be able to move the skin without sliding over it. Using a short up-and-down and side-to-side motion, move the skin over the underlying tissues (Fig. 5-17). Work in small sections, covering the entire back. This procedure can also be performed with a rolled up towel to move the skin.

2. *Myofascial Spreading on the Back*. Standing at the side of the table, sink into the tissues with your fingers or knuckles. Glide through the tissues with a spreading motion, moving as the fascia softens, pausing at resistance. Begin the stroke at the spine and move outward in horizontal motions across the back (Fig. 5-18). If using the fingers, work on the opposite side of the client's back from the side of the table you are standing on, stroking from the spine away from yourself. When using knuckles, work on the same side of the back, stroking from the spine toward yourself.

3. *Myofascial Release of the Tissues over the Bones*. Roll the myofascial tissue over the bones, using a circular friction motion. In the upper back, roll the tissues over the ribs and scapulae. In the lower back, roll against the 12th rib, the lumbar spine, and the iliac crest.

4. *Back Stretch*. Have the client lift up onto hands and knees while under the sheet and then sit back on the heels, resting the chest on the thighs and the forehead on the table in front of the knees to stretch the muscles of the back (Fig. 5-19).

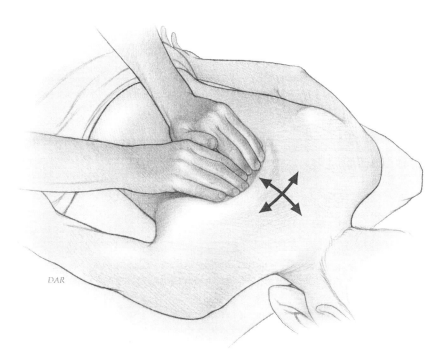

FIGURE 5-17   Myofascial mobilization of the back.

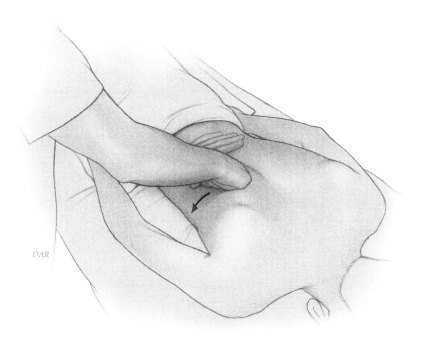

FIGURE 5-18   Myofascial spreading on the back.

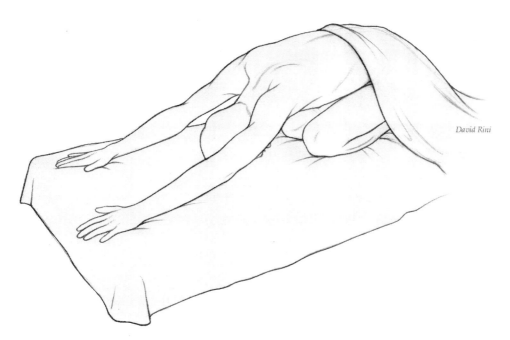

David Rini

FIGURE 5-19   Back stretch.

FOOT

POSITION

- The client is lying supine.
- The therapist is standing at the side of the table next to the client's foot, facing away from the client's head.

1. *Myofascial Spreading of the Plantar Surface of the*

Foot. Stand at the side of the table, facing the dorsal side of the client's foot. Curve the fingers of both hands around the underside of the foot. Sink your fingers into the sole of the foot until mild resistance is felt. Slowly spread your fingers from the midline to the outer edges of the foot (Fig. 5-20).

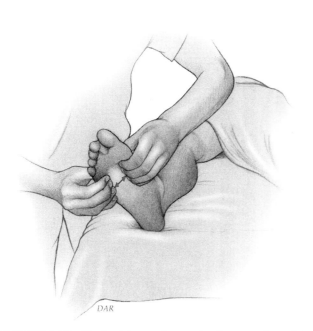

FIGURE 5-20   Myofascial spreading on the plantar surface of the foot.

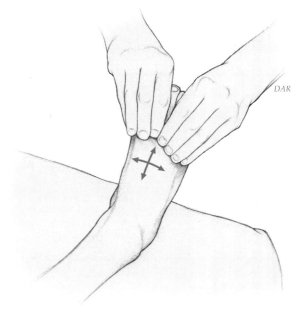

DAR

FIGURE 5-21   Myofascial mobilization on the dorsal side of the foot.

b. Hold both sides of the client's foot with your hands. Shift the bones of the foot back and forth by alternately moving one hand toward you and the other hand away from you in a continuous motion (Fig. 5-23).

LEG

POSITION

- The client is lying supine.
- The therapist is standing at the side of the table next to the client's ankle.

1. *Myofascial Spreading of the Leg.* Place the hands around the tibia with the heels of the hand meeting at the midline of the leg. Slowly spread the hands apart, with pressure against the base of the palms (Fig. 5-24). Begin the sequence at the ankle. Moving in horizontal strips, work your way up the leg to the knee.
2. *Myofascial Mobilization of the Leg.* Using the fingers or knuckles, roll across the lateral leg muscles until they slide freely over the bone (Fig. 5-25). Begin at the ankle. Work in horizontal strips, up to the knee.
3. *Fascial Stretches for the leg.* With one hand on the ankle and the other hand on the metatarsal, alternately flex and extend the client's foot. Place one palm on the dorsal surface of the foot and the other palm on the plantar surface of the foot. Invert the foot and hold, allowing the myofascial tissues to stretch. Evert the foot and hold.

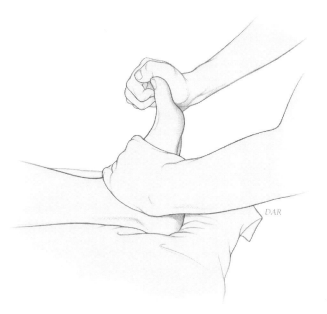

FIGURE 5-22 Position for foot stretch.

2. *Myofascial Mobilization on the Dorsal Side of the Foot.* Standing at the base of the table, place your fingers on the dorsal surface of the foot. Slide the tissues up and down and side to side in small sections (Fig. 5-21). Cover the entire surface of the foot.
3. Fascial Stretching of the Foot
   a. Grasp the client's toes with one hand while holding the metatarsal portion of the foot with the other hand. Flex the toes forward and back to stretch the foot (Fig. 5-22).

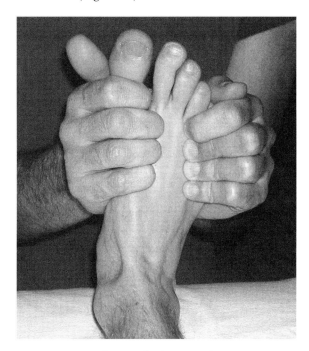

FIGURE 5-23 Position for foot stretch.

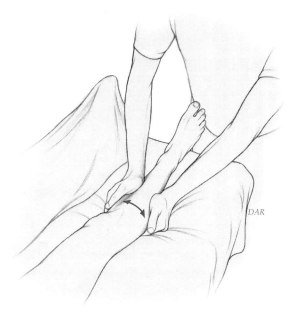

FIGURE 5-24 Myofascial spreading on the leg.

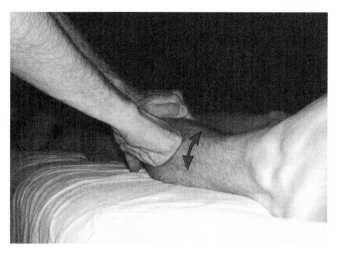

FIGURE 5-25   Myofascial mobilization on the leg.

ANTERIOR THIGH

POSITION

- The client is lying supine.
- The therapist is standing at the side of the table next to the client's knee.

1. *Lift and Roll the Myofascial Tissue of the Thigh.* Place your hands in the skin rolling position on the thigh, parallel to the muscle fibers. Lift and roll the tissues of the thigh (Fig. 5-26). Move from the knee to the hip. Work in horizontal strips, covering the entire thigh.

2. *Myofascial Spreading of the Thigh.* Place the hands around the thigh with the heels of the hand meeting at the midline. Applying pressure with the base of the palm, slowly slide the hands apart, spreading the tissues of the thigh. Begin the stroke at the knee. Repeat the spreading action in horizontal strips to the hip.

3. *Myofascial Mobilization of the Thigh.* Using the fingers of both hands, roll the muscles of the thigh over the bone until they slide freely (Fig. 5-27).

MEDIAL THIGH

POSITION

- The client may be positioned supine with the leg to be worked on bent at the knee and turned out, or in side posture with the top leg flexed 90° and the bottom leg straight. The underneath leg is the one to be massaged.
- The therapist is standing at the side of the table next to the client's knee.

1. *Myofascial Spreading of the Medial Thigh.* Place the sides of the thumbs next to each other on the midline of the medial thigh. Slowly spread the thumbs apart, stretching the myofascia (Fig. 5-28). Begin the stroke at the knee. Working in horizontal strips, continue to the groin.

2. *Myofascial Mobilization of the Medial Thigh.* Using your finger pads, roll the muscles against the bones, helping them to slide freely.

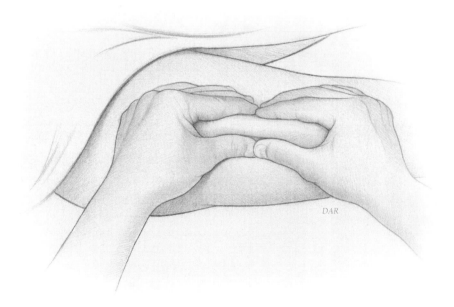

FIGURE 5-26   Lifting and rolling the myofascial tissue of the thigh.

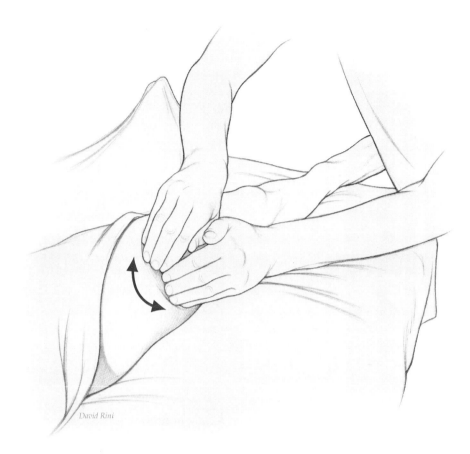

David Rini

FIGURE 5-27 Myofascial mobilization on the thigh.

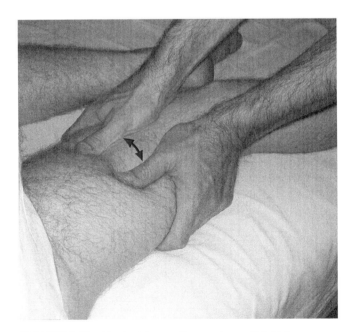

FIGURE 5-28 Myofascial spreading on the medial thigh.

LATERAL THIGH

POSITION

- The client is placed in side posture. The upper leg is flexed, with a bolster under the knee. This is the leg that will be massaged.
- The therapist is standing on the front side of the table facing the thigh of the client's top leg.

1. *Lift and Roll the Myofascial Tissues.* Place the hands in the skin rolling position along the lateral thigh, parallel to the muscle fibers. Lift and roll the muscles (Fig. 5-29).

   Start at the knee. Continue, in horizontal strips, to the hip.

2. *Myofascial Spreading of the Lateral Thigh.* Place the heels of the hands against the midline of the lateral thigh. Slowly spread the hands apart (Fig. 5-30). Begin the first stroke at the knee. Repeat, in horizontal strips, to the hip.

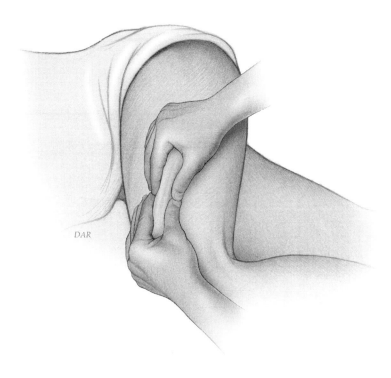

FIGURE 5-29   Lifting and rolling the tissues on the lateral thigh.

Variation—Spread each half of the thigh individually. Place the hands parallel along the midline of the thigh. Using the fingertips, spread from the midline outward. Work in horizontal strips, to the hip. Repeat on the other side.

3. *Myofascial Mobilization of the Hip.* Standing behind the client, place the forearm across the hip area. Roll the muscles in a back and forward motion slowly (Fig. 5-31). Place the forearm further back into the gluteal area and repeat.

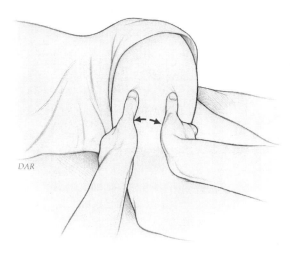

FIGURE 5-30   Myofascial spreading on the lateral thigh.

CALF

POSITION

- The client is lying in a prone position.
- The therapist is standing at the side of the table next to the client's calf.

1. *Fascial Lift and Roll Technique.* Lift and roll the skin and muscles of the calf, the gastrocnemius and soleus, moving in horizontal strips (Fig. 5-32).
2. *Myofascial Spreading of the Calf.* Placing the heels of the hands on the midline of the calf, spread laterally.
   Variation—Use the fingertips to spread each side of the calf separately, from the midline laterally (Fig. 5-33).
3. *Myofascial Mobilization.* Using your fingers, roll the muscles against the underlying muscles and bones. Work to release areas that feel adhered.
4. *Flex the Knee, Bringing the Leg Perpendicular to the Table.* Dorsiflex the foot. Hold the stretch.

POSTERIOR THIGH

POSITION

- The client is lying prone.
- The therapist is standing at the side of the table next to the client's thigh.

1. *Fascial Lift and Roll Technique.* Lift and roll the skin and muscles, working parallel to the fibers. Begin the

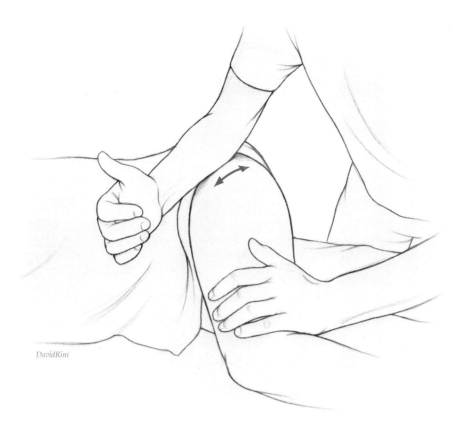

FIGURE 5-31   Myofascial mobilization on the hip.

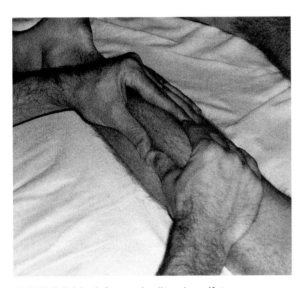

FIGURE 5-32   Lifting and rolling the calf tissues.

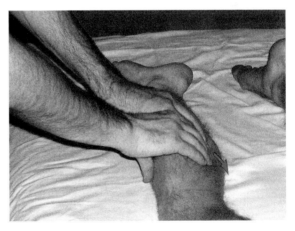

FIGURE 5-33   Myofascial spreading on the calf.

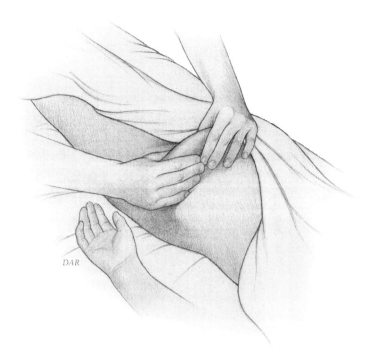

DAR

FIGURE 5-34 Lifting and rolling the gluteal tissues.

stroke slightly above the knee joint. Move in horizontal strips to the hip.

2. *Myofascial Spread.* Use either the heels of hands or knuckles. Place your hands on the midline of the thigh, just above the knee. Spread the hands apart slowly and evenly. Move in horizontal strips, from the knee to the hip.

Variation—Stand at the side of the table, facing the client's thigh. Place the fingertips of both hands on the midline of the thigh. Allow the fingers to sink into the tissues until mild resistance is felt. As the tissues soften, let the fingers slide slowly in a medial direction. Walk around to the other side of the table and repeat the stroke on the posterior thigh in the opposite direction.

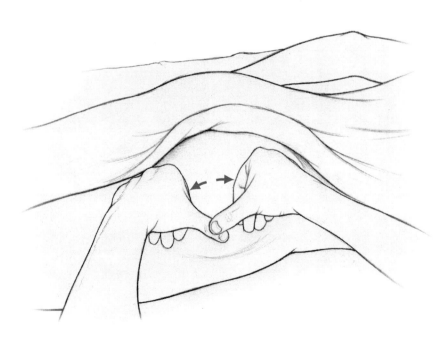

FIGURE 5-35 Myofascial spreading on the gluteal area.

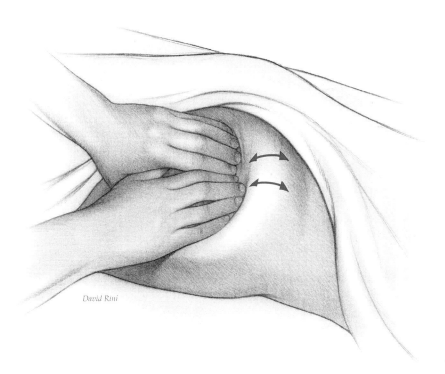

David Rini

FIGURE 5-36 Myofascial mobilization on the gluteal tissues.

3. *Myofascial Mobilization.* Using the fingers, roll the muscles of the thigh over each other and against the femur. Work to free the individual muscles from adhering.

POSTERIOR HIP

POSITION

- The client is lying prone.
- The therapist is standing at the side of the table next to the client's pelvis.

1. *Fascial Lift and Roll Technique.* Lift and roll the gluteal muscles in a superior direction (Fig. 5-34).
2. *Myofascial Spread.* Spread the tissues from the sacrum to the trochanter, using your knuckles or the heels of the hands (Fig. 5-35).
3. *Myofascial Mobilization.* Using your fingers, roll the muscles to re-establish individual action (Fig. 5-36).

REFERENCE

1. Julian D. Connective tissue. In: Job's body: a handbook for bodywork. Barrytown, NY: Station Hill Press, 1987.

The Basis—Breath and Support

THE CHEST

INTRODUCTION

The deep tissue series begins with the chest. Since the overall goal of deep tissue therapy is to bring a person's body to a condition of better balance and function, the logical place to begin is with the breathing mechanism. It is primarily through the breath that the body receives and metabolizes the energy necessary to carry on its vital processes. The first breath we take marks our entry into this world, and the last breath signals our departure. How we manage all the breaths in between has much to do with determining the quality of the life we lead.

The movement of the breath in and out establishes a primary rhythm, or flow, through the body. It represents our ability to take in and assimilate and to give out and let go. The smooth flow of breath is also crucial to the body work process. During a deep tissue session, the recipient is called on to absorb pressure, process change, and release stored tension. If the breath is inhibited, this sequence of events is blocked and consequently the person cannot obtain the full effects of the deep tissue work.

Tension in the muscles of the chest inhibits the movement of the lungs and constricts the capillaries, diminishing the amount of oxygen taken into the body. Decreased oxygen affects metabolism all the way to the cellular level. With less oxygen available, the body's connective tissues become less pliable, restricting muscular action. Over time, a person becomes encased in muscular tension that severely limits full interaction with the surrounding environment and diminishes the capacity to feel. Through observation and palpation, the deep tissue therapist evaluates the patterns of myofascial constriction that are limiting full breathing capacity and focuses on reducing or eliminating them.

The effects of open, full breathing are many. The amount of stress and tension stored in the body is reduced while endurance levels are often substantially increased. The body's ability to eliminate toxins is greatly improved. As much as 70% of the body's toxins are released through the breath. When breathing capacity is reduced, other organs of elimination, such as the skin and kidneys, have to overwork to flush toxins out of the system. This can leave the body in a weakened state and more vulnerable to disease. Full breathing helps to keep blood pressure normalized. A structure in the brain called the medulla oversees the size and tone of the arteries. The medulla responds to the condition of the blood circulating through it. If the carbon dioxide level is high, the blood pressure becomes elevated as well. Full, rhythmic breathing also plays an important role in managing states of anxiety and panic, which can positively influence conditions like depression and asthma.

MUSCULOSKELETAL ANATOMY AND FUNCTION (ESSENTIAL ANATOMY BOX 6-1 AND FIG. 6-1A—C)

The chest, or thoracic cage, is one of the three major weight segments supported by the spine. It consists of 12 pairs of ribs, the 12 thoracic vertebrae, costal cartilage, and sternum. The thoracic portion of the spine is its least moveable segment, providing a stable attachment for the ribs in the back of the body. The ribs join the sternum on the anterior side by means of the costal cartilage. The cylindrical, cage-like design of the chest forms a protective housing for the heart and lungs.

The **pectoralis major** muscle is made up of three overlapping sections that fan across the anterior chest cavity. They all attach on the lateral side of the upper humerus, on the lateral side of the bicipital groove. The upper section originates on the medial half of the clavicle. It is the most superficial of the three sections. The middle section attaches along the sternum. The lower section, which is also the deepest, attaches to the costal cartilages. The broad fan-like arrangement of the pectoralis major fibers allows it to act on the arm from numerous angles. This design also distributes force coming from the arm over the entire anterior ribcage, minimizing impact stress to the thorax.

All three sections of pectoralis major contribute to horizontal flexion and internal rotation of the arm. It is opposed by the latissimus dorsi in these actions, which extends and laterally rotates the arm. Both muscles work together to adduct the arm and lift the thorax toward the arm in pull-ups. Chronically contracted pectoralis major muscles are characterized posturally by a collapsed chest with the arms drawn forward and rolled inward when hanging at the sides of the body. The **subclavius** muscle lies deep to the clavicular section of pectoralis major. It attaches on the first rib and to a groove on the underside of the clavicle. It fixes the clavicle to the chest wall and depresses it.

Breathing is a vital and complex activity, involving not only all the bones and muscles of the chest area, but also accessory muscles in the abdomen, shoulder girdle, and neck. The respiratory muscles function continuously throughout life. These muscles must be freed to carry out the coordinated actions necessary to achieve full breathing.

Although 46 muscles are involved in the breathing process, the primary breathing muscle is the **diaphragm**. This dome-shaped muscle is connected to the lower ribs, sternum, and lumbar spine in a rim around the body. The bases of the lungs attach to the upper surface of the diaphragm. The diaphragm forms the floor of the chest cavity and the roof of the abdominal cavity. The movement of the diaphragm creates a bellows action in the chest and lungs that allows air to be drawn in and out of the body.

ESSENTIAL ANATOMY BOX 6–1

The Chest Routine

Muscles	Bones and Landmarks
Pectoralis major	Ribs
Subclavius	Sternum
Intercostals	Manubrium
Diaphragm	Xiphoid process
Serratus posterior superior	Sulcus intertubercularis
Serratus posterior inferior	Locations of vertebrae T1-T3, T11-L2
	Clavicle

FIGURE 6-1 (**A**) Muscles of the chest with areas of possible trigger point formation. (**B**) Posterior breathing muscles with areas of possible trigger point formation. (**C**) Bones and landmarks of the chest.

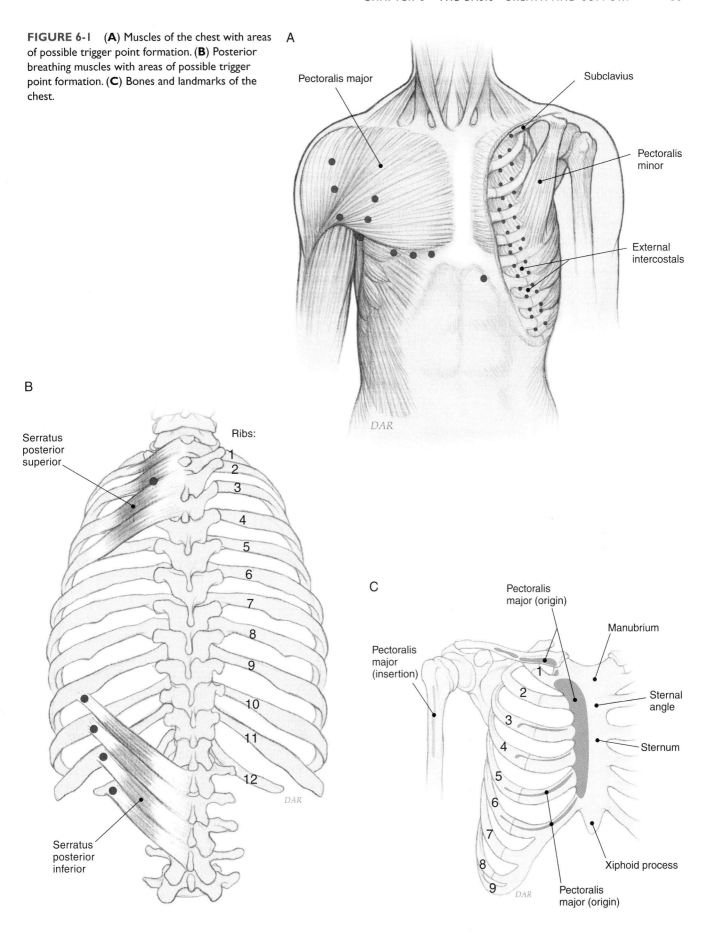

The diaphragm has two main portions. The central tendon, which is noncontractile tissue, forms the central roof of the dome. It blends with the pericardium. Being firm, the central tendon helps the diaphragm maintain its shape.

Surrounding the central tendon are muscular fibers arranged in a radial design, like spokes on a wheel. This muscular portion of the diaphragm consists of two sections, the crural part and the costal part. The crural portion forms a muscular extension of the diaphragm that runs in two sections down the anterior surface of the lumbar spine, attaching on the vertebral bodies and discs of L1–L3 and on the aponeurotic arcuate ligament. The crura form a connection for the breathing apparatus between the upper and lower spine.

As the diaphragm contracts on the inspiration phase of breathing, the fibers are drawn downward toward the crura. The dome flattens, causing the lungs to be stretched downward, increasing their surface area and diminishing the internal air pressure in the lungs. Air from outside the body rushes in to fill the vacuum, thus equalizing the internal and external pressure. As the diaphragm descends, the amount of space in the abdominal cavity is decreased, increasing internal abdominal pressure and causing the abdominal wall to distend to make room for the squeezed abdominal contents.

During inspiration, the **external intercostal** muscles contract, elevating the ribs and causing the lower portion of the ribcage to lift and extend laterally. The intercostal muscles attach to adjacent ribs all the way around the circumference of the ribcage. They are extensions of the abdominal oblique muscles into the chest cavity. The fibers of the external intercostals angle obliquely downward and inward. The fibers of the internal intercostals angle obliquely upward and outward.

The **serratus posterior superior** also contributes to inspiration. It lies deep to the rhomboids in the upper back. Serratus posterior superior connects C7–T3 vertebrae and ribs 2–5 at a 45° downward angle. When the serratus posterior superior contracts it lifts the upper ribs, thus expanding the chest. This muscle can be strained when a person engages in too much forceful high chest breathing without incorporating the abdominal muscles.

On exhalation, the abdominal muscles contract, pushing the abdominal contents inward and upward, thus causing the diaphragm to be lifted back to its dome-shaped position. This diminishes the size of the lungs and decreases internal air pressure, causing the air to rush out of the lungs to re-establish air pressure equalization. The **internal intercostals** contract, causing the ribs to move downward and inward, assisting in diminishing the size of the lungs.

The **serratus posterior inferior** muscle attaches to T11–T12 and L1–L2 vertebrae. Its fibers angle upward at about a 45° angle, mirroring serratus posterior superior, to attach to ribs 8–12. It serves to stabilize the lower ribs and assists in expiration. Serratus posterior inferior can be strained during lifting, twisting, and reaching actions (such as stretching to grasp an item located on a high shelf).

As mentioned previously, many other muscles are involved in the breathing process, assisting in the essential movements and stabilizing muscles and bones. Full, unrestricted breathing is actually a full-body phenomenon. The breath is experienced as a pressure wave moving throughout the entire body. Watching a small baby breathe demonstrates this effect beautifully. The deep tissue massage therapist should be aware of how the client's body is moving as he or she breathes and where breath is inhibited. The reintegration of full-body breathing is a primary goal of deep tissue massage.

CONDITIONS (INDICATIONS/CONTRAINDICATIONS BOX 6-1)

1. *Asthma* is a respiratory disorder characterized by periodic bouts of difficulty in breathing, accompanied by coughing and a buildup of mucus secretion. Attacks are precipitated by an inflammation of the bronchial

INDICATIONS/ CONTRAINDICATIONS BOX 6-1 *Conditions Affecting Chest Massage*	**Indications**	**Contraindications**
	Shallow breathing	Inflammatory conditions of chest tissues
	Tightness in the chest	Broken ribs
	Chronic cough	Tuberculosis
	Pain in the chest	Recent surgery
	Difficult or painful breathing	High fever
	Heaviness around the heart	Severe illness

tubes triggered by factors such as allergens, strenuous exertion, or emotional factors. Massage is beneficial if performed between attacks when the bronchial tubes are not inflamed. It can help to expel excess mucus, release tension in the chest muscles, and reduce stresses that may contribute to attacks.

2. *Emphysema* is a condition affecting the lungs. The alveoli or air sacs are overexpanded to the point at which the walls begin to break down, making breathing difficult. Cigarette smoking is a major contributing factor. Breathing exercises and massage can be helpful if the condition is not too advanced.

3. *Acute bronchitis* is an inflammation of the tubes leading from the trachea to the lungs in the upper respiratory tract that is short in duration but severe. It is accompanied by coughing and heavy mucus production, along with a low-grade fever and constriction behind the sternum. Because it is an inflammatory condition, deep massage is contraindicated until it begins to subside and the patient starts to expel built-up mucus.

4. *Pleurisy* is an inflammation of the pleurae, the membranes covering the lungs. It is accompanied by difficulty in breathing and sharp pain under the ribs, extending into the abdomen. It is a contraindication for massage.

5. *Cracked ribs* are best left alone. They usually heal easily, but taping is sometimes required.

6. *Weak respiratory tract due to pollution.* The toxic substances floating around in the air, from industry, aerosols, cigarette smoke, and many other sources are irritants to the lungs and can generate the respiratory conditions listed above as well as many others. Good diet, breathing exercises, stretching of the chest muscles, and regular massage greatly benefit the respiratory tract.

THE MIND/BODY CONNECTION

The chest region has two primary functions: it serves as a container and a pump. The heart is housed and protected by the chest. We identify the heart with feeling, primarily with our capacity to experience and radiate love. Love is considered a warm emotion. It is often associated with fire. We feel the fires of passion burning or the warm glow of a smoldering ember in our chest when we are in love. When the chest is open, our feeling expands outward to others and is returned to nourish our heart center.

A chest that is tight, closed, and shut off squeezes the heart and reduces its capacity to produce warm, loving emotions. The fire has died and we are left with the experience of cold-heartedness, a lack of warmth. As chronic tightness in the muscles of the chest cavity is released, one often feels an energizing of the heart-felt emotions. Tears may accompany the reconnection to the capacity for joy, sadness, affection, and intimacy.

The chest also serves as a pump for the oxygen and blood that flow through the body. The heart is situated between the lungs. Therefore, each breath we take massages the heart and helps increase circulation. The outward, expansive movement of the body that accompanies inspiration represents our capacity to give outwardly of ourselves, to share. The inward, contractive movement of expiration denotes our ability to receive, to surrender, and to take in.

Balance of the mind/body system is reflected in a full, integrated breathing rhythm that allows us to shift easily between these two phases. The ribcage and abdomen are mobile, with the ability to change shape and size easily.

POSTURAL EVALUATION (TABLE 6-1)

1. Describe the general shape of the chest.
   - Do the right and left halves match?
   - Are the upper and lower portions symmetrical?

2. Check the position of the sternum.
   - Is it lifted?
   - Is it depressed?

3. Observe the position of the ribs.
   - Do the ribs hang from the manubrium?
   - Where do the ribs appear to be squeezed together?
   - Where are the spaces between the ribs expanded?

4. Observe the breathing pattern.
   - Which phase of breath (inhalation or exhalation) is favored, if any?
   - What portions of the chest appear to move easily with the breath?
   - What portions of the chest appear to be rigid and not moving with the breath?

5. Look at the region of the diaphragm, at the level of the lower ribs.
   - Are the lower ribs spread apart and pulled up?
   - Do the lower ribs appear to be relaxed and hanging downward?
   - Are the lower ribs squeezed or drawn together?

EXERCISES AND SELF-TREATMENT

1. Stand in a doorway with your arms spread apart, hands or forearms resting against the sides of the door frame (Fig. 6-2). Shifting your weight forward from

TABLE 6–1	Body Reading for the Chest	
Conditions		**Muscles that May Be Shortened**
Overexpanded chest—the sternum is lifted, ribs are expanded, shoulders drawn back		Scalenes External intercostals Rhomboids
Hollow chest—the sternum is depressed, upper ribs are compressed, shoulders are pulled forward		Pectoralis major Pectoralis minor Subclavius Internal intercostals Anterior deltoid Diaphragm Rectus abdominus

your pelvis, allow the back to arch slightly and the chest to lift and stretch. Breathe deeply. Positioning the arms higher or lower along the sides of the door frame will alter the muscle fibers being stretched.

2. Lie on your back across a bed with the mid-thoracic spine on the side edge of the mattress, so that your upper body can hang down toward the floor, with the arms extended. This position stretches the chest and abdomen. Take deep breaths. Alternative surfaces are an exercise ball (Fig. 6-3), the arm of a large couch, or several blankets rolled up tight into the shape of a cylinder at least 18 inches in diameter and fastened with belts or rope.

3. Lie on your back on the floor. Place two tennis balls on either side of the low back, at the level of the 12th rib. Slowly allow your weight to sink into the balls as you relax and breathe fully. This exercise helps to release the diaphragm and the serratus posterior inferior muscle.

CHEST ROUTINE

OBJECTIVES

- To restore the chest cavity to its full volume.
- To release inhibiting factors in the breathing muscles.
- To integrate effective breathing patterns.
- To realign the shoulders and ribs.

ENERGY

Position

The client is lying supine on the table, with a bolster under the knees.

The therapist is standing at the side of the table next to the client's chest.

Polarity

The left palm is placed over the manubrium, and the right palm slides under the back and is positioned between the

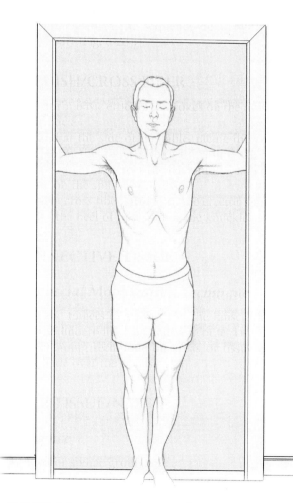

FIGURE 6-2   Stretching the pectoral muscles.

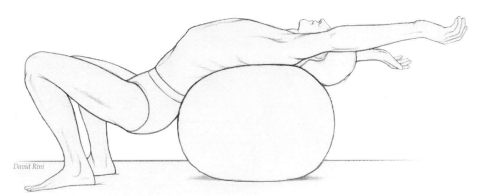

FIGURE 6-3   Stretching the chest and abdominal muscles.

shoulder blades. The therapist's hands move in accordance with the rising and sinking of the client's thorax with each breath, envisioning the smooth, pump-like motion of the lungs. The position is held for at least 1 minute, allowing the client to relax and focus on the breath.

Shiatsu

Moving to the head of the table, the therapist presses the finger pads into the intercostal spaces on both sides of the upper chest simultaneously to stimulate points on the lung, stomach, and kidney channels (Fig. 6-4). The fingers move to different spaces, covering the upper chest area thoroughly. Each set of fingertip compressions is held for the length of the client's exhale and released as the client inhales.

SWEDISH/CROSS FIBER

1. *Shingles stroke on the pectoralis major muscles.* The therapist stands on the side of the table at the client's shoulder level. One hand is placed on the opposite side of the upper chest from the side the therapist is standing, with the heel of the hand against the sternum and the fingers facing the client's shoulder. Perform short, alternate strokes with the palms across the chest to the client's shoulder. Repeat several times.
2. *Pétrissage strokes on the pectoralis major muscles.* Each side of the chest may be worked individually or both sides simultaneously.
3. *Fingertip raking across the upper chest muscles.* Slide the fingers in both directions perpendicular to the direction of the pectoralis major muscle. The breast tissue is avoided when working on a woman.

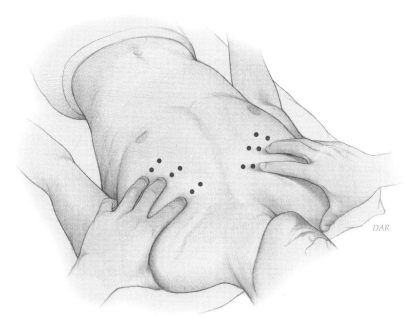

FIGURE 6-4   Fingertip compressions in the intercostal spaces.

CONNECTIVE TISSUE

Perform the fanning stroke on the upper portion of the chest. Begin with the sides of the thumbs touching. Slowly spread them apart, stretching the tissues. Keep the strokes small, spreading the thumbs 2 or 3 inches apart with each stroke.

Start at the midline of the chest over the sternum, just above the level of the breasts. The fanning strokes move upward toward the clavicles. Repeat the stroke a number of times, covering the entire upper segment of the chest. The intention is to free the fascia of the upper thorax, creating a sense of lift in the chest.

DEEP TISSUE/NMT

Sequence

1. Pectoralis major (attachments and belly)
2. Subclavius
3. Intercostal muscles (from supine and side position)
4. Diaphragm
5. Back muscles (serratus posterior superior and inferior)

Commonly Found Trigger Points
It is likely that the chest muscles will be restricted in many areas, as the breathing mechanism is compromised in the majority of the adult population due to stress and the lack of encouragement of full expression of feeling and sensation. The release of trigger points not only assists in opening up the breathing, it is also instrumental in rebalancing the shoulder girdle and freeing the ribs.

1. Pectoralis Major (Attachments and Belly)
Origin: Clavicular—medial half of the clavicle. **Sternal**—sternum to the 7th rib, cartilages of upper 6 ribs.
Insertion: Lateral lip of the bicipital groove of the humerus.
Action: Adduction of shoulder. Medial rotation of shoulder. **Clavicular**—shoulder flexion, medial rotation of shoulder, horizontal adduction of humerus. **Sternal**—adduction of humerus diagonally downward, anterior shoulder stabilizer.

Pectoralis Major (Origin)
- Elongation stroke on the sternum, just lateral to the midline, from the xiphoid process to the manubrium, using the fingers or the thumb (Fig. 6-5).
- Elongation stroke along inferior border of the medial half of the clavicle, using fingers or thumb. Move medial to lateral. Feel for small knots and stringy fibers. If they are tender or refer pain, work on them with cross fiber strokes and direct compression.
- Insertion of pectoralis major. Perform the side-to-side stroke and static compression with the fingers on the lateral lip of the bicipital groove of the humerus (Fig.

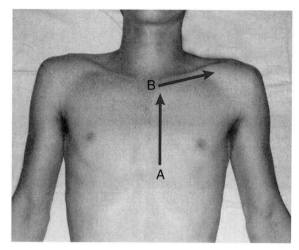

FIGURE 6-5 Directions of elongation strokes on the sternal and clavicular attachments of pectoralis major.

6-6). To locate it, take the client's arm to an abducted position. Slide your fingers along the border of the pectoralis major and the anterior deltoid to reach the point of attachment on the humerus. It is superior to the deltoid tuberosity. Check for trigger points. If any are found, hold them for 8 to 12 seconds while checking with the client about the level of pain reduction.

Pectoralis Major (Belly)
There are three sections to the pectoralis major muscle. They are named after their sites of origin: clavicular, sternal, and costal. Trigger points in the upper or clavicular portion may be found along the lateral border, underneath the edge of the anterior deltoid muscle. They refer pain throughout the anterior deltoid and into the area of the pectoralis major near the trigger point.

Trigger points in the sternal section tend to accumulate in the medial and lateral portions between ribs 3, 4, and 5, near the insertion points of pectoralis minor. Check along the inferior border of the costal section of the muscle for

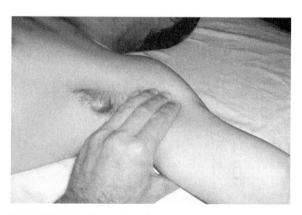

FIGURE 6-6 Contacting the insertion of pectoralis major on the lateral lip of the bicipital groove of the humerus.

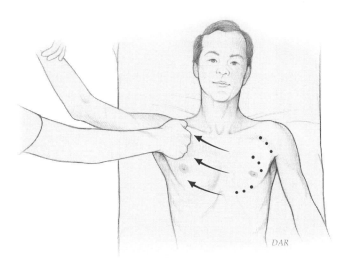

FIGURE 6-7 Elongation stroke on the clavicular, sternal, and costal sections of pectoralis major.

trigger points. The pain pattern is into the front of the chest and down the arm.

Trigger points in the lower section of the muscle tend to form along the lateral border. They refer pain into the breast and nipple.

Heavy lifting, prolonged holding of the arms in an abducted position, and emotional stress may all contribute to the formation of trigger points in this muscle.

■ The client's arm is still in the abducted position. Using your knuckles, perform the elongation stroke from the sternum to the insertion on the humerus in several strips (Fig. 6-7). Begin the first strip just inferior to the clavicle. Begin the last strip across the muscle at the xiphoid process.

■ With a female client, the knuckle stroke should only be done on the upper chest, superior to the breast tissue. At the level of the breast, stroke outward from the sternum to the medial border of the breast, using the fingers or thumb.

2. Subclavius (Fig. 6-8)
Origin: Upper border of the first rib.
Insertion: Groove on the inferior surface of the clavicle.
Action: Depresses and moves clavicle forward, stabilizes clavicle during shoulder movements.

A commonly occurring trigger point is found on the medial side of the muscle near the manubrium. Its referral zone is along the inferior border of the clavicle and down the arm into the thumb side of the hand.

■ Stand at the side of the table, facing the inferior border of the client's clavicle. The client's arm is flexed at 90°. Hold it slightly inferior to the elbow. Traction the arm

toward the ceiling, drawing the clavicle slightly away from the chest wall for easier access to the subclavius muscle.

■ Using the pads of the index and middle fingers or the thumb pad, stroke under the inferior border of the clavicle from the medial to lateral end.

3. Intercostal Muscles
Origin: External—from lower border of each of the upper 11 ribs. **Internal**—from the cartilages to the angles of the upper 11 ribs.
Insertion: External—superior border of rib below the origin. **Internal**—superior border of rib below the origin.
Action: External—elevation of ribs during inspiration. **Internal**—depression of ribs during exhalation.

Intercostals (Supine Position)
Trigger points are likely to be found in concentration along the borders of the ribs where the intercostal muscles attach. Contracted muscles related to inhibited breathing are the probable cause of their formation.

■ Begin at the base of the ribcage, in the rib space between the 10th and 9th rib. Place your fingers between the two ribs. Allow the fingers to sink into the tissues until resistance is met (Fig. 6-9).

■ Perform a short side-to-side stroke, feeling for deviations in the tissues (i.e., stringy fibers, tiny knots). Hold with static compression on tender points until pain

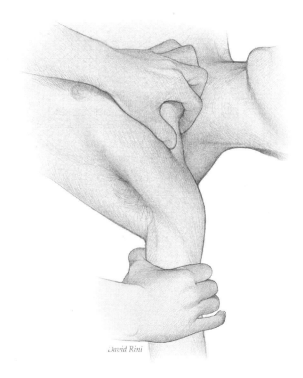

FIGURE 6-8 Accessing the subclavius.

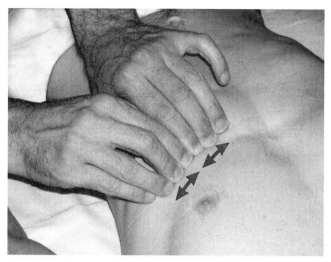

FIGURE 6-9 Releasing the intercostals (supine position).

diminishes. The thumbs may be used instead of the fingers if more pressure is required.
■ Continue with this procedure, working between each pair of ribs, to the clavicle. Be thorough.

Intercostals (Side Posture)

Position
The client is put in side posture, with the knees flexed and a pillow placed between them. The top arm is positioned in front of the client, allowing access to the side of the chest. A pillow may be placed under the side of the head for comfort.
 The therapist stands behind the client.

■ Perform fanning strokes with fingers or heels of the hand in a superior direction on the side of the chest, from the base of the ribcage to the axilla, to soften the superficial fascia and prepare the tissues for deeper work.

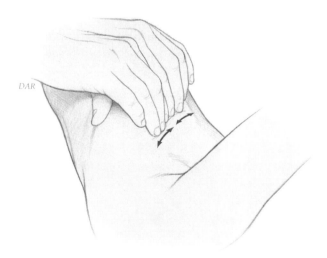

FIGURE 6-10 Releasing the intercostals from side posture.

■ Find the space between ribs 10 and 9 (Fig. 6-10). Sink the fingers into the tissues until resistance is met and begin short side-to-side strokes, working the intercostals in sections. Continue, working in each rib space, to the top of the axilla, to reach the spaces between the upper ribs.

4. Diaphragm
Origin: Sternal part—inner surface of xiphoid process.
Costal part—inner surfaces of cartilages of ribs 7–12.
Lumbar part—L1–L3 vertebrae.
Insertion: Central tendon.
Action: Increases volume of thoracic cavity on inspiration by drawing the central tendon down.
An active trigger point along the diaphragm attachment on the underside of the costal cartilage may be found approximately 1 inch lateral to the xiphoid process.

Position
The client is placed back in a supine position with a bolster under the knees.
 The therapist is standing at the side of the table facing the client's rib cage.

■ With the palm supinated, slide your fingers under the border of the costal cartilage of ribs 7–10, just lateral to the xiphoid process. The finger pads must stay in contact with the underside of the costal cartilage to avoid pressing into the underlying organs. Take time to let the fingers sink into the tissues (Fig. 6-11).
■ Do short side-to-side motions with your fingers, feeling for tightness and trigger point activity. Move laterally along the border. Place the palm of your non-working hand over the lower ribs to give additional support to the upward pressure of your working hand.
■ Work with the client's breath. On the exhalation, sink into the tissues with your fingers until resistance is felt. On the inhalation, allow the client's abdomen to push your fingers out from under the ribs.

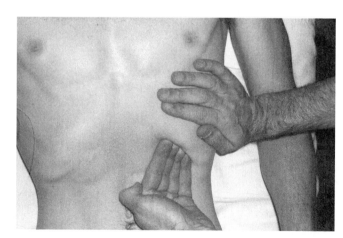

FIGURE 6-11 The diaphragm release.

5. Back Muscles

Position
The client is lying supine.

The therapist is standing or sitting at the side of the table.

Serratus Posterior Superior
Origin: Spinous processes of C7 and T1–T3 vertebrae, ligamentum nuchae.

Insertion: Upper borders of ribs 2–5 just lateral to their angles.

Action: Elevates upper ribs, possible assistance in inspiration.

This muscle may house a trigger point just medial to the superior angle of the scapula. It is a common cause of shoulder pain. The pain is felt deep, under the upper portion of the scapula. It can also extend over the posterior deltoid and down the triceps.

■ Slide your hands under the client's back at the level of the upper thoracic spine (T1–T3). Beginning at the spinous processes, perform short back-and-forth motions with your finger pads moving toward the vertebral border of the scapula.

■ Hold static compression over sensitive points as the client breathes deeply.

■ As an alternative move, use the knuckles instead of the fingers.

Serratus Posterior Inferior
Origin: Spinous processes of T11–T12 and L1–L2 vertebrae.

Insertion: Inferior borders of ribs 9–12, lateral to their angles.

Action: Depresses lower ribs and moves them dorsally; possible assistance in expiration.

To locate trigger points, examine its attachments along the inferior borders of ribs 9–12. The pain pattern is throughout the muscle itself and over the lower ribs.

■ Slide your hands under the client's back at the level of the lower thoracic and upper lumbar vertebrae (T11–12 and L1–L2). (If the client is too large or heavy to effectively slide your hands under his or her trunk, you may position the client in side posture to release the serratus posterior superior and inferior muscles.) Beginning at the spinous processes, perform short back-and-forth motions with your finger pads in a diagonally upward direction toward the muscle's insertion on the inferior borders of ribs 9–12 (Fig. 6-12).

■ Hold with static compression over sensitive points as the client breathes deeply.

■ As an alternative procedure, use the knuckles instead of the fingers.

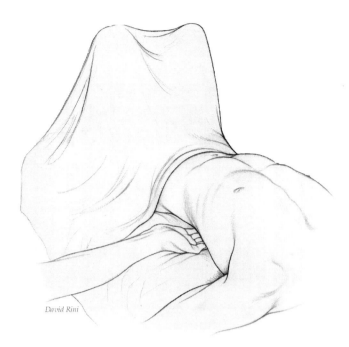

David Rini

FIGURE 6-12   Hand position for accessing serratus posterior inferior along ribs 9–12.

Stretch

1. The therapist stands at the head of the table. The client extends the arms overhead toward the therapist. Take hold of the client's arms slightly superior to the elbow joints. Pull the arms toward you and slightly downward while the client takes full breaths, focusing on expanding the chest (Fig. 6-13).

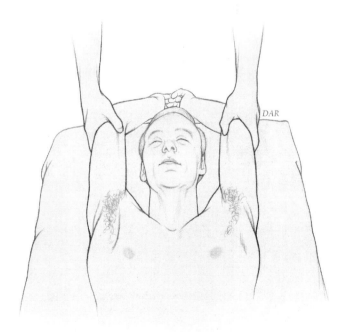

DAR

FIGURE 6-13   Thoracic stretch with the client supine.

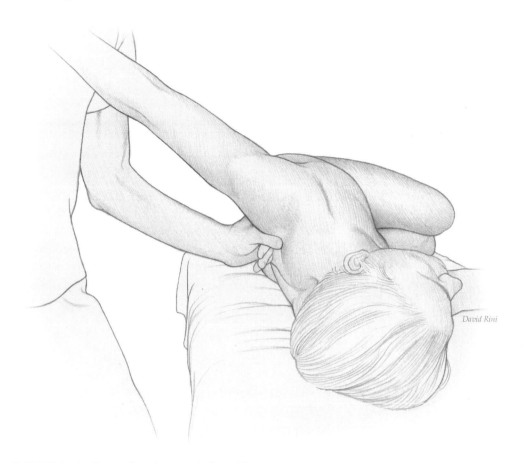

David Rini

FIGURE 6-14   Pectoralis major stretch from side posture.

2. The client turns onto his or her side, with the knees flexed. The client's straightened superior arm reaches behind him. The therapist stands behind the client's shoulder. Hold the extended arm and slowly increase the stretch, while your fist is placed against the client's scapula, to prevent the client from rolling backward too far (Fig. 6-14). This position stretches the pectoralis major muscle.

Accessory Work

1. Perform an elongation stroke on the erector spinae and paraspinal muscles. Using the forearm, begin the stroke between the scapula and spinous processes on one side of the back. The forearm is parallel to the

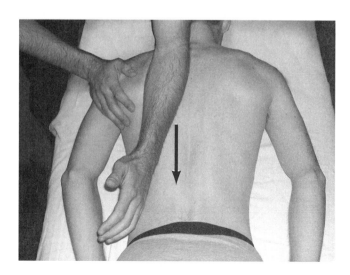

FIGURE 6-15   Elongation stroke for the erector spinae muscles.

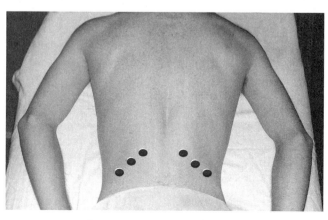

FIGURE 6-16   Pressure points for diaphragm release.

spine until you clear the inferior angle of the scapula. Then it is rotated perpendicular to the spine to make contact with a broader section of the back. Continue the stroke to the iliac crest of the pelvis (Fig. 6-15). Repeat on the other side of the back.

2. Press points along the inferior border of the 12th rib, which is near the attachment of the diaphragm muscle (Fig. 6-16). Both sides may be palpated simultaneously. Begin with the thumbs on either side of T12 and move them apart laterally.

3. Diaphragm reflex points on the foot (Fig. 6-17). Press points along the diaphragm line on the plantar surface of the foot, moving medial to lateral. The line is located slightly inferior to the metatarsal bones and runs all the way across the surface of the foot. It is easy to distinguish because the color of the skin is darker above the diaphragm line and lighter below it.

Closing

Sitting at the foot of the table, lightly hold the heels of the client's feet in your hands for 30 to 60 seconds. Remove your hands slowly.

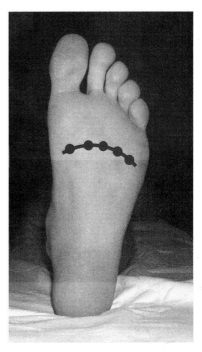

FIGURE 6-17   Reflex zone for the diaphragm.

THE BACK/SPINE

INTRODUCTION

The spine acts as the primary support structure for the entire body. Proper alignment of the spine is essential so that it can carry the weights that are connected to it (the head, ribcage, and pelvis) without producing stress in the muscles of the trunk. A poised, balanced spine results in the effortless elongation of the trunk associated with correct posture. The muscles attached to the spine must be freed of restrictions to achieve the equalization of forces along the spinal column necessary for a balanced relationship between its components. This is the next goal in the deep tissue series.

The spine is constructed so that many muscles and ligaments attach to it in a lattice-like pattern, allowing for a

Muscles	Bones and Landmarks	
Trapezius	Vertebral column	**ESSENTIAL ANATOMY BOX 6–2**
Latissimus dorsi	Spinous processes	
Erector spinae	Transverse processes	
Rhomboid minor	Lamina groove	
Rhomboid major	Scapula	
Intercostals	Ribs	
Quadratus lumborum	Iliac crest	*The Back/Spinal*
Sacral ligaments	Sacrum	*Column Routine*
	Coccyx	

great deal of mobility and flexibility. The spinal column is capable of the movements of forward and side flexion, extension, and rotation. One reason for this tremendous movement versatility is to protect the spinal cord. The spinal column's high degree of flexibility reduces the risk of spinal cord and nerve injuries.

MUSCULOSKELETAL ANATOMY AND FUNCTION (ESSENTIAL ANATOMY BOX 6-2 AND FIG. 6-18A—C

The spinal column consists of 33 bones. There are 7 cervical vertebrae, 12 thoracic vertebrae, 5 lumbar vertebrae, and at birth, 5 modified sacral vertebrae and 4

small vertebral remnants forming the coccyx. The bones of both the sacrum and coccyx fuse later in life, leaving 24 functional vertebrae in the adult. There are also 23 intervertebral discs sandwiched between the vertebral bones.

Most vertebrae are composed of two parts, a round body and a posterior segment called the vertebral arch. The vertebral arch is a complex structure. It includes the spinous and transverse processes, which provide attachment sites for many muscles and ligaments. The opening between the vertebral body and arch is called the vertebral foramen. Lined up within the spinal column the foramen form a tunnel, called the vertebral canal, within which the spinal cord is located.

The vertebral bodies are separated by collagenous discs. The two components of the disc are a central, compressed fluid core called the nucleus pulposus, and a

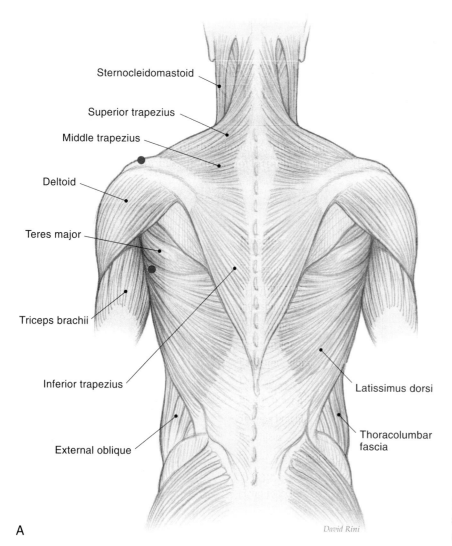

Sternocleidomastoid

Superior trapezius

Middle trapezius

Deltoid

Teres major

Triceps brachii

Inferior trapezius

External oblique

Latissimus dorsi

Thoracolumbar fascia

David Rini

A

FIGURE 6-18 (**A**) Muscles of the back—superficial layer with areas of possible trigger point formation. *(continued)*

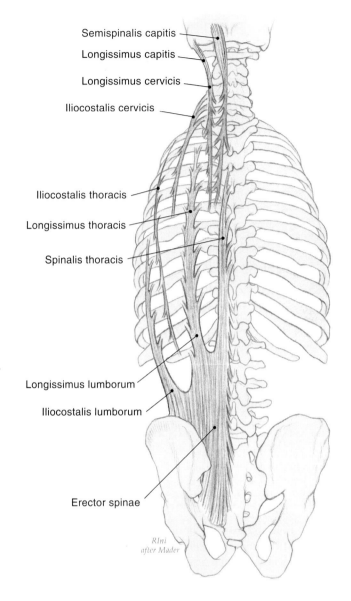

Semispinalis capitis

Longissimus capitis

Longissimus cervicis

Iliocostalis cervicis

Iliocostalis thoracis

Longissimus thoracis

Spinalis thoracis

Longissimus lumborum

Iliocostalis lumborum

Erector spinae

*RJni
after Mader*

B

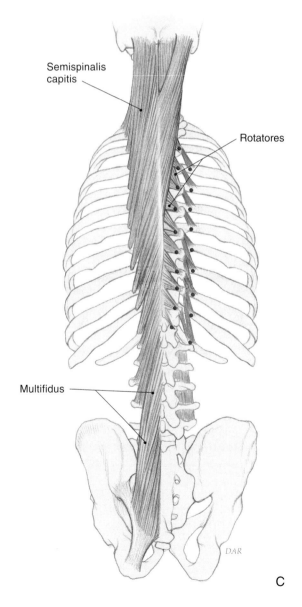

Semispinalis
capitis

Rotatores

Multifidus

DAR

C

FIGURE 6-18 *Continued.* (**B**) Muscles of the back—middle layer. (**C**) Muscles of the back—deep layer, with areas of possible trigger point formation. *(continued)*

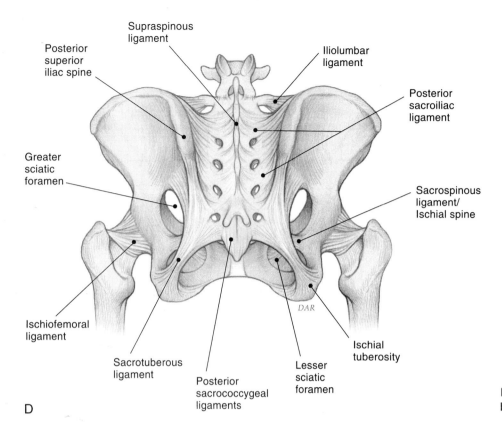

D

FIGURE 6-18 *Continued.* (**D**) Sacral ligaments.

fibrous covering called the annulus fibrosus. The discs act as cushions, helping to transfer weight evenly between the vertebrae and preventing adjacent bones from rubbing against each other. The discs in the lumbar and cervical segments of the spine are thicker in relation to the height of the vertebrae, allowing for greater movement between the individual vertebrae, while the discs in the thoracic segment are smaller, decreasing the amount of possible motion. When adjacent vertebrae are properly aligned, compression on the intervertebral disc is distributed evenly, allowing for a smooth downward transfer of weight.

Vertebrae that are chronically displaced put uneven pressure on the intervertebral disc that is sandwiched between them, causing it to bulge and to possibly slip out of position. This can produce pain if the disc presses against a nerve. It also diminishes the ability of the disc to maintain space between the vertebral bodies, another major source of spinal pain.

One of the spinal column's primary functions is to provide an anchor of support and stability for the cranium, thorax, and pelvis. These body segments are displaced along the spinal column in the sense that none of them falls directly through the body's central line of gravity. Therefore, to support them effectively the spinal column is composed of a series of four opposing curves that offset the uneven size and placement of these three weights (Fig. 6-19).

There are two concave curves, the cervical and lumbar, and two convex curves, the thoracic and sacral. It is an ingenious design, creating continuity of weight transfer throughout the spinal column. The vertebrae where the curves change (C7–T1, T12–L1, L5–S1) bear the greatest weight load and must remain aligned for the spine to act as an integrated, stress-free unit.

Mechanically speaking, all the bony weights of the trunk should be placed as close to the central axis of the body and as close to each other as possible to minimize stress on the weight-bearing spine. This is an important factor in determining correct posture and movement. For this balance to occur, the soft tissues of the back must be able to contract and lengthen freely to accommodate all the shifts of weight and movements necessary to maintain this dynamic equilibrium.

Although the spine is referred to as a column, this is not a completely accurate description. A column transfers weight vertically through its central axis by internal compression of its structural components. It does not rely on outside forces to distribute weight. The spine does not function this way. Because of its curved design, it is not aligned to the body's central axis and therefore cannot maintain balance on its own. It must rely on the aid of the muscles attached to it, which constantly transfer and redistribute forces to maintain equilibrium of the trunk.

The concept of tensegrity provides a more precise description of the relationship between the bones and

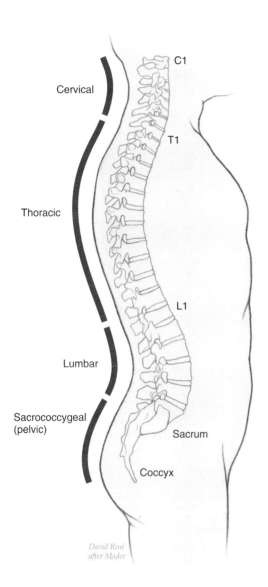

Cervical

Thoracic

Lumbar

Sacrococcygeal
(pelvic)

C1

T1

L1

Sacrum

Coccyx

David Rini
after Mader

FIGURE 6-19   The four counter-balancing spinal curves.

muscles of the back.[1] In a tensegrity structure, weight is transferred through the tension members, or stretching components of the structure, rather than through the compression members. The compression members act as spacers and points of attachment for the tension components to maintain the necessary shape and distribution of force in the structure. An example of this design in architecture is the geodesic dome.

In the back, the bones serve as the compression members. The spine, ribs, cranium, and pelvis act as spacers, maintaining the proper lengths for the muscles attached to them, which serve as the tension members. Thus, the bones are suspended in a web of soft tissue support. When the muscles become chronically shortened and dysfunc-

tional, they are unable to distribute weight effectively. The spine begins to act more as a compression-style column, setting the stage for breakdown and injury.

Chronic compression of the spine is the cause of many back difficulties. The ligaments, which are the reinforcing supports for the spine, and the intervertebral discs take over the job of transferring weight, which should be done by the muscles. The ligaments may become inflamed and tear, as they have to reinforce and carry weight beyond the maximum load they were designed to support. The discs become chronically compressed, losing their springiness and ability to cushion the vertebrae.

The muscles that move the spine consist of two groups, the superficial and deep paraspinal muscles. The superficial group is called the **erector spinae**. It is made up of three muscles, the **iliocostalis, longissimus,** and **spinalis**. Depending on their location along the spine, these muscles are subdivided into segments called cervicis, thoracis, and lumborum. They span the entire length of the back with iliocostalis lumborum extending all the way down to the sacrum.

The longissimus and iliocostalis muscles are the strongest of the group and the most likely to be injured and to develop trigger points. The spinalis is a smaller and weaker muscle. It is the most medially placed, attaching to the spinous processes of L2–T2 vertebrae. Collectively, the erector spinae muscles extend the vertebral column. The iliocostalis and longissimus are also responsible for lateral flexion of the spinal column.

The **deep paraspinal muscles**, also known as the transversospinalis muscles, connect the transverse processes of the vertebrae to the spinous processes in a layered, upwardly angled pattern. From the most superficial to the deepest-lying they are the **semispinalis, multifidi,** and **rotatores**. The semispinalis span five to six vertebrae. The multifidi span three vertebrae, and the rotatores connect adjacent vertebrae. All three muscles extend, laterally flex, and rotate the vertebrae. They also serve to elongate the spinal column. These muscles are active most of the time, as they are responsible for maintaining the alignment of the spinal column as the body shifts its position.

A primary purpose of deep tissue therapy on the back is to relieve compression and other stresses along the spine by re-establishing effective muscle function. Massage work, along with exercise and proper spinal mechanics, can help to relieve the majority of back problems.

SOURCES OF BACK PROBLEMS

Improper standing and sitting posture contributes to strain in the soft tissues around the spine. Many people wear shoes with high heels, which throws the body forward of the line of gravity. To remain upright, the upper back is brought backward, causing an increased lumbar curve, with resulting compression in the soft tissues.

Sitting in a slumped position with the low back

rounded is a common habit. This position eliminates the proper lumbar curve. The vertebrae are no longer aligned, placing stress on the surrounding ligaments and muscles.

Incorrect lifting techniques are a major cause of back strain. The spine should always maintain its integrity as a unit during any kind of lifting activity. The only flexing of the upper body that should occur during lifting is at the hip joints. Many people bend at the waist when reaching to pick up something. Bending at the waist throws a tremendous amount of pressure onto the discs and soft tissues of the low back, which are not designed to pull heavy weight when bringing the spine upright. To lift properly, persons should always bend from the legs rather than the low back, bringing the object as close to the body as possible before lifting it. They should then push up to standing, using the thigh muscles and keeping the back straight.

Lack of exercise causes weakness in the abdominal muscles, which help to support the low back. If the psoas muscle is tight, it will also cause tightness and compression in the low back. Short, restricted hamstring muscles pull the pelvis downward, which reduces the lumbar curve and places stress on the ligaments of the low back.

A sudden, unexpected movement or force, such as slipping on a wet floor or even sneezing (particularly if the back is already in a weakened condition), can result in muscle spasms and tears. Unfortunately, most furniture is not designed to position the spine properly. Most people find themselves slumping in it, again compromising the lumbar curve and weakening the low back.

CONDITIONS (INDICATIONS/ CONTRAINDICATIONS BOX 6-2)

1. *Scoliosis* is a lateral curve or curves of the spine.

   a. Functional scoliosis originates from factors other than structural deformity in the spinal column itself. Imbalances in the feet and legs, like a pronated foot or one leg being shorter than the other, can cause a lateral pelvic tilt, which leads to lateral spinal curvature. Unequal degrees of strength in the right and left psoas muscles will cause them to pull on the pelvis unevenly, resulting in pelvic rotation, which also leads to lateral spinal curvature. Muscular asymmetry due to dominant handedness also creates scoliosis. Functional scoliosis disappears when the distorting factors to the spine are eliminated.

   b. Structural scoliosis is a permanent condition, indicating a bony deformity, usually congenital. In severe cases the vertebrae rotate, causing the ribcage to distort. The curvature remains no matter what position the person assumes.

   There may or may not be pain accompanying scoliosis. If the curve is long-standing, the person's musculature has probably adapted to the condition. Muscles on the concave side of the curve will be shortened. Muscles on the convex side of the curve will be stretched.

2. *Kyphosis* is an exaggerated posterior thoracic spinal curve causing a rounded or humpbacked look in the upper back. The myofascial tissues of the upper back tend to become hardened and adhere to each other due to chronic compression. Contributing factors can include poor postural habits, poor nutrition, osteoporosis, or systemic disorders causing a deterioration of the spine.

3. *Lordosis* is an abnormal curvature in the lumbar portion of the spine. It results in compression of the lumbar intervertebral discs and the surrounding musculature. Some contributing factors are wearing high-heeled shoes, having shortened iliopsoas muscles, and having tight rectus femoris muscles. Most children exhibit a degree of lordosis that they outgrow.

INDICATIONS/ CONTRAINDICATIONS BOX 6-2 *Conditions Affecting Back Massage*	Indications	Contraindications
	Tension	Inflammation
	Chronic back pain	Sunburn
	Scoliosis	Rashes
	Pelvic tilt	Recent trauma
	Back injury	Severe hypertension
	Back surgery	High fever
	Open heart surgery	Severe bruises
	Fatigue	

4. *Damage to intervertebral discs.* Disc injuries can occur due to a variety of causes. Structural imbalances, such as leg length differences, pelvic rotation, and scoliosis, may lead to wear and tear on the discs. Muscle imbalance, poor posture, incorrect lifting habits, excess weight, and trauma due to accidents are other common causes of disc problems. Disc injury is accompanied by pain that can be sudden or gradual in onset. Progressive weakness on one side of the body in muscles that control the lower limb along with sensations of tingling, numbness, or pain are characteristic of disc injury.

Some common types of disc injury are as follows:

a. Degeneration. This is a deterioration of the material of the disc. It is often caused by dehydration, due to chronic squeezing of the disc, and inadequate intake of water.
b. Rupture. This condition is also referred to as a herniated or protruding disc. It means that either the internal nucleus or the surrounding fibers of the disc have moved out of position.

The lay term for this condition is "slipped disc."

5. *Muscle spasm.* This is a protective reaction to damage in the back, rather than its cause. Causative factors can include torn ligaments, damage to discs, muscle sprain (refers to injury to muscle fibers), or stretching of the joints. Left untreated, muscle spasm will contribute to back pain. Treatment includes massage, ice application, and mild stretching.

THE MIND/BODY CONNECTION

As mentioned previously, the spine is the major support structure of the body. Strength of character is often judged by the degree of strength exhibited by the back. We speak of a courageous, forthright person as "having a strong backbone." Someone who is considered to be weak or cowardly is labeled "spineless."

A baby's spine is extremely flexible because the muscles around it have not yet developed the strength to support it, and the balancing spinal curves have not formed.

Newborn infants are almost completely helpless. They cannot sit up or hold the weight of the head and thorax through the spine. Children's early movements of kicking and squirming are necessary to develop the musculature of the pelvis and low back. Through exploring and exerting themselves through movement, infants are gradually developing the core strength of support. Even the actions of crying and screaming are important in building up the muscles that will stabilize the necessary lumbar curve, so that the child can hold the head up and eventually be able to sit and stand without aid.

When lying on the abdomen, a very young baby cannot lift his or her head off the floor. It is a great accomplishment when infants can finally pull the trunk up and be able to look around. They are beginning the first stages of asserting themselves as individuals as they survey the world around them. Contractions of the extensor muscles control the lift and arching motion of the spine. The stance of opening the chest and stretching the arms back is associated with joy, expansion, and self-expression. Moshe Feldenkrais[2] called the extensor muscles the happy muscles because their use tends to elicit a happy response in individuals throughout life.

When the body is open and lifted, we make ourselves available to receive and interact with the world around us. By contrast, contraction of the flexor muscles causes the body to be pulled forward and the spine to flex. This position tends to produce feelings of withdrawal, fear, and lack of initiative. Opening and lifting the spine through deep tissue massage can do much to improve a person's self-esteem and tends to improve his or her outlook in general.

As a child develops and grows, it is hoped that the spine and the muscles around it will become strong and supple. The child will gain a sense of independence and self-reliance. Dr. Ida Rolf[3] referred to the spine and its intrinsic support muscles as the inner core of the body. This core represents our sense of security and our will. When the spine and its associated muscles are weak, there may be a feeling of not being able to stand up for one's self, or lack of trust that one has the inner resources to handle all the conflicts or problems that may arise in life.

The lower back acts as a bridge between two solid bony structures, the pelvis and thorax. It is responsible for mediating feelings between these two areas. The lumbar spine is rather vulnerable, having no bony protection around it. Pain and tightness in this area may reflect areas of vulnerability within a person. When weakness and degeneration in the lumbar spine is present, it may be beneficial to look at areas in one's life where security and support are not present. This could relate to a person's finances, job, home life, or relationships.

The upper back has a direct structural relationship to the shoulders. Feelings of anger or even rage can lodge in this segment. We tend to "hold back" aggressive actions of the arms, like punching, with the upper back muscles. The thoracic curve corresponds to the heart center. It is usually when the heart center is shut down that hostile and resentful feelings arise.

POSTURAL EVALUATION (TABLE 6-2)

The client is standing, facing away from the therapist, so the back may be observed.

TABLE 6–2	Body Reading for the Back
Conditions	**Muscles that May Be Shortened**

Scoliosis	Muscles on concave sides of the spinal curves:
	    Erector spinae
	    Paraspinal muscles
	Check for lateral imbalances in:
	    Iliopsoas
	    Quadratus lumborum
	    Biceps femoris

Kyphosis	Capital extensors Neck extensors Pectoralis minor Anterior deltoid
Lordosis	Iliacus Psoas major Rectus femoris Quadratus lumborum

1. Imagine a vertical line running down the spine, or have the person's spine lined up to a plumb line, dividing the back into left and right segments.
   - Check for balance of the musculature on the right and left sides.
   - Observe underdevelopment and/or overdevelopment of muscles.

2. Check for exaggeration or underdevelopment of the spinal curves.
   - Sacral.
   - Lumbar.
   - Thoracic.
   - Cervical.

3. Note if any vertebrae are protruding or sunken. This is determined by observing or palpating the spinous processes.

4. Check for evenness in the height of the iliac crests.

5. Look for scoliosis. Lack of symmetry in the musculature on the left and right sides may be an indication of scoliosis. To confirm this, run your fingers down the back over the spinous processes. Check for lateral deviations.

EXERCISES AND SELF-TREATMENT

1. Back strengthener (extensor muscles–lumbar region).
   - *Position*—Lie on the floor prone, legs extended, ankles and knees touching. The arms are against the sides of the body, with the palms touching the thighs. The chin is tucked under, with the forehead resting on the floor.
   Preparation—Exhaling, squeeze the legs together, tighten the gluteal muscles, tuck the pelvis under, and contract the abdominal muscles.
   Execution—Inhaling, lift the head and chest a few

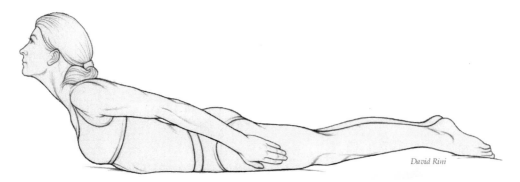

David Rini

FIGURE 6-20 Back strengthening exercise.

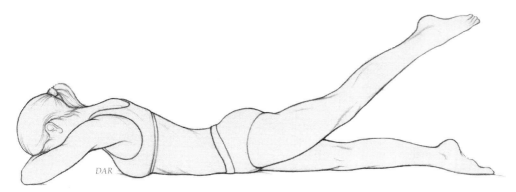

FIGURE 6-21   Single leg lift.

inches off the floor, keeping the pelvic muscles contracted (Fig. 6-20). Hold for the length of the inhalation, then lower the upper body to the floor. Rest for a few moments, then repeat. The movement may be repeated two or three more times.

Position—Lie on the floor prone, legs extended. The arms are positioned on the floor under the head. The elbows are flexed, palms down, with one hand placed on top of the other, the chin resting on the hands.

Preparation—Inhaling, tuck the pelvis under slightly, contracting the gluteal muscles.

Execution

■ Exhaling, lift the right leg a few inches off the floor, keeping the gluteal muscles contracted (Fig. 6-21). Inhaling, lower the right leg to the floor. Repeat with the left leg. The sequence may be repeated several times.

■ Repeat the exercise, lifting both legs a few inches off the floor as you exhale. Hold for the length of the exhalation.

2. Back stretches.

■ Lying on your back, bring the right knee to your chest and hold it with your right hand. Then bring the left knee to your chest, holding it with the left hand. As you inhale, extend the arms, moving the thighs away from the chest. Exhaling, bring the thighs close to the chest using your arms. Hold the

squeeze for the length of the exhalation. Repeat several times.

■ From the above position, squeeze both thighs toward your chest (Fig. 6-22). Then rock the legs from side to side using your arms, letting the back muscles roll against the floor.

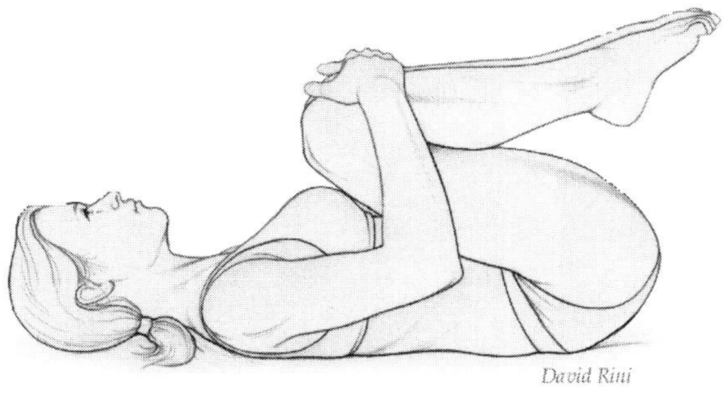

3. Place two tennis balls under your back, one on either side of the spine, beginning between the shoulder blades. Take deep breaths, allowing the muscles to sink into the balls, visualizing the tension melting. Reposition the balls farther down the spine and repeat the procedure. Continue, down to the sacrum.

BACK/SPINAL COLUMN ROUTINE

OBJECTIVES

■ To relax the back area, which tends to hold excessive tension.
■ To lengthen the spine by releasing the muscles that control the position and movement of the vertebrae.
■ To release the posterior breathing muscles.
■ To balance the weight segments along the spine: the head, thorax, and pelvis.
■ To treat tissues that have been strained by back injuries and/or poor postural habits.

ENERGY

Position

The client is lying prone on the table. A bolster may be placed under the ankles and/or the pelvis.

Polarity

Contact the sacrum and occiput with the palms of your hands. Imagine the spine decompressing and lengthening between your hands. Hold for at least 30 seconds.

FIGURE 6-22   Back stretch.

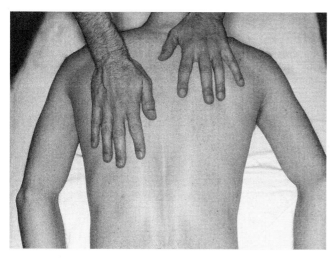

FIGURE 6-23 Cat's paws.

Shiatsu

Cat's Paws

With your hands placed on either side of the spine at the level of the upper back, alternately press your palms down the back, as if walking on your hands. When you reach the iliac crests, bring your hands back to the shoulders and perform the sequence again with the hands wider apart (Fig. 6-23).

SWEDISH/CROSS FIBER

1. Perform basic effleurage strokes on the musculature of the back.
2. Stand at the side of the table, facing the client's back. Perform the **swim stroke** by rolling and spreading your forearms across the back muscles, avoiding pressure on the spinous processes.
3. Apply cross fiber strokes to the erector spinae muscles with the heel of the hand or the knuckles.

CONNECTIVE TISSUE

Myofascial Mobilization Technique

Using the fingers or palms, roll the muscles of the back over the underlying ribs and vertebrae. Use the myofascial spreading technique on areas of tissue that do not easily slide over the bones.

DEEP TISSUE/NMT

Sequence

1. Erector spinae group
2. Deep paraspinal muscles (the lamina groove)
3. Iliac crest

4. Sacral ligaments
5. Intercostals

Commonly Found Trigger Points

Trigger points may be located in any of the musculature of the back, particularly where injuries have occurred and tissues have been damaged. Observe the client's posture and movement patterns. Note where bending and reaching are initiated along the spine. These are stress points and are likely candidates for trigger point formation and connective tissue build-up.

1. Erector Spinae Group
(Spinalis, Longissimus, Iliocostalis)
Origin: Iliocostalis lumborum—external lip of the iliac crest; posterior surface of sacrum. **Iliocostalis thoracis**—upper borders of ribs 12–7. **Longissimus thoracis**—transverse processes of L1–L5 vertebrae. **Spinalis thoracis**—spinous processes of T11–T12 and L1–L2 vertebrae.
Insertion: Iliocostalis lumborum—angles of ribs 6–12. **Iliocostalis thoracis**—transverse process of C7, angles of ribs 1–6. **Longissimus thoracis**—accessory processes of L1–L3 vertebrae, transverse processes of T1–T12 vertebrae, between tubercles and angles of ribs 2–12. **Spinalis thoracis**—spinous processes of T1–T4 vertebrae.
Action: Iliocostalis lumborum and thoracis; longissimus thoracis—extension and lateral flexion of vertebral column, depression of ribs. **Spinalis thoracis**—extension and rotation of vertebral column.

The longissimus and iliocostalis muscles are the most likely sites for trigger point activity. Trigger points in the iliocostalis thoracis at its upper level tend to refer along the scapular border and between the shoulder blades. In the lower portion of the muscles, pain may be referred downward into the lumbar and hip region and into the abdomen.

- Perform elongating strokes down the back, parallel to the spine, beginning at the level of T1 and ending at the iliac crest. Use the base of the palm, forearm, or knuckles (Fig. 6-24). Cover each of the three erector spinae muscles.
- Stroke along the borders of the muscles using the elbow or thumbs. Begin at the level of T1 and end at the iliac crest.

2. Deep Paraspinal Muscles
Origin:
  Semispinalis thoracis—transverse processes of T6–T10 vertebrae.
  Semispinalis cervicis—transverse processes of T1–T5 vertebrae.
  Semispinalis capitis—transverse processes of C4–C7 and T1–T6 vertebrae.
  Multifidi—sacrum to S4 foramen, erector spinae

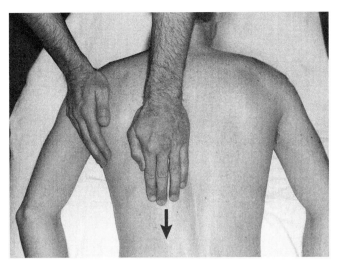

FIGURE 6-24 Elongation stroke on the erector spinae muscles using the base of the palm.

aponeurosis, posterior superior iliac spine, posterior sacroiliac ligaments, mamillary and transverse processes of T1–T12 vertebrae, articular processes of C4–C7 vertebrae.

Rotatores—transverse process of all vertebrae.

Insertion:

Semispinalis thoracis—spinous processes of C6–C7 and T1–T4 vertebrae.

Semispinalis cervicis—spinous processes of C2–C5.

Semispinalis capitis—occiput, between superior and inferior nuchal lines.

Multifidi—spinous process of two to four vertebrae above origin.

Rotatores—base of spinous process of next highest vertebra.

Action: Extend and rotate vertebral column.

Trigger points in the semispinalis thoracis often register as a continuous, aching sensation. In the next lower layer, the multifidi, the referral pattern tends to be across the vertebra at the level of the trigger point. At the lowest level, the rotatores, trigger points may be found along the entire length and often create a band of pain across the back at the level of involvement.

- Perform elongating strokes down the spine in the space between the spinous processes and the transverse processes of the vertebrae, from T1 to the sacrum (Fig. 6-25). Use the thumbs or the elbow.
- Use static compression and/or short spreading techniques in muscular areas that feel dense, fibrous, or unyielding.

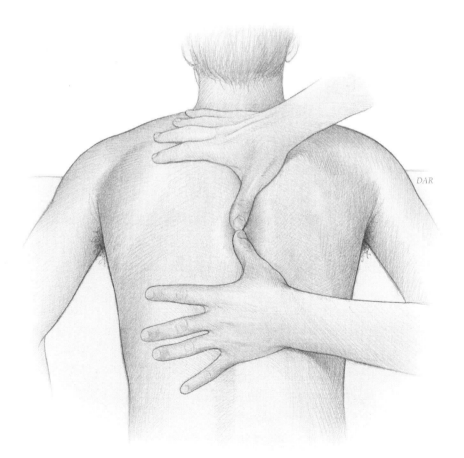

DAR

FIGURE 6-25 Placement of the thumbs next to the spinous processes to release the deep paraspinal muscles.

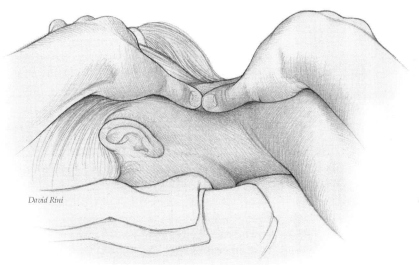

David Rini

FIGURE 6-26 Hand placement for releasing the cervical paraspinal muscles.

- Place the thumbs end to end at C7 (Fig. 6-26). Do an elongating stroke along the lamina groove of the cervical spine to the occiput. Repeat, using the side-to-side strokes, along the muscle fibers.

3. Iliac Crest, Iliolumbar Ligament

Position
Place a pillow under the client's pelvis for the next three sections (iliac crest, iliolumbar ligament, sacral ligaments).

Superior Border of the Iliac Crest
- Trace the edge of the iliac crest using the thumbs or elbow. Feel for congested areas of tissue and/or tender spots.

- Use static compression on tender spots. Do the side-to-side spreading technique across the congested tissues to release them.

Thoracolumbar Fascia
This broad band of fascia, covering the low back, attaches to the iliac crest and covers the sacrum. Examine it carefully, as trigger points may be formed anywhere.

Iliolumbar Ligament
Find the junction formed by the lumbar spine and the pelvis. Place your elbow into it, pressing inward and downward, at approximately a 45° angle toward the iliac crest (Fig. 6-27). Hold, with static compression. Perform short cross fiber strokes.

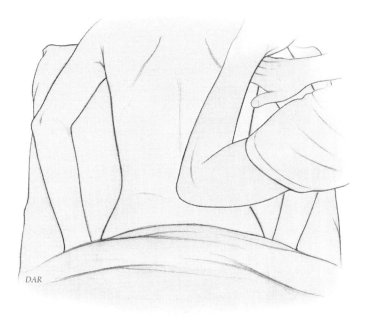

DAR

FIGURE 6-27 Elbow position for contacting the iliolumbar ligament.

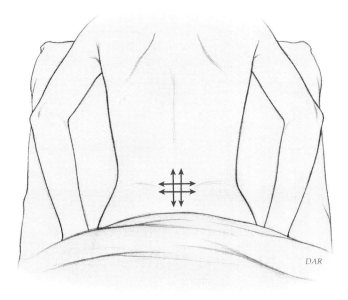

FIGURE 6-28   Directions of strokes on the sacrum.

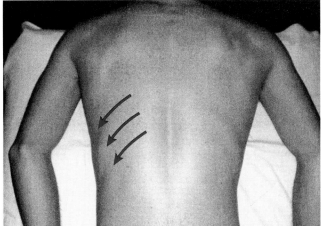

FIGURE 6-29   Direction of strokes on the intercostal muscles.

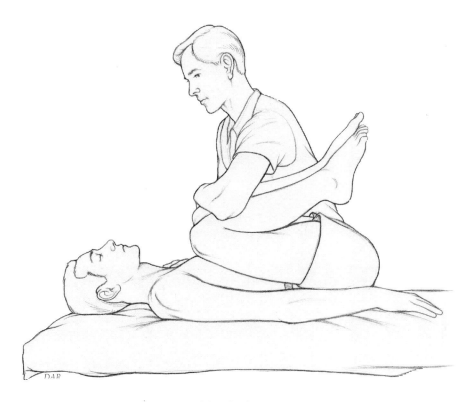

FIGURE 6-30   Stretching the client's low back.

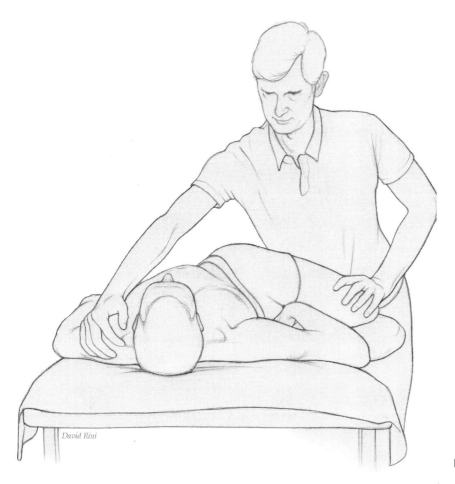

David Rini

FIGURE 6-31 The spinal twist.

4. Sacral Ligaments

■ Warm up the sacral area by applying fingertip friction over the entire sacrum.
■ Do all the deep tissue spreading techniques over the sacrum (up-down, side-side, and combination) (Fig. 6-28) using the thumbs or fingers.

5. Intercostals

■ Stand on the opposite side of the table from the section of ribs on which you are working. Place your fingers just below the inferior angle of the scapula. Moving your fingers back and forth and up and down, feel for the spaces between the ribs.
■ Using short back-and-forth motions, feel for restricted areas in the soft tissues between the ribs (i.e., knots, strings, lumps) (Fig. 6-29). Check for trigger point activity. The thumbs or a knuckle may be used in the intercostal spaces where more pressure is required.
■ Continue to the 12th rib.

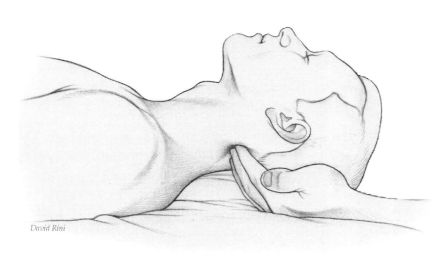

David Rini

FIGURE 6-32 Hand position for the occipital release.

Stretch

1. Bring the client's knees to his or her chest. Holding the client's knees with your hands or by pressing your forearm against them, slowly lean forward, flexing the thighs to the chest (Fig. 6-30). This stretches the client's low back muscles.
2. Reaching across the table, press the client's shoulder down to stabilize it against the table. With your other hand, slowly pull the client's knees toward you and down toward the table, creating a twist for the spine and back muscles (Fig. 6-31).
3. Have the client hold the knees to the chest. Standing at the head of the table, hold the client's head in your hands. Traction the neck very slightly by drawing the head toward you, then lifting the head off the table, bringing the forehead toward the knees. This stretches the upper back muscles.

Accessory Work

1. Occipital release. Sitting at the head of the table, slide your fingers under the client's occipital ridge, lifting the head slightly (Fig. 6-32). Wait for the muscles to soften and for the sensation of an even pulse on both sides of the occiput.
2. Spinal reflex points on the foot. With your thumb, press points along the medial border of the foot, beginning at the big toe and working down to the heel. The curves of the instep correspond to the curves of the spine (Fig. 6-33). Hold sensitive spots for 8 to 12 seconds.

Closing

Sitting at the foot of the table, lightly hold the heels of the client's feet in your hands for 30 to 60 seconds. Remove your hands slowly.

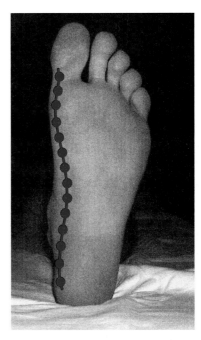

FIGURE 6-33   The spinal reflex zone.

REFERENCES

1. Heller J, Henkin W. The body as a tensegrity structure. In: Bodywise. Berkeley, CA: Winbow Press, 1991: 47–52.
2. Feldenkrais M. Body and mature behavior. New York: International Universities Press, 1970.
3. Rolf IP, Feitis R, ed. Rolfing and physical reality. Rochester, VT: Healing Arts Press, 1990: 211.

7

Aligning the Upper Extremity

THE SHOULDER, ARM, AND HAND

INTRODUCTION

The shoulder, arm, forearm, and hand form the upper extremity. This is an extremely important area because it is largely through the shoulder-arm complex that we express ourselves bodily and make contact with the world. The ways in which persons hold their shoulders and arms say much about their attitudes and characters in general.

Functionally, the pectoral girdle forms a base of support for the arms that allows almost unlimited range of motion. It also protects the lungs and heart from damage due to impact stress arising from the use of the arms by diverting force away from the chest cavity.

The pectoral girdle and pelvic girdle share a similar function in that they both support and anchor the limbs. The major difference between the two is that the pelvis is a more rigid structure. Unlike the pectoral girdle, all of its bones are joined together, limiting its movement. The shoulder girdle is open in the back because the scapulae do not connect to each other. This design allows the arms much greater freedom of individual motion at the shoulder joints than the legs are capable of at the hip joints.

For proper balance and integration of the body, the pectoral girdle and pelvis need to be aligned to each other. The muscles of the pectoral girdle and arms should be free to adjust to weight shifts that occur from movements in the lower body. By design, the pectoral girdle acts like a yoke, suspended over the ribcage by muscles attaching to the neck and head. The arms should hang loosely from the shoulder joints, with freedom to swing. Tension in the muscles of the shoulders produces rigidity in the upper back and neck that contributes to imbalance and stress throughout the body.

When the muscles of the upper extremity are working in a coordinated fashion, the centers of the shoulder joints will be directly at the sides of the body, creating maximum width in the upper torso. As the arms hang to the sides, the lateral aspects of the elbows should slightly turn out and the palms of the hands face posteriorly, according to Dr. Ida

Rolf. Rolf's opinion that the hands should face in a posterior direction in a properly aligned body is a controversial one. She claimed that this position affords the greatest width across the shoulder girdle. Illustrations of her views of correct vertical standing alignment can be found on page 72 of her book, "Rolfing The Integration of Human Structures."[1]

When all the joints of the upper extremity are balanced, a force applied through the fingers and hand will pass cleanly through the wrist, up the forearm and humerus, and through the scapula to the spine. From there, the force will pass down the vertebrae to the sacrum and flare out across the ilium to the hip joints. Then it will pass down the bones of the legs to the ankles and across the feet. In this way, forces are transferred smoothly through the body, eliminating strains caused by soft tissues having to brace uneven forces around misaligned joints.

Integrated deep tissue therapy on the shoulder girdle, arms, and hands helps to remove uneven pulls on the scapula and clavicle and balances the humerus in the shoulder joint. Soft tissue reorganization at the shoulder girdle improves movement of the arms, increases breathing capacity, and reduces the risk of injury to the area.

MUSCULOSKELETAL ANATOMY AND FUNCTION (ESSENTIAL ANATOMY BOX 7-1)

The shoulder girdle consists of the clavicles, the scapulae, and the humerus bones. It does not attach to the spine at all; its only connection to the rest of the skeleton is where the clavicles attach to the sternum. The lateral ends of the clavicles join the scapulae via the acromioclavicular joint. The clavicles support the shoulder joints and keep the scapulae away from the chest wall, so that they may move freely and independently. In maintaining this distance from the thorax, the clavicle prevents the shoulder girdle from interfering with the important functions of circulation and respiration, and protects the nerves passing through the upper ribs. It also absorbs shocks coming through the shoulder and arm, protecting the sternum and ribs from the force of direct impact.

The humerus and scapula are joined via a ball-and-socket type joint. The rounded head of the humerus fits into a concave depression on the side of the scapula, called the glenoid fossa. This fossa is shallow and does not fit around the humerus, as the acetabulum of the pelvis does with the femur. The humerus is held in the joint by a ligamentous capsule and supporting muscles.

This design allows for greater range of motion than is possible at the hip. When the arms no longer have to function solely for support of body weight, as they do in most animals, they become free to develop other capabilities. Early humans learned to fashion tools with their hands, which allowed them to rise far above the level of the rest of the animal kingdom.

The motions of the arms are controlled by a series of muscles attached around the shoulder joint and along the humerus (Fig. 7-1A). These muscles form a wheel-like design, fanning out from the shoulder joint to connect to the skeleton over a broad area. Thus, the action of the

ESSENTIAL ANATOMY BOX 7-1	Muscles	Bones and Landmarks
	Trapezius	Scapula
	Supraspinatus	Spine of scapula
	Infraspinatus	Acromion process
	Teres minor	Humerus
	Teres major	Olecranon process
The Shoulder and Arm Routines	Latissimus dorsi	Olecranon fossa
	Deltoid	Deltoid tuberosity
	Biceps brachii	Lateral epicondyle
	Triceps brachii	Medial epicondyle
	Brachialis	Ulna
	Forearm extensors and flexors	Radius
	Hand muscles	Carpals metacarpals
		Phalanges

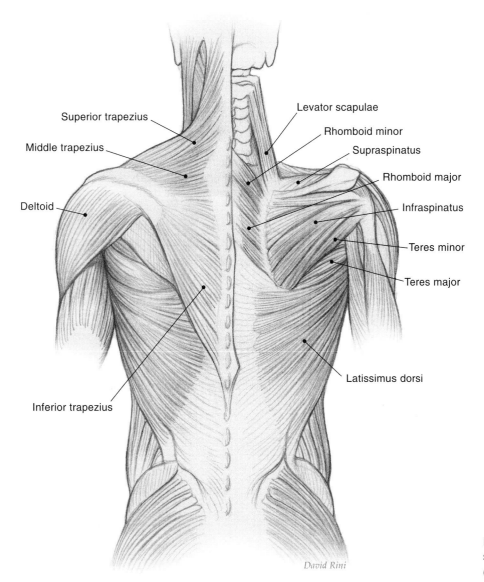

Superior trapezius

Middle trapezius

Deltoid

Inferior trapezius

Levator scapulae

Rhomboid minor

Supraspinatus

Rhomboid major

Infraspinatus

Teres minor

Teres major

Latissimus dorsi

David Rini

FIGURE 7-1   (A) Muscles of the scapula and arm—posterior view. *(continued)*

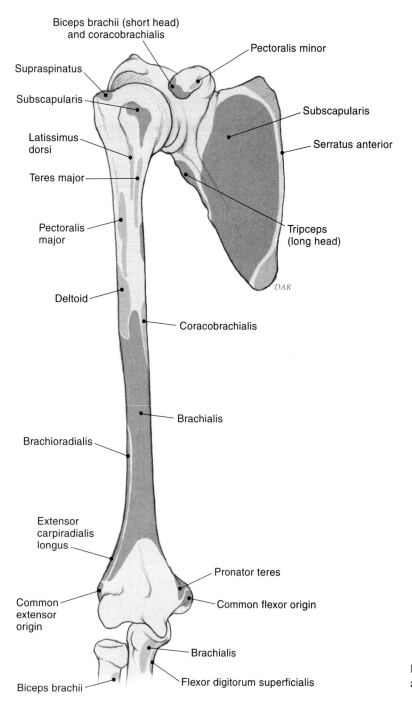

Biceps brachii (short head)
and coracobrachialis

Pectoralis minor

Supraspinatus

Subscapularis

Subscapularis

Latissimus
dorsi

Serratus anterior

Teres major

Pectoralis
major

Tripceps
(long head)

DAR

Deltoid

Coracobrachialis

Brachialis

Brachioradialis

Extensor
carpiradialis
longus

Pronator teres

Common
extensor
origin

Common flexor origin

Brachialis

Flexor digitorum superficialis

Biceps brachii

FIGURE 7-1   *Continued.* (**B**) Muscles of the scapula
and arm—anterior view. *(continued)*

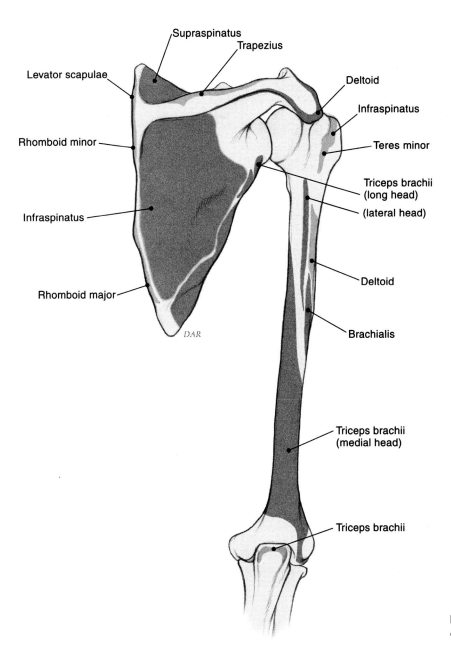

Supraspinatus

Trapezius

Levator scapulae

Deltoid

Infraspinatus

Rhomboid minor

Teres minor

Triceps brachii
(long head)

(lateral head)

Infraspinatus

Deltoid

Rhomboid major

DAR

Brachialis

Triceps brachii
(medial head)

Triceps brachii

FIGURE 7-1 *Continued.* **(C)** Posterior muscles of the scapula and arm. *(continued)*

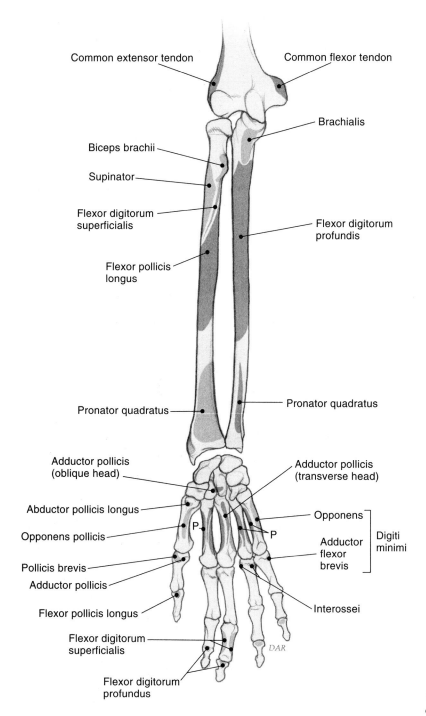

Common extensor tendon

Common flexor tendon

Brachialis

Biceps brachii

Supinator

Flexor digitorum
superficialis

Flexor digitorum
profundis

Flexor pollicis
longus

Pronator quadratus

Pronator quadratus

Adductor pollicis
(oblique head)

Adductor pollicis
(transverse head)

Abductor pollicis longus

Opponens

Opponens pollicis

Adductor
flexor
brevis

Digiti
minimi

Pollicis brevis

Adductor pollicis

Flexor pollicis longus

Interossei

Flexor digitorum
superficialis

DAR

Flexor digitorum
profundus

FIGURE 7-1 *Continued.* (**D**) Anterior muscles of the forearm and hand.

arms is dependent on coordination of movement coming through the trunk and legs. Isolated movement of the arms, without support of the body, creates strain that can lead to injury.

The muscles that control movements of the arm include those that must also stabilize the scapula. It is important that the scapula is free to move in combination with all movements of the humerus, but it must also remain anchored to the body wall through muscular action to provide leverage for the head of the humerus.

In the back, the **trapezius** and rhomboids help support the scapulae (Fig. 7-1A). The upper trapezius, with assistance from the lower trapezius, elevates the shoulders. It can become strained when the arms are held in elevated positions for long periods, as when carrying a bag of groceries home.

A tender point that frequently develops near the attachment point of the **levator scapula** muscle on the superior angle of the scapula is often attributed to holding the shoulders in an elevated position. However, this soreness is more likely due to a chronic forward head position. When the head is held forward, the levator scapulae are constantly active drawing the neck posterior to bring the head back toward the vertical axis of gravity. The scapulae must be held steady to stabilize the pulling action of the muscles, causing the scapular attachments of the levator scapulae to become strained. The stress on these muscles is relieved by properly positioning the head on the neck, thus reducing the pulling action by the levator scapulae.

The **rhomboids**, which retract the scapulae, are opposed by the **serratus anterior** muscles, which protract them. When the musculature controlling the placement of the scapulae is balanced, they lie on the horizontal plane along with the clavicles (e.g., when a man is standing with his arms at his sides). When the rhomboids are weak, they cannot fix the vertebral borders of the scapulae to the body wall, and the lower portion of the scapulae will lift away from the back, or wing.[1]

Several large muscles emanating from the spine, sternum, and ribs contribute to arm movements. These muscles include the trapezius, latissimus dorsi, and pectoralis major. This is an advantageous arrangement, as it distributes forces generated from the arms throughout the length of the spine, helping to stabilize the spine against large, peripheral motions.

The ligamentous capsule surrounding the head of the humerus is quite loose to allow for increased range of motion of the arm. Because of this laxity of the capsule, it cannot maintain the head of the humerus in the joint. This support is accomplished by the tendons of four muscles positioned around the shoulder joint, known as the rotator cuff. The muscles that comprise the rotator cuff are the **supraspinatus, infraspinatus, teres minor,** and **subscapularis.** They are joined in their function of reinforcement by the tendon of the long head of the **biceps brachii** on the top of the joint and the long head of the **triceps brachii** on the underside of the joint. The balance of all these muscles is crucial to proper positioning of the humerus in the shoulder joint.

The primary abductors of the humerus are the **deltoids.** However, due to their position at the superior end of the humerus, they lack the leverage to initiate abduction when the arm is against the side of the body. The supraspinatus muscle initiates abduction, which is taken over by the deltoids when the arm is abducted about 12 inches from the side of the body.

The infraspinatus muscle is responsible for external rotation of the humerus. It is opposed by the subscapularis, which internally rotates the arm. Both of these muscles help to stabilize the humerus in the glenoid fossa. They are easily strained by swinging the arm forward or backward from a horizontal position. Sleeping on one's side with full body weight resting on the folded underneath arm can also aggravate strain in both of these muscles. Placing a small pillow under the side of the head takes some weight off the arm when lying on one's side.

The teres minor assists the infraspinatus in external rotation and stabilization of the head of the humerus against the scapula. **Teres major** assists the **latissimus dorsi** in external rotation and extension of a flexed arm. The teres major and latissimus dorsi muscles form the posterior axillary fold, which is the back of the armpit.

Pectoralis minor connects the scapula to the anterior side of the ribcage. It brings the scapula forward, downward, and medial. Shortened pectoralis minor muscles are characterized by rounded or stooped shoulders. The lateral bundle of nerves of the **brachial plexus** and the axillary artery pass underneath the pectoralis minor. When this muscle is chronically contracted, it may impinge blood flow and nerve supply to the arm when the arm is abducted and externally rotated. In this position, the pectoralis minor is unable to lengthen and presses against these structures. The most common symptom of this form of impingement is numbness in the forearm and on the palmar side of the first 3.5 digits of the hand.

The forearm consists of two bones, the ulna and radius (Fig. 7-1D). The radius is capable of rotation around the ulna at its proximal end, via a ligamentous ring that joins the two bones. This ring also prevents the radius from being pulled away from the ulna by the action of the biceps muscle as it supinates the forearm and hand and flexes the elbow. The radius and ulna are tied together by an interweaving interosseus membrane. This gives additional strength to the forearm while keeping it much lighter than if it were composed of one large bone.

The **brachialis** is deep to the biceps and is a stronger flexor of the forearm. Both of these muscles are opposed by the triceps, which extends the forearm. The triceps is usually much weaker than the biceps and brachialis and is prone to overuse injuries from actions that require repetitive flexing and straightening of the forearm (e.g., hammering). It often requires strengthening to balance movement at the elbow joint.

The hand connects to the forearm by the wrist joint, formed between the radius and ulna and the eight small carpal bones. The number of small gliding joints this design creates allows for great mobility and flexibility at the wrist. A unique feature of the human hand is that the thumb is opposable, meaning it is capable of touching each of the fingers. This allows for an oppositional type grip and a superior degree of control and refinement of movement.

INDICATIONS/ CONTRAINDICATIONS BOX 7-1 *Conditions Affecting Shoulder*	**Indications** Pain in the shoulder Limited range of motion Subacute injuries Poor posture Headaches Carpal tunnel syndrome Fatigue in arms and hands	**Contraindications** Inflammation Bursitis Acute injury Bad bruising Broken bones

Most of the muscles that control the hand lie along the forearm. The extensor muscles merge at the **common extensor tendon**, which attaches on the lateral epicondyle of the humerus. The flexor muscles merge at the **common flexor tendon**, attaching to the medial epicondyle of the humerus.

CONDITIONS (INDICATIONS/ CONTRAINDICATIONS BOX 7-1)

1. *Bursitis* is an inflammation of the bursa sac, which is a cushioning, fluid-filled sac in the shoulder joint. Bursitis is characterized by achiness and pain when lifting the arm.

   a. *Acute bursitis* can be an extremely painful condition that usually starts mildly and gets progressively worse over a period of days. A blow to the shoulder can cause the bursa sac to become irritated and then to swell to a much larger-than-normal size. Pain in the shoulder will be intense for days or weeks, making it very difficult to lift the arm or lie on the shoulder. Massage and exercise are contraindicated; both will worsen the condition. Rest is the treatment of choice.
   b. *Chronic bursitis*, although not nearly as debilitating as acute bursitis, can still be an annoyance. Lifting the arm to shoulder height becomes painful due to compression and irritation to the bursa sac within the humeral joint. As the arm is lifted overhead, the pain diminishes as pressure on the sac is relieved. Pain comes in bouts, lasting anywhere from weeks to years if untreated. Massage is contraindicated. Cortisone injections have been found to be effective.

2. *Arthritis* is a general term covering a broad range of ailments. Osteoarthritic conditions indicate a degener-

ation of the joint, either from a deformation of the bones or irritation due to shrinkage or compression of the soft tissue components of the joint. Arthritis can be brought on by chronic misuse of the arm or by misalignment of the shoulder. It may also be aggravated by trauma to the shoulder resulting in irritation to the joint capsule.

Another common form of arthritis is rheumatoid arthritis. It is a chronic systemic disease believed to be related to an antigen-antibody reaction that leads to crippling deformation of joints. Rheumatoid arthritis is characterized by periods of painful, inflammatory flare-ups of joints. Massage is contraindicated during these times. A physician can prescribe anti-inflammatory compounds that may be helpful. Light massage can be performed on the muscles between periods of flare-up. Affected joints should always be avoided.

Proper assessment of the cause of the arthritis is necessary for correct treatment. Stretching or corrective movement work may be indicated. Massage of irritated tissues is contraindicated.

3. *Injuries to muscles and tendons.* It is often difficult for a client to tell exactly where a shoulder injury is originating. To pinpoint injury sites in this area, the therapist should apply resistive tests to the suspected muscles. Once located, the injured muscle or tendon may be treated with a combination of ice and massage. If massage treatments are not helping, they should be discontinued; ice and rest should then be recommended.

4. *Shoulder separation.* The source of this injury is usually a tear in the ligament that binds the clavicle and the acromion. It is caused by trauma to the joint, such as a fall. Massage is contraindicated. Initial treatment should be rest, followed by stretching exercises when the injury begins to heal.

5. *Shoulder dislocation.* The humerus is held in place at the glenoid fossa mainly through ligamentous binding. It is fairly easy to knock the humerus out of the

socket. This is painful and results in irritation and possible chronic stretching of the ligaments. The injury tends to be repeated as the ligaments lose their integrity. Surgery to tighten the ligaments may be the only solution.

6. *Tennis elbow.* This term describes an injury to the extensor tendon that connects the extensor muscles of the hand to the elbow. It may be caused by incorrect form when swinging a tennis racquet or baseball bat, or during any other action that involves the use of the wrist extensor muscles. Rest and ice are appropriate treatments. Massage to the forearm to increase blood flow to the injured tendon is indicated.

7. *Carpal tunnel syndrome* is a painful condition in the wrist area caused by a compression of the median nerve. The site of irritation is usually the carpal tunnel through the wrist, which forms a passage for the nerve and the tendons of the hand muscles. If these tendons swell due to overuse or improper use of the hand, they will put pressure on the median nerve. The result is pain and perhaps a numbing sensation in the thumb and index finger. Other causes of the tunnel becoming restricted include fracture of the wrist, endocrine disorders such diabetes, menopause, tumors, and body fluid retention. Treatment consists of rest, ice, elevation of the arm, and massage to the forearm.

8. *Painful weak grip.* This is a condition in which a person loses the ability to close the hand powerfully. It is attributed to overuse and trigger point development in the extensor carpi radialis longus, extensor carpi radialis brevis, and extensor digitorum muscles. Activities that involve grasping with the hand (e.g., gripping a steering wheel, digging with garden tools, or holding a hammer) aggravate the condition. Massage and trigger point deactivation are the recommended treatment protocols. If inflammation is present, the client should apply ice and rest the affected muscles until the inflammation subsides before massage therapy is attempted.

THE MIND/ BODY CONNECTION

By design, the shoulder girdle is similar to an old-fashioned yoke, which was a weight-carrying device balanced across the shoulders. A yoke consisted of a broad piece of wood, with ropes or chains attached at either end from which hung buckets or bundles of some sort. Although in the Western world we no longer use yokes to carry things, the shoulders themselves often continue to serve that function psychologically, in that in our minds and emotions we do often carry heavy loads across our shoulders.

The muscles of the shoulder girdle often receive the brunt of our concerns and worries about our ability to carry all the responsibilities and burdens that accompany us in life. It is not uncommon to see a person literally stooped over as if weighted down by some tremendous, invisible load.

As explained previously, the position of the shoulders is dependent on muscle action, perhaps more than any other joint. As muscles are controlled by the nervous system, which is controlled ultimately by the mind, there is an obvious relationship between the way a person positions the shoulders and his or her beliefs and attitudes in general. An interesting experiment is to stand in front of a mirror and put your shoulders and arms into different poses. Observe how each position changes the way you feel and how the image you project changes based on your body posture.

The shoulders and arms reflect how we interact with the world. The arms can act as a barrier, pushing people away, or they can draw people in with an embrace. Being on the same plane as the heart center, the arms physically manifest the state of the heart's energy. The hands give and receive energy. It is through the medium of the hands that healing therapeutic touch is administered. The Chinese qi gong and Indian yoga systems both refer to the existence of energy centers in the hand. The Bill Moyers PBS series, "The Healing Mind," available on video, includes a demonstration of a qi gong master's ability to move a candle flame utilizing qi directed from his hand.

POSTURAL EVALUATION (TABLES 7-1 AND 7-2)

1. Check the position of the clavicles. How close are they to being horizontal?
2. Compare the height of the right and left shoulders. Observe the distance from the shoulder to the ear.
3. Compare the length of both arms. Where do the fingertips reach on the thigh?
4. Make note of any hollow spaces around the clavicles.
5. Have the client raise the arms to the sides. Do the arms move independently of the shoulder girdle? (They should.)
6. Note any areas of restriction or muscle tension around the shoulder girdle.
7. How do the arms hang?
   - Straight or flexed at the elbow?
   - In what direction do the hands face?
   - What is the distance of the arms from the sides of the body? Is it the same on both sides?
8. From a side view, observe the alignment of the tip of the shoulder to the ear, hip, knee, and ankle.
9. From the posterior view, check the position of the scapulae.
   - Protracted.

TABLE 7–1	Body Reading for the Shoulder Girdle

Conditions	Muscles that May Be Shortened
Raised shoulder(s)—one or both shoulders are elevated	Scalenes Upper trapezius Lower trapezius
Rounded shoulders—shoulders are rotated medially	Trapezius Pectoralis major Pectoralis minor Anterior deltoid Teres major Serratus anterior
Retracted shoulders—shoulder blades are pulled back, scapulae winged	Rhomboids Trapezius Teres minor Infraspinatus Latissimus dorsi

- Retracted.
- Depressed.
- Elevated.
- Upward or downward rotation.
- Relaxed and properly positioned.

10. Observe the condition of the musculature affecting the scapulae.

EXERCISES AND SELF-TREATMENT

SHOULDERS

1. Standing in a doorway, extend your arms upward and open them slightly wider than shoulder width. Placing your palms against the top of the door frame, lean your body forward leading with the hips and chest, until you feel a stretch in the shoulders. Hold for a few seconds as you breathe deeply into the stretch. (Stretches pectoralis minor, clavicular division of pectoralis major.)
2. Stand in front of a dresser or table, facing away from it. Reach your arms behind you with the elbows flexed, placing your palms on top of the flat surface, fingers facing you. Squeezing your shoulder blades and elbows towards each other, slowly flex your knees and sink down as if sitting into a chair, until you feel a stretch in the shoulder area. Hold as you breathe deeply and focus on releasing tension in the shoulders. (Stretches anterior deltoid, sternal division of pectoralis major.)

3. The following shoulder exercises may be performed from a seated position:
   - As you inhale, raise both shoulders toward your ears. Hold for a few seconds. (Contracts upper trapezius.)
   - Exhaling, lower your shoulders slowly, feeling the tension flowing out of the muscles. (Stretches upper trapezius.)
   - Inhaling, draw both shoulders back, squeezing the vertebral borders of the scapulae toward each other. (Contracts rhomboids.)
   - Exhaling, press the outside edges of the shoulders forward, feeling the space between the scapulae stretching. (Stretches rhomboids.)
   - Slowly circle the shoulders, inhaling for half of the circle, exhaling for half of the circle. Repeat a few times and then reverse the direction of the circle. (Stretches rotator cuff muscles.)
4. Lie on your side with both knees flexed. Your head may rest on the arm closest to the floor. The uppermost arm is straight and placed on the floor in front of your chest with the palm facing downward. Slowly circle the arm around your body, tracing the circle on the floor with your fingers. As the arm moves overhead, allow it to rotate naturally so that the palm is facing upward. Pause in positions that feel tight or restricted and imagine breathing into the shoulder. Repeat a few times, then reverse the direction of the circle. Turn onto your other side and repeat the entire exercise. (Stretches rotator cuff muscles, pectoralis major, latissimus dorsi.)

TABLE 7–2   Range of Motion (ROM) for the Shoulder and Arm

Action	Muscles
Shoulder	
Flexion (ROM 170°)	Anterior deltoid
	Biceps brachii
	Pectoralis major
	Coracobrachialis
Extension (ROM 60°)	Posterior deltoid
	Teres major
	Latissimus dorsi
	Triceps brachii
Abduction (ROM 170°)	Supraspinatus
	Deltoids
	Biceps brachii
Adduction (ROM 50°)	Biceps brachii
	Pectoralis major
	Teres major
	Coracobrachialis
	Latissimus dorsi
	Triceps brachii
Medial rotation (ROM 70°)	Anterior deltoid
	Pectoralis major
	Subscapularis
	Teres major
	Latissimus dorsi
Lateral rotation (ROM 90°)	Infraspinatus
	Teres minor
	Posterior deltoid
Elbow	
Flexion (ROM 150°)	Biceps brachii
	Brachialis
	Brachioradialis
	Extensor carpi radialis
	Pronator teres
	Flexor carpi ulnaris
	Flexor carpi radialis
Extension (ROM 0°)	Triceps brachii
	Anconeus
Forearm	
Supination (ROM 90°)	Biceps brachii
	Brachioradialis
	Supinator
Pronation (ROM 90°)	Brachioradialis
	Pronator teres
	Pronator quadratus
Wrist	
Flexion (ROM 80°)	Flexor carpi radialis
	Flexor carpi ulnaris
Extension (ROM 70°)	Extensor carpi radialis
	Extensor carpi ulnaris

ARMS

1. Stand facing a wall with your arms extended so that your palms are against the wall. Lean into the wall, flexing only your arms, like doing a push-up. Keep your body straight. Vary the speed of the push and the degree of lean to strengthen the arm muscles effectively. Repeat several times. (Strengthens biceps, brachialis, triceps.)

WRISTS

1. To strengthen your wrists, hold a broom handle out in front of you as if shaking hands with it. Slowly raise the broom upward and downward with the motion of your wrist. To work with less weight, hold the broom closer to the broom head. To use more weight, hold the broom closer to the end of the handle. (Strengthens wrist flexors and extensors.)
2. Sitting cross-legged on the floor, lean forward slightly from the hip joints. With your arms fully extended in front of you, place the palms on the floor with the fingers turned toward your ankles. Gently press the heel of the palm toward the floor. Hold for at least 10 seconds. (Stretches wrist flexors.)
3. In the same position as above, place the back of the hands on the floor and press down very gently until you feel a mild stretch in the back of the wrist. Hold for 5 to 10 seconds. (Stretches wrist extensors.)

HANDS

1. Exhaling, squeeze the fingers and thumbs of both hands into fists. Inhaling, slowly open them all the way against resistance, as if a rubber band were wrapped around the fingers. (Alternately strengthens and stretches the muscles of the hand.)

THE SCAPULA ROUTINE

OBJECTIVES

- To balance the scapula in relation to the clavicle and humerus.
- To release tension in muscles affecting the scapula.
- To help alleviate painful conditions in the scapular region arising from dysfunction and imbalance.
- To explore movement patterns and habits that might be generating stress in the scapular muscles.

ENERGY

Position

The client is lying prone on the table. A bolster may be placed under the ankles.

The therapist is standing at the side of the table next to the client's shoulder.

Polarity

Contact the superior angle of the scapula with the index finger of one hand (negative pole on the hand) and the inferior angle of the scapula with the middle finger of the other hand (positive pole on the hand). Envision the scapula floating freely over the underlying ribs. Allow any subtle movements of the scapula to occur. Hold the position for 30 seconds or longer.

Shiatsu

1. Press points along the vertebral border of the scapula with the thumbs or elbow. The outer branch of the bladder channel runs slightly medial to the border of the scapula.
2. With your outside hand holding the shoulder, place the fingers of your inside hand along the lower portion of the vertebral border of the scapula near the inferior angle. The palm of your hand is facing upward. As you circle the shoulder with your outside hand, slide the fingers of your inside hand under the border of the scapula, pointing them toward the shoulder joint (Fig. 7-2). Attempt this move only if the musculature feels fairly relaxed.

SWEDISH/CROSS FIBER

1. Use a three-stroke effleurage pattern over the scapula. Beginning at the upper thoracic region of the spine, stroke outward over the upper, middle, and lower scapular region, alternating hands with each stroke.
2. Apply cross fiber strokes over the upper back and shoulder area using fingertips and the broad side of the thumb.

CONNECTIVE TISSUE

1. Myofascial mobilization technique. Using the fingers or palms, slide the muscles of the upper back over the scapula and ribs, noting areas that are not moving freely.
2. Apply the myofascial spreading technique to tight, unyielding musculature.

DEEP TISSUE/NMT

Sequence

1. Trapezius (upper, middle, lower)
2. Levator scapula (attachment)
3. Rhomboids

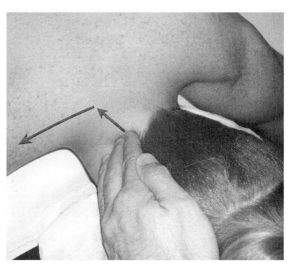

FIGURE 7-3 Elongation stroke on the upper trapezius from the occiput to the acromion process.

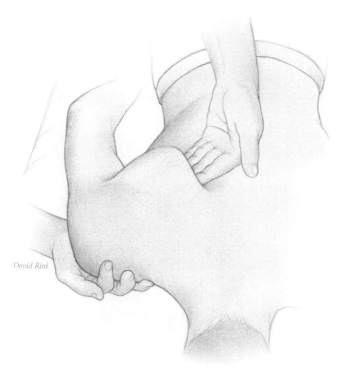

David Rini

FIGURE 7-2 Scapula release.

4. Subscapularis
5. Pectoralis minor
6. Serratus anterior

1. Trapezius

Upper Trapezius
Origin: Medial third of the superior nuchal line and external occipital protuberance, ligamentum nuchae, and the spinal processes of C1–C5 vertebrae.
Insertion: Lateral third of the clavicle.
Action: Elevation and upward rotation of scapula, capital extension.

Trigger points are best located using the sifting technique. Flexing the client's head in the direction of the side being examined may make palpation of the muscle fibers easier. Trigger points may be found along the border of the muscle, slightly above the lateral portion of the clavicle. Pain is referred up the posterior neck to the mastoid process. Trigger point activity in this muscle is a major source of tension headaches. Complementary trigger points may be located in the supraspinatus and levator scapulae muscles.

■ Perform an elongation stroke down the posterior portion of the neck from the occiput to C7, using the fingers. At the base of the neck, switch to knuckles or heel of hand and continue stroking outward to the acromioclavicular joint (Fig. 7-3).

■ Sift the upper trapezius by grasping the belly of the muscle between the thumb and fingers and roll the fibers, feeling for taut bands. Treat any trigger points that are found (Fig. 7-4).

Middle Trapezius
Origin: Interspinous ligaments and spinous processes of C6–T3 vertebrae.
Insertion: Acromion and superior lip of spine of the scapula.
Action: Adduction (retraction) of scapulae.

A commonly occurring trigger point in the middle trapezius may be located on the superior edge of the spine of the scapula near the acromion process. It shoots pain to the top of the shoulder.

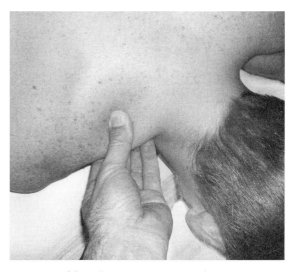

FIGURE 7-4 Sifting the upper trapezius to locate trigger points.

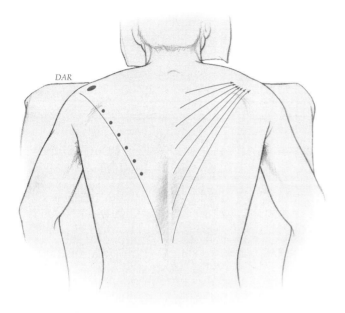

FIGURE 7-5   Elongation strokes on middle and lower trapezius from origins (T1–T12) to insertion (spine of the scapula).

Stand at the side of the table, facing the client's shoulder that is to be treated. Perform an elongation stroke using the knuckles. Covering the space between T1 and T3, stroke laterally across the middle trapezius, ending on the lateral edge of the superior lip of the spine of the scapula.

Lower Trapezius
Origin: Interspinous ligaments and spinous processes of T4–T12 vertebrae.
Insertion: Tubercle on medial end of the spine of the scapula.
Action: Depression and upward rotation of scapula.

The lateral border of the middle and lower trapezius should be examined carefully for trigger points. Trigger points in these muscles are best located by rubbing the fibers over the underlying ribs.

■ Stand at the side of the table facing toward the client's head. Perform a series of elongation strokes using the forearm. Beginning at T4, stroke diagonally upward to the medial end of the spine of the scapula.
■ Repeat the stroke, in strips. The final stroke begins at T12. Cover the muscle completely (Fig. 7-5).

2. Levator Scapula (Insertion)

Levator Scapula
Origin: Posterior tubercles of the transverse processes of C1–C4
Insertion: Vertebral border of the scapula between the superior angle and the root of the spine.
Action: Elevation and adduction of scapula, rotation causing lateral angle to move downward.

To find a trigger point, palpate the fibers slightly lateral to the superior angle (0.5 inches). This trigger point is one

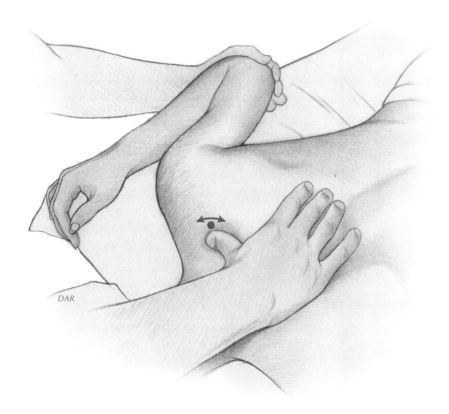

FIGURE 7-6   Cross fiber stroke on the insertion of levator scapula (superior angle of scapula).

of the most common and is usually very tender. It refers pain to the surrounding area of the neck.

Sit or stand at the head of the table. The client's arm is flexed at the elbow with the palm resting against the table next to the shoulder. Hold the client's elbow with your outside hand. The thumb of your other hand is placed against the inferior end of the edge of the superior angle of the scapula. Draw the client's arm toward the head of the table, which lifts the superior angle of the scapula. Apply cross fiber strokes with your thumb pad to the attachment of the levator scapula, just inferior to the superior angle, palpating the tendon for tenderness (Fig. 7-6).

3. Rhomboids

Rhomboid Minor
Origin: Ligamentum nuchae and spinous processes of C7–T1 vertebrae.
Insertion: Medial border of the scapula at the root of the spine.

Action: Adduction of scapula; elevation of scapula; rotates scapula so that lateral angle faces downward.

Rhomboid Major
Origin: Supraspinous ligament and spinous processes of T2–T5 vertebrae.
Insertion: Medial border of the scapula below the root of the spine.
Action: Adduction of scapula; elevation of scapula; rotates scapula so that lateral angle faces downward.

To locate trigger points check just medial to the vertebral border of the scapula. The pain pattern for these trigger points is local, along the edge of the scapula.

- Using thumbs or elbow, do short up-and-down strokes along the origin of the rhomboids at the sides of the spinous processes of C7–T5 (Fig. 7-7A).
- Perform an elongation stroke with the knuckles along the belly of the muscle from the upper thoracic spine to

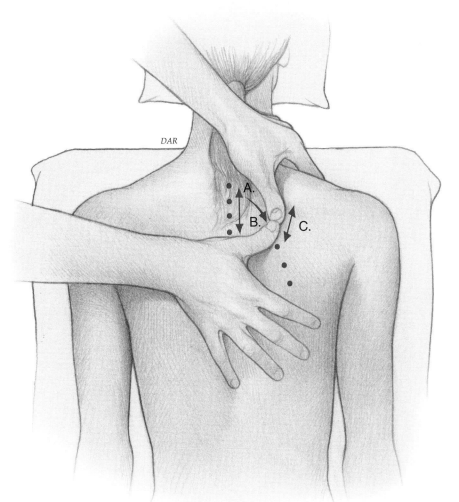

FIGURE 7-7 Strokes on the rhomboids. (A) Origin (C7–T5). (B) Belly (spinous processes to vertebral border of scapula). (C) Insertion (vertebral border of scapula).

the vertebral border of the scapula (Fig. 7-7B). Cover the area from C7–T5.

- Face the client's scapula from the opposite side of the table. The scapula may be raised by placing the client's forearm across the back, or sliding a folded towel under the shoulder of the arm being massaged. Using thumbs or elbow, do short up-and-down strokes on the insertion of the rhomboids (Fig. 7-7C) along the vertebral border of the scapula. Release any trigger points that are found.

4. Subscapularis

Origin: Subscapular fossa along axillary margin of the anterior surface of the scapula.

Insertion: Lesser tuberosity of the humerus and anterior capsule of the shoulder joint.

Action: Medial rotation of shoulder; stabilizes shoulder (glenohumeral) joint by keeping head of humerus in glenoid fossa.

The lateral fibers are the most likely to contain trigger points. They send pain into the posterior part of the shoulder and sometimes down the arm.

Position

The client is resting in side posture with the bottom leg extended and the top leg flexed 90° at the hip and knee. A bolster is placed under the knee. A small pillow or folded towel may be placed under the side of the head.

The therapist is standing behind the client at shoulder level.

- To reach the muscle on the client's right side, place the fingers of your right hand on the ribs just in front of the medial side of the scapula, the left hand grasping the client's upper forearm near the elbow. Pull the client's arm upward to protract the scapula, exposing more of the medial surface (Fig. 7-8). Reverse hand positions for the left side.

- Move the fingers posteriorly along the ribs until the anterior surface of the scapula is felt. Apply short side-to-side strokes with the fingers, along the bone, seeking out tender areas. There are often painful spots in these fibers, so move slowly and elicit client feedback often.

 Move slowly and stay close to the edge of the scapula. The axilla contains several arteries and nerves that are not well protected by muscle, including the axillary, brachial, and cephalic arteries and nerves of the brachial plexus.

- This muscle can also be treated with the client supine. The humerus is abducted 90°, with the forearm flexed 90°. Slide your fingers posteriorly along the ribs until the medial surface of the scapula is felt. Slowly press the fingers into the front side of the scapula and apply short side-to-side and up-and-down strokes to treat the subscapularis muscle.

5. Pectoralis Minor

Origin: Upper and outer surfaces of ribs 3, 4, and 5.

Insertion: Coracoid process of the scapula.

Action: Protraction of scapula (moves scapula forward

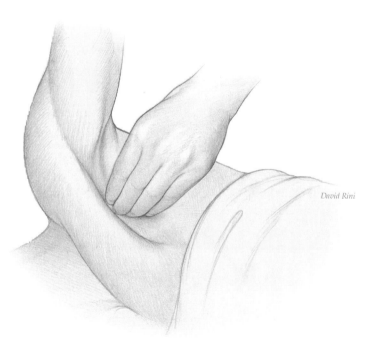

David Rini

FIGURE 7-8   Contacting the subscapularis along the lateral anterior surface of the scapula.

with a downward tilt); elevation of ribs in forced inhalation with scapulae fixed.

Position
The client's top arm rests over a bolster placed in front of the chest.

The therapist stands behind the client at chest level.

Trigger points will most likely be found in the section of the pectoralis minor that attaches to the 5th rib. This is the easiest portion of the muscle to palpate.

The referral zone is the anterior deltoid. When trigger points are found in this muscle, there are almost always complementary trigger points located in the pectoralis major.

- To relax the pectoralis major, perform circular friction with the fingers on the muscle.
- Position your fingers under the pectoralis major muscle and palpate the ribs (Fig. 7-9). Slide slowly along the length of the muscle from its insertions on ribs 3, 4, and 5 to its origin on the coracoid process. Move slowly and pause at painful areas with static pressure. Lift the client's arm that is resting on the bolster and hold it in your non-working hand to gain better access to the muscle.

6. Serratus Anterior
Origin: Outer surfaces of ribs 1 to 8 or 9.
Insertion: Anterior (costal) surface of the vertebral border of the scapula.
Action: Abduction (protraction) of scapula; upward rotation of scapula; fixes medial border of scapula to thoracic wall.

Examine the section of the muscle that lies over the 5th and 6th ribs, in an approximate line with the nipple. The pain referral zone is surrounding the trigger point. Expect much tenderness in this muscle, even when trigger points are not present.

Position
The client's top arm rests on a bolster placed in front of the chest or is extended overhead.

The therapist stands behind the client.
- Perform circular friction strokes using the heel of the hand over the side of the chest.
- Perform an elongation stroke with the heel of the hand from the axillary border of the scapula to the muscle's insertion on the ribs (ribs 1–8). Repeat the stroke several times to cover the entire muscle.
- Perform short up-and-down and side-to-side strokes on the fibers of the muscle over the ribs (Fig. 7-10).
- Pause to treat trigger points.

Stretch

Position
The client is supine.

The therapist stands at the side of the table facing the client's shoulder.

1. Hold the client's arm on the upper forearm, just below the elbow. Place the client's arm perpendicular to the

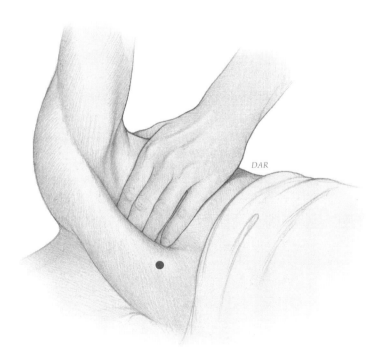

FIGURE 7-9 Reaching pectoralis minor from underneath pectoralis major.

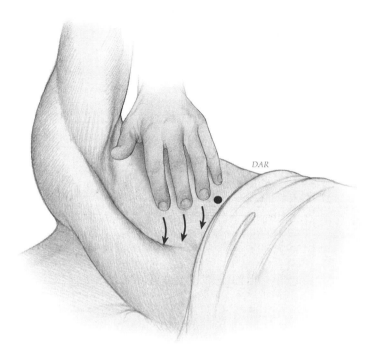

FIGURE 7-10   Contacting serratus anterior over ribs 1–8.

table, with the forearm at a right angle to the humerus and facing across the client's chest (Fig. 7-11).

2. Pull up on the arm, protracting the scapula. The humerus may be adducted to stretch the scapular muscles.

Accessory Work

1. Shiatsu in the chest region (fingertip compression in the intercostal spaces).

2. Trigger point work on the pectoralis major muscle.

3. Circumduction of the arm in both directions.

Closing

Sitting at the foot of the table, lightly hold the heels of the client's feet in your hands for 30 to 60 seconds. Remove your hands slowly to complete the session.

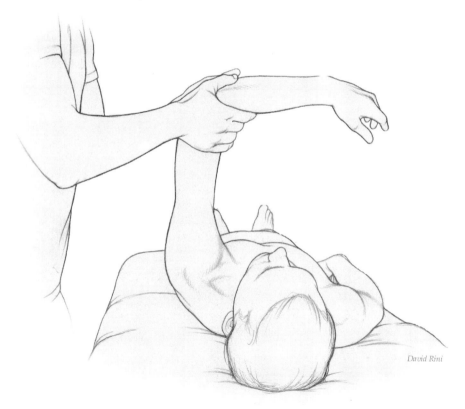

FIGURE 7-11   Stretch for the scapular muscles.

SHOULDER AND UPPER ARM ROUTINE

OBJECTIVES

- To relieve muscular pulls that may be causing misalignment of the shoulder.
- To achieve full range of motion of the humerus in the shoulder joint.
- To reduce stress caused by poor posture and movement.
- Reduction or elimination of pain due to soft tissue damage/dysfunction.

ENERGY

Position

The client is lying supine on the table with arms at the sides of the body.

The therapist is standing at the side of the table next to the client's shoulder.

Polarity

Place the right palm (positive pole) on the posterior side (negative pole) of the shoulder joint; place the left palm (negative pole) on the anterior side (positive pole) of the shoulder joint. Align the two hands along the vertical axis that passes through the center of the shoulder joint. Sense any subtle movements or adjustments that occur in the shoulder and allow your hands to follow them. Hold for 1 minute or more.

Shiatsu

Wrap the hands around the upper arm at the shoulder. Compress the arm and roll it slightly medially, from the shoulder to the wrist (Fig. 7-12). This procedure stimulates the yin channels (lung, pericardium, heart) and the yang channels (large intestine, triple heater, small intestine) of the arm.

SWEDISH/CROSS FIBER

1. Perform effleurage strokes on the arm, from the wrist to the shoulder.
2. Perform pétrissage strokes from the elbow to the shoulder.
3. Perform circular friction with the heel of hand on the shoulder area.

CONNECTIVE TISSUE

Myofascial Spread

Place the client's upper arm slightly away from the body. Wrap your hands around the upper arm, just above the elbow, with the base of the palms at the midline of the arm. Slowly slide the palms apart as the fascia softens, spreading the tissues of the arm with the heels of the hand. Continue, in horizontal strips, to the top of the shoulder.

DEEP TISSUE/NMT

Sequence

1. Deltoids
2. Supraspinatus
3. Infraspinatus
4. Teres minor
5. Teres major and latissimus dorsi
6. Triceps brachii
7. Biceps brachii
8. Brachialis

Position

The shoulder sequence is performed with the client in side posture. Place a pillow between the client's knees and a small support under the side of the client's head. The top arm rests along the client's side.

The therapist stands at the head of the table, cupping both hands around the client's shoulder (Fig. 7-13).

1. Deltoids

Posterior Deltoid

Origin: Lower lip of the posterior border of the spine of the scapula.

Insertion: Deltoid tuberosity on the lateral midshaft of the humerus.

Action: Extension and lateral rotation of humerus.

To locate trigger points, check along the posterior portion, near the border of the muscle. The referral zone is throughout the posterior deltoid and sometimes down the arm.

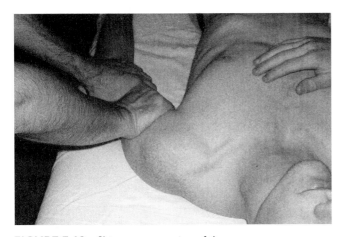

FIGURE 7-12   Shiatsu compression of the upper arm.

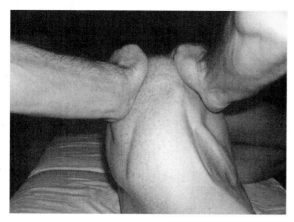

FIGURE 7-13 Beginning hand position for releasing the deltoids (posterior, medial, and anterior).

- Apply elongation strokes with the knuckles or heel of hand from the inferior border of the spine of the scapula to the deltoid tuberosity on the humerus. The hand on the front of the shoulder stabilizes it and provides support.
- To palpate trigger points stand behind the client's shoulder, with both hands grasping the shoulder with the fingers in front and the thumb tips touching each other at the level of the posterior deltoid (Fig. 7-14). Perform short back-and-forth and side-to-side strokes along the entire length of the muscle, seeking taut bands.

Medial Deltoid
Origin: Lateral border of the acromion process.
Insertion: Deltoid tuberosity on the lateral midshaft of the humerus.
Action: Abduction of humerus.

This muscle does not develop trigger points as commonly as the other two deltoid muscles. Trigger points may be found in the upper portion just below the acromion.

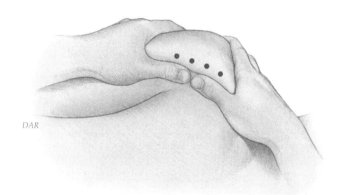

DAR

FIGURE 7-14 Locating trigger points in the posterior deltoid along the medial border.

- Stand at the head of the table, with both hands cupped around the shoulder. Using the knuckles or heel of the hand, stroke down the middle of the upper humerus, from the acromion process to the deltoid tuberosity.
- To palpate trigger points, the hands should remain cupped around the shoulder, with the sides of the thumbs touching. Perform short back-and-forth and side-to-side strokes along the entire length of the muscle, from the acromion to the deltoid tuberosity (Fig. 7-15).

Anterior Deltoid
Origin: Anterior surface of lateral third of the clavicle.
Insertion: Deltoid tuberosity on the lateral midshaft of the humerus.
Action: Flexion and medial rotation of humerus.

Check for trigger points in the front portion of the muscle, high up where the muscle covers the head of the humerus. Pain can refer over the anterior and medial deltoid and down the arm.

- Apply elongation strokes with the heel of hand from the lateral third of the clavicle to the deltoid tuberosity.
- To palpate trigger points stand in front of the client's shoulder, with both hands grasping the shoulder and with the fingers wrapped around the back and the thumb tips touching in front, over the anterior deltoid (Fig. 7-16). Perform the trigger point searching techniques over the entire length of the muscle.

2. Supraspinatus
Origin: Supraspinous fossa of the scapula.
Insertion: Superior facet of the greater tuberosity of the humerus, capsule of the shoulder joint.

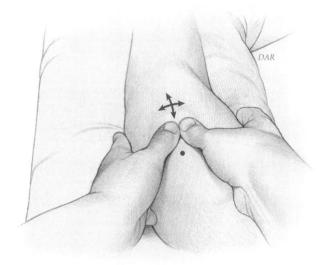

DAR

FIGURE 7-15 Locating trigger points in the medial deltoid.

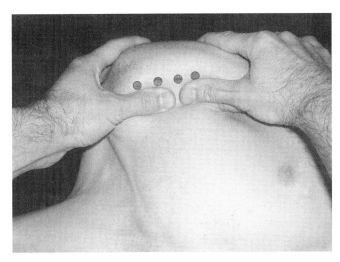

FIGURE 7-16 Locating trigger points in the anterior deltoid beginning along the anterior border.

Action: Abduction of shoulder; stabilizes head of humerus in shoulder joint.

Search for trigger points along the superior border of the spine of the scapula. They refer pain into the medial deltoid and down the side of the arm. A trigger point is often located in the space between the clavicle and scapula, just before they meet at the acromioclavicular joint. The pain referral zone is over the deltoid.

Position

Stand at the head of the table facing the client's shoulder. Cup your hands around the shoulder near the base of the neck. The thumbs are placed against the superior border of the spine of the scapula, with one thumb on top of the other to reinforce it.

■ Perform an elongation stroke along the superior border of the scapula, to the acromioclavicular joint (Fig. 7-17). Repeat the stroke, with the thumbs placed slightly superior to the spine of the scapula.
■ Palpate trigger points in the muscle using the trigger point seeking strokes. Treat any that are found.

3. Infraspinatus

Origin: Infraspinous fossa of the scapula.
Insertion: Middle facet of greater tuberosity of the humerus, capsule of the shoulder joint.
Action: Lateral rotation of shoulder; stabilizes head of humerus in shoulder joint.

Trigger points tend to accumulate readily in this muscle. Pay close attention to the fibers that run about 0.5 inches below the spine of the scapula. They refer pain to the deltoid and down the arm. Another trigger point is found about halfway down the vertebral border of the scapula. It refers pain along the medial edge of the scapula.

■ Perform an elongation stroke using the knuckles or elbow, from the vertebral border of the scapula to the head of the humerus. The stroke is repeated several times, in strips, over the body of the scapula to cover the entire muscle. Place your non-working hand on the front of the client's shoulder to provide stability (Fig. 7-18).
■ A bolster can be placed in front of the client's chest to prevent the upper body from rolling forward when pressure is applied to the infraspinatus muscle.
■ To locate trigger points more effectively, turn the client to the prone position with the upper arm abducted 90° and the forearm hanging off the table. Use thumb strokes to palpate and treat trigger points.

4. Teres Minor

Origin: Upper two-thirds of the dorsal surface of axillary border of the scapula.
Insertion: Lowest facet of greater tuberosity of the humerus, capsule of the shoulder joint.
Action: Lateral rotation of humerus; weak adduction of shoulder; stabilizes humeral head in shoulder joint.

This muscle is often clear of trigger points. Trigger points are more likely to form in the synergistic muscle to teres minor, the infraspinatus.

Position

The client is lying in side posture, with the side to be treated uppermost.

The therapist stands at the side of the table, behind the client's shoulder. If treating the right side of the client, the therapist's right thumb is placed along the axillary border of the scapula. The therapist's left thumb is placed over the top of the client's right shoulder. (When working on the left side, hand positions are reversed.)

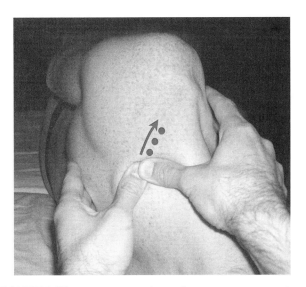

FIGURE 7-17 Elongation stroke on the supraspinatus muscle from origin to insertion.

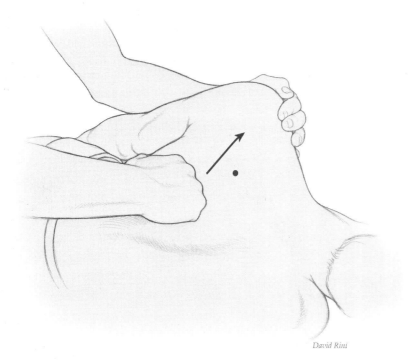

David Rini

FIGURE 7-18   Elongation stroke on the infraspinatus from origin to insertion.

Beginning with the thumb one-third of the way up along the axillary border, stroke along the edge of the bone, following the muscle fibers out to the head of the humerus (Fig. 7-19). Pause at tender areas and treat.

5. Teres Major and Latissimus Dorsi

Teres Major

Origin: Dorsal surface of the scapula near the lateral side of the inferior angle.

Insertion: Medial lip of the bicipital groove of the humerus.

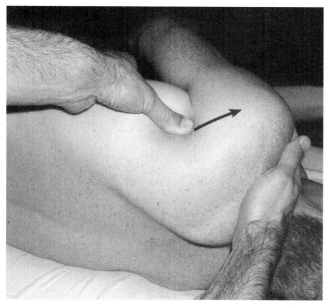

FIGURE 7-19   Elongation stroke on teres minor from origin to insertion.

Action: Medial rotation, adduction, and extension of the arm.

Easily confused in palpation with the latissimus dorsi, the teres major is closer to the border of the scapula and more medial. Trigger points are usually close to the scapular border. The pain referral zone is over the posterior deltoid and the long head of the triceps.

Latissimus Dorsi

Origin: Spinous processes of T6–T12 vertebrae, spinous processes of L1–L5 vertebrae and sacral vertebrae, supraspinal ligament, posterior one-third of iliac crest of ilium, ribs 9–12, inferior angle of the scapula.

Insertion: Floor of bicipital groove of the humerus.

Action: Extension, adduction, and medial rotation of the arm (most powerful when arm is in overhead position); active in strong inspiration and expiration.

When using the sifting technique, the latissimus dorsi is the most superficial muscle felt. Check the upper portion, in particular, near the posterior deltoid. This trigger point, found in the axillary fold, refers pain to the mid-back region.

Standing behind the client's shoulder, grasp the muscles along the posterior border of the axilla, thumbs on the surface, fingers underneath in the axilla. Sift the muscle fibers thoroughly, feeling for taut bands and adhered tissues (Fig. 7-20). Treat any trigger points that are found.

Stretch for Teres Major and Minor, Latissimus Dorsi, and Subscapularis

The client is in side posture. Lift the client's arm overhead so that the upper arm is resting along the ear, with the forearm flexed. Holding the arm near the elbow, rotate

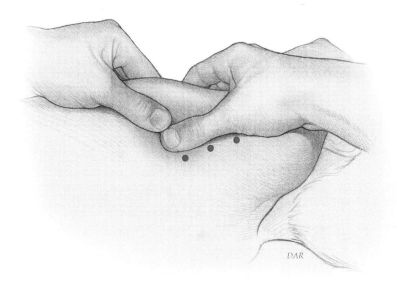

FIGURE 7-20   Sifting the latissimus dorsi and teres major.

the humerus medially and allow the forearm and hand to hang off the back of the table (Fig. 7-21). If further stretch is needed, press down on the humerus until an adequate stretch is felt.

6. Triceps Brachii
Origin: Long head—infraglenoid tuberosity of the scapula. **Lateral head**—upper half of posterior shaft of the humerus. **Medial head**—lower half of posterior shaft of the humerus.
Insertion: Posterior surface of olecranon process of the ulna.
Action: Extension of forearm; when arm is abducted, long head aids in adduction.

Trigger points may be found along the lateral border of the triceps near the elbow. A trigger point that contributes to

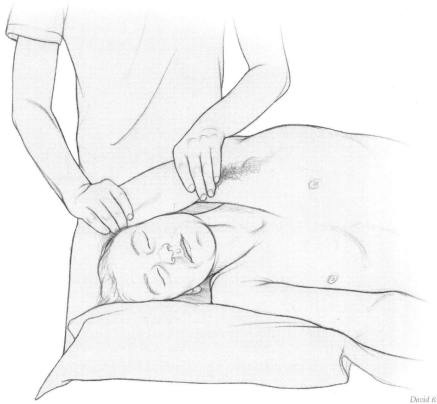

David Rini

FIGURE 7-21   Stretch for teres major and minor, latissimus dorsi, and subscapularis.

tennis elbow pain is located in the medial portion of the muscle from 1.5 to 2.5 inches above the lateral epicondyle. Using the thumb, snap across a taut band in that area to find the trigger point. Pain is referred to the lateral epicondyle and may continue down the radial side of the forearm.

Position

The client is placed in prone position. The arm to be worked on is abducted 90°, with the forearm hanging off the side of the table.

The therapist is standing at the side of the table next to the client's shoulder.

- Apply elongation strokes from the elbow to the head of the humerus, using heel of hand or knuckles.
- With the thumbs, stroke up the middle of the triceps between the heads of the muscle (Fig. 7-22).
- Grasp the edges of the triceps between the thumb and fingers. Lift the muscle away from the bone and squeeze. Check for trigger points along its length.

7. Biceps Brachii

Origin: Short head—apex of coracoid process of the scapula. **Long head**—supraglenoid tubercle of the scapula.

Insertion: Radial tuberosity of the radius, bicipital aponeurosis fusing with deep fascia over forearm flexors.

Action: Flexion and supination of forearm; weak flexion of arm at shoulder joint when forearm is fixed.

The lower third of the biceps brachii may contain a trigger point in each head. They may refer pain throughout the biceps and upward into the anterior deltoid. These trigger points are most easily palpated by stretching the biceps fibers. Hold the client's arm at the wrist and extend it slightly off the table, keeping the forearm fully extended. With your other hand, feel for taut bands in the biceps muscle.

Position

The client is placed in supine position. The arm to be treated is resting on the table next to the client's side, with the palm supinated.

The therapist is standing at the head of the table, superior to the client's shoulder.

- Apply elongation strokes from the elbow to the shoulder joint, using the heel of the hand or the knuckles.
- With the thumbs, stroke up the center of the biceps between the two heads (Fig. 7-23).
- Grasp the edges of the biceps between the fingers and thumb. Lift the muscle away from the bone and squeeze. Check for trigger points along its length.

8. Brachialis

Origin: Lower two-thirds of anterior shaft of the humerus.

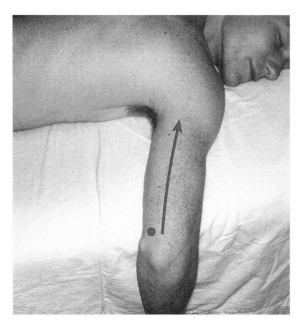

FIGURE 7-22   Direction of strokes on the triceps from the insertion (olecranon process) to origin (upper portion of humerus).

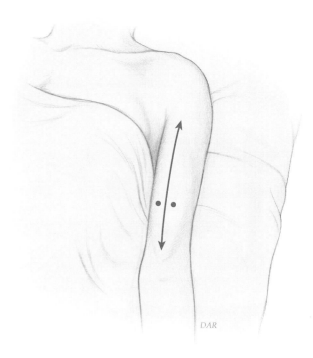

FIGURE 7-23   Direction of strokes on the biceps from insertion (tuberosity of radius) to origin (coracoid process of scapula).

Insertion: Tuberosity and coronoid process of the ulna.
Action: Flexion of forearm.

Trigger points are usually located in the distal portion of the brachialis, near the elbow. They refer pain chiefly to the base of the thumb.

Position

The client is supine, with the arm to be worked on flexed at the elbow about 45°.

The therapist is standing at the side of the table, holding the wrist of the flexed arm.

- The brachialis muscle is deep to the biceps. To reach it, slide your fingers under the biceps brachii muscle, on the medial side of the humerus, about halfway down the upper arm (Fig. 7-24).
- Do the side-to-side stroke with your fingers along the muscle fibers to the elbow, allowing the muscle to lengthen and relax.

Stretch

Position
The client is lying supine.

The therapist is standing at the head of the table.

1. Triceps. Lift the client's arm overhead, with the humerus next to the ear, and the forearm hanging over the end of the table. Holding the humerus near the elbow, press the arm toward the table while the client flexes the forearm further by reaching the palm toward the underside of the table (Fig. 7-25).
2. Biceps and brachialis. The client slides to the edge of the table. Bring the client's straight arm off the side of the table and, holding at the wrist, extend it downward toward the floor as the client reaches down and back with the hand (Fig. 7-26).

Accessory Work

1. Circumduct the shoulder, hip, and ankle joints on both sides of the body to help balance the muscles acting on the joints.
2. Press the shoulder line on the feet with your thumb tips (Fig. 7-27). It runs horizontally across the foot at the base of the toes.

Closing

Sitting at the foot of the table, lightly hold the heels of the client's feet in your hands for 30 to 60 seconds. Remove your hands slowly to complete the session.

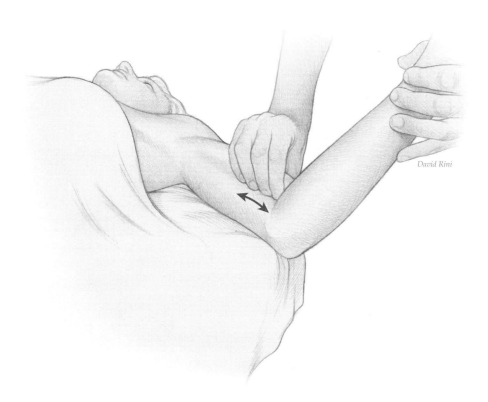

David Rini

FIGURE 7-24 Contacting the brachialis deep to the biceps brachii.

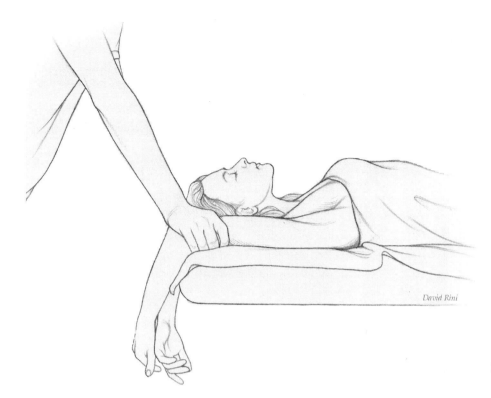

FIGURE 7-25   Stretch for the triceps muscle.

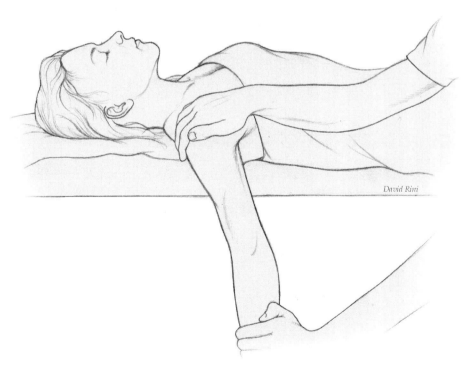

FIGURE 7-26   Stretch for the biceps brachii.

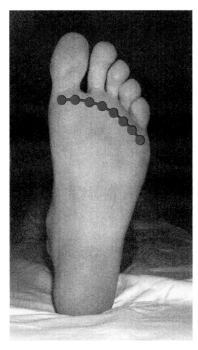

FIGURE 7-27 Reflex zone for the shoulder.

FOREARM AND HAND ROUTINE

OBJECTIVES

- To reduce stress and pain in the muscles of the forearm and hand brought about by extended use of the hand in work-related and other activities.

- To improve dexterity and coordination skills of the hand.
- To promote relaxation through the reflexive effects of hand massage.

ENERGY

Position

The client is lying supine with the arms to his or her sides.

The therapist is standing at the side of the table facing the client's forearm.

Polarity

Lightly contact the wrist and elbow with the palms of the hands. Envision the forearm lengthening and relaxing. Hold for at least 30 seconds.

Shiatsu

1. Grasping the client's forearm just below the elbow joint with both hands, compress the forearm from the elbow to the wrist. This move stimulates the same meridians as the upper arm Shiatsu procedure.
2. Flex the client's forearm 90°. Interlace your fingers with your client's fingers.

    Holding the client's forearm slightly inferior to the wrist with your other hand, flex, extend, and circumduct the hand in both directions (Fig. 7-28).

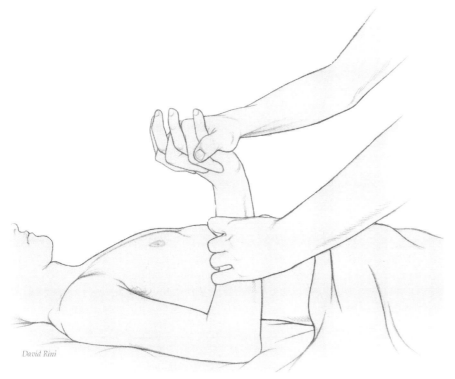

David Rini

FIGURE 7-28 Hand position for performing Shiatsu wrist movements.

Opening up the wrist area stimulates the flow of energy (qi) through the arm channels.

SWEDISH/CROSS FIBER

1. Perform effleurage strokes from the wrist to elbow.
2. Perform thumb gliding on the palm and back of the hand.
3. Perform pétrissage strokes on the muscles of the forearm.
4. Perform cross fiber strokes with the broad side of the thumb on the hand and forearm muscles.

CONNECTIVE TISSUE

Myofascial Spread

1. Grasping both sides of the client's hand, curve your fingers and press them into the center of the palm. Slowly slide the fingers of each hand away from each other, stretching the tissues of the palm.
2. Flex the client's forearm 90° at the elbow. Place your hands around the forearm at the wrist, with the fingers sinking into the midline of the palmar side of the forearm. Slowly spread the fingers away from the midline, stretching the fascia. Continue, in horizontal strips, to the elbow. Repeat on the other side of the forearm.

DEEP TISSUE/NMT

Sequence

1. Palm—superficial muscles, lumbricales, and interossei
2. Thenar eminence—adductor pollicis brevis, flexor pollicis brevis, opponens pollicis
3. Fingers—digital flexors and extensors, ligaments, retinacula
4. Dorsal surface of the hand—extensor digitorum tendon, interossei
5. Wrist—flexor tendons and retinaculum, extensor tendons and retinaculum, pronator quadratus
6. Forearm

   a. Anterior surface—pronator teres, flexor carpi radialis, palmaris longus, flexor carpi ulnaris, flexor digitorum superficialis, flexor pollicis longus, flexor digitorum profundus, and brachioradialis.
   b. Dorsal surface—extensor carpi radialis longus, extensor carpi radialis brevis, extensor carpi ulnaris, extensor digitorum, extensor digiti minimi, supinator, abductor pollicis longus, extensor pollicis brevis, extensor pollicis longus, and extensor indicis.

7. Elbow

   a. Lateral epicondyle—attachments of extensor carpi radialis longus and brevis, extensor digitorum, and supinator.
   b. Medial epicondyle—attachments of the common flexor tendon, brachialis, and pronator teres.

1. The Palm

Position

The client is lying supine with the arm to his or her side, the palm supinated.

The therapist is standing at the side of the table next to the client's hand.

Interossei Muscles

a. Palmar

   Origin:

   1st—entire ulnar side of 2nd metacarpal.

   2nd—entire radial side of 4th metacarpal.

   3rd—entire radial side of 5th metacarpal.

   Insertion:

   1st—index finger at base of proximal phalanx on ulnar side.

   2nd—ring finger at base of proximal phalanx on radial side.

   3rd—entire radial side of 5th metacarpal.

   Action: Adduction of index, ring, and pinkie fingers toward the middle finger.

b. Dorsal

   Origin:

   1st—lateral head: 1st metacarpal of thumb on proximal half of ulnar border, medial head: 2nd metacarpal of index finger on entire radial border.

   2nd—adjacent sides of metacarpals of index and middle fingers.

   3rd—adjacent sides of middle and ring fingers.

   4th—adjacent sides of metacarpals of ring and pinkie fingers.

   Insertion:

   1st—radial side of index finger at base of proximal phalanx.

   2nd—radial side of proximal phalanx of middle finger.

   3rd—ulnar side of proximal phalanx of middle finger.

   4th—ulnar side of proximal phalanx of ring ringer.

   Action: Abduction of fingers away from middle finger.

   To locate trigger points, have the client spread the fingers wide apart to separate the metacarpal bones. Using your thumb and index finger, squeeze the spaces between the bones. Nodules are often found around active trigger points in these muscles. Pain usually refers into the finger of the adjacent tendon.

■ Perform an elongating stroke with the fist, lengthwise, from the base of the palm to the fingers, then horizontally across the palm from the pinkie side to the thumb side (Fig. 7-29).

■ Lumbricales. Perform an elongating stroke along the

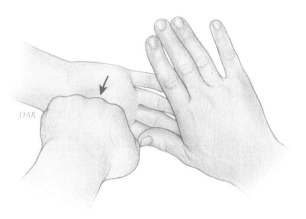

FIGURE 7-29 Elongation stroke from the fifth metatarsal to the first metatarsal.

sides of the finger tendons using the thumb or tip of the index finger (Fig. 7-30).

2. Muscles of the Thenar Eminence (Adductor Pollicis Brevis, Flexor Pollicis Brevis, Opponens Pollicis)
Apply up-and-down and side-to-side strokes over the mound with your thumb, checking for tenderness and taut bands (Fig. 7-31).

Locating and Treating Trigger Points in Thumb Muscles

Adductor Pollicis
Origin: Oblique head—bases of 2nd and 3rd metacarpals, capitate, trapezoid. **Transverse head**—distal two-thirds of palmar side of 3rd metacarpal.
Insertion: Base of thumb at ulnar side of proximal phalanx.
Action: Adduction of thumb.

Trigger points may be located in this muscle by squeezing the webbing between the thumb and index finger. The

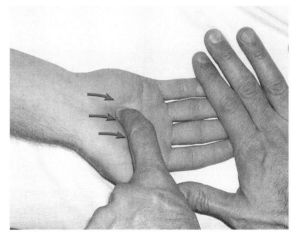

FIGURE 7-30 Contacting the lumbricales muscles between the finger tendons.

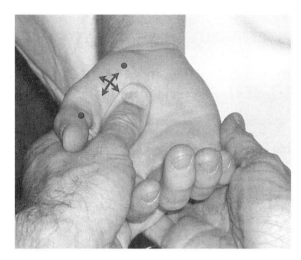

FIGURE 7-31 Deep tissue strokes on the thenar eminence.

referral zone is on the thumb, particularly on the lower outside edge near the wrist.

Flexor Pollicis Brevis
Origin: Flexor retinaculum and trapezium, first metacarpal bone.
Insertion: Base of proximal phalanx of thumb.
Action: Flexion of metacarpophalangeal joint of thumb.

Place the tip of your thumb against the head of the metacarpal bone. As the client flexes the thumb several times, feel for the tendon and press. The referral zone is local, around the trigger point.

Opponens Pollicis
Origin: Flexor retinaculum, tubercle of trapezium.
Insertion: Entire radial side of first metacarpal bone.
Action: Draws first metacarpal bone forward and medial, bringing thumb into opposition to the other fingers.

Using the thumb tip, roll across the muscle fibers on the thenar eminence, feeling for taut bands and tenderness. Pain is referred to the inside portion of the thumb and to a spot on the radial side of the wrist.

3. Fingers

Preparation
Begin the following sequence at the base of the proximal phalanx of the thumb. Continue to the tip of the thumb and then repeat, sequentially, on each of the four fingers.

■ Grasp the digit with the tip of the thumb on one side, tip of the index finger on the other side. Alternately move the thumb and index finger up and down along the sides of the bone, between the joints.
■ Repeat the stroke, grasping the front and back of the bone.

4. Dorsal Surface of the Hand
■ Apply the fanning stroke with thumbs over the entire dorsal surface of the hand.

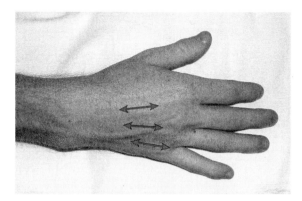

FIGURE 7-32   Direction of strokes on the dorsal interossei.

- Perform short up-and-down strokes with the tip of the index finger on the interosseus muscles between the tendons of extensor digitorum muscle (Fig. 7-32).

5. Wrist (Tendons of Flexor and Extensor Muscles of Fingers)

- Apply the fanning stroke with thumbs on the palmar and dorsal surfaces of the wrist (Fig. 7-33A).
- With the sides of your thumbs touching, do short up-and-down and side-to-side strokes on the palmar and dorsal surfaces of the wrist (Fig. 7-33B).

6. Forearm

Hand and Finger Extensor Muscles
Trigger points will lodge in the distal portion of the muscles, near the elbow. Pain is referred to the lateral epicondyle and down the forearm to the wrist and hand area.

Hand and Finger Flexor Muscles
Trigger points tend to be located in a line across the muscles, about one-third of the way down the forearm from the elbow. They are best palpated with cross fiber strokes, feeling for taut bands in the fibers. They refer pain to the wrist and into the fingers.

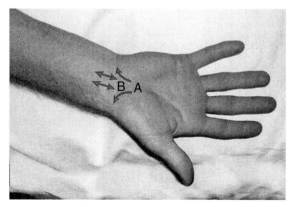

FIGURE 7-33   (A) Fanning and (B) up-and-down strokes on tendons of finger flexor muscles at the wrist.

- Perform elongation strokes with the knuckles from the wrist to the elbow (A in Fig. 7-34). Work in strips, with the palm supinated and then pronated, to cover the forearm thoroughly.
- Separate the muscles of the forearm by stroking between them with a thumb, knuckle, or elbow (B in Fig. 7-34)
- Perform short up-and-down and side-to-side strokes on the bellies of the muscles using thumbs or elbows (C in Fig. 7-34) Treat areas of tenderness and trigger points.
- Turn the client's forearm so that the thumb side of the hand is up. Grasp the brachioradialis muscle between the thumb and fingers, on the forearm, below the lateral epicondyle of the elbow. Roll the muscle fibers, checking for tenderness and trigger point activity (Fig. 7-35).

7. Elbow

Supinator
Origin: Lateral epicondyle of humerus, radial collateral ligament of elbow joint, annular ligament of radioulnar joint, supinator crest of ulna on dorsal surface of shaft.
Insertion: Dorsal and medial surfaces of upper one-third of the radial shaft.
Action: Supination of forearm and hand.

A trigger point may be located near its attachment on the lateral epicondyle. The referral zone is the lateral epicondyle. Pain may also shoot to the webbing of the thumb.

Pronator Teres
Origin: Humeral head—distal supracondylar ridge, medial epicondyle of humerus. **Ulnar head**—coronoid process of medial ulna.
Insertion: Pronator tuberosity on lateral surface of radius.
Action: Pronation and flexion of forearm.

A trigger point may be located near its attachment on the medial epicondyle. Pain is felt deep in the radial side of the wrist and may spill over into the forearm

- With the thumb, apply up-and-down, side-to-side, and static compression strokes around the lateral epicondyle. Treat the attachments of extensor carpi radialis longus and brevis, extensor digitorum, and supinator muscles (Fig. 7-36). Having the client extend the hand makes these tendons easier to palpate.

 Be careful when treating these attachments due to the close proximity of the radial nerve. If the client experiences a sharp, radiating sensation characteristic of nerve stimulation, release the pressure immediately and shift the location of your thumb.

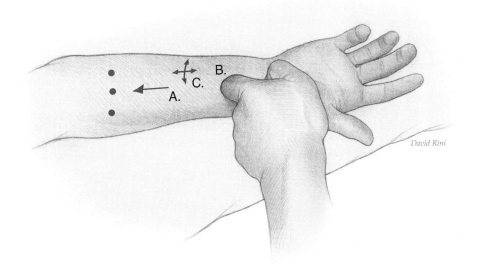

David Rini

FIGURE 7-34   Location and direction of strokes on the hand and finger flexor muscles along the forearm.

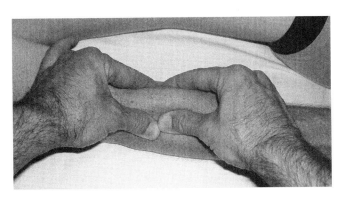

FIGURE 7-35   Rolling the fibers of the brachioradialis muscle.

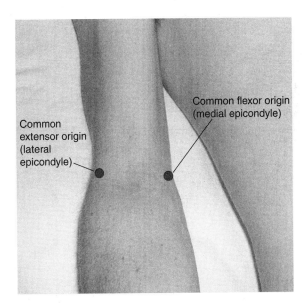

FIGURE 7-36   Location of forearm muscle attachments.

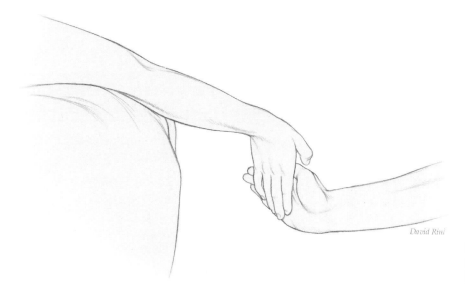

David Rini

FIGURE 7-37   Stretch for the flexor muscles of the fingers and hand.

■ With the thumb, apply up-and-down, side-to-side, and static compression strokes around the medial epicondyle. Treat the attachments of the common flexor tendon, brachialis, and pronator teres muscles. Having the client flex his hand makes these tendons easier to palpate. Use the same caution as above due to the position of the median nerve at the medial epicondyle.

Stretch

1. With both hands facing each other in front of him or her, the client cups the palms and spreads all the fingers. Touching the tips of the fingers of both hands together, the client begins to push the hands toward each other, keeping the fingers apart and resisting somewhat with the cupped palms. The client continues to press the hands toward each other until a stretch is felt in the fingers and palms. The stretch is held for a minimum of 10 seconds.

2. Place your palm across the palmar surface of the client's fingers and extend the client's hand until a stretch is felt in the flexor muscles of the fingers and hand (Fig. 7-37). (This and the following stretch are more effective if the client's arm is kept fully straight.)

3. Place your palm across the dorsal surface of the client's fingers and flex the client's hand until a stretch is felt in the extensor muscles of the fingers and hand (Fig. 7-38).

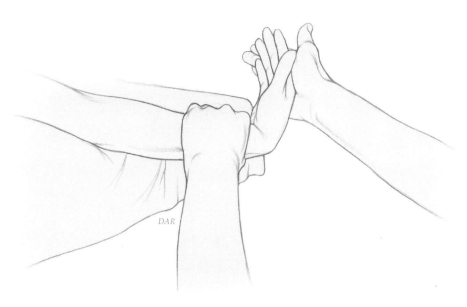

DAR

FIGURE 7-38   Stretch for the extensor muscles of the fingers and hand.

Accessory Work

1. "Snapping off" the fingers (a Shiatsu technique) will help to draw off accumulated energy that has built up from release of the hand and forearm muscles. An indication of this build-up is sweaty hands. To perform the move, hold the anterior and posterior sides of the client's finger at the base between your index and middle fingers. Gently slide down the finger, gliding straight off at the tip (Fig. 7-39). Begin with the thumb. Continue with each finger in succession to the pinkie.
2. A thorough foot massage is a good accompaniment to hand and forearm work. It gives the client a sense of integration between the upper and lower extremities.

Closing

Sitting at the foot of the table, lightly hold the heels of the client's feet in your hands for 30 to 60 seconds. Remove your hands slowly to complete the session.

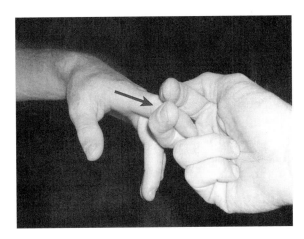

FIGURE 7-39   The Shiatsu technique, "snapping off."

REFERENCE

1. Rolf IP. Rolfing: the integration of human structures. New York: Harper and Row, 1977: 72

Establishing a Firm Foundation

THE FOOT, LEG, AND KNEE

INTRODUCTION

The legs and feet are responsible for efficiently transferring weight from the upper body to the ground with minimal stress. They are also the locomotive structures of the body, providing the means for its movement through space. To perform the multiple tasks of weight transfer and movement, the knees and feet are necessarily complex in design. Balance of muscle, tendon, and ligament in the lower extremity is essential to enable its effective operation without breakdown. The focus of deep tissue work on the knees, lower legs, and feet is to re-establish the precise integration of muscle action with correct bony alignment. Lack of harmony among these body parts will result in tension and instability throughout the rest of the body.

The feet form a horizontal platform on which the entire weight of the vertical body rests. The feet are small in proportion to the load they carry, which can create problems for effective weight distribution and support. This dilemma is solved by a series of arches located throughout the feet. Architecturally, the arch is used to distribute weight evenly from a smaller, concentrated area over a broad surface. In the case of the feet, the body forms a vertical column whose weight is focused at the ankle joints and then spread out through the feet and transferred to the ground.

When the body's weight is properly balanced on the foot, it radiates out from the talus through the bones of the foot. This even distribution of weight can be observed in the symmetrical shape of a footprint in the sand. (Photographs of footprints in the sand demonstrating various patterns of weight distribution can be found in Rolf.[1]) When the arches break down, the body's weight is more concentrated on the outside or inside of the foot, causing a distortion in the footprint and an uneven wearing down of the soles of shoes. Whether the initial breakdown occurs in the foot itself or further up in the body, it results in a redistribution of weight throughout the body segments in an effort to compensate for lack of balance. This creates stress and pain around joints, particularly the knee, and loss of full function in the muscles.

The arches of the foot are supported and stabilized by muscles of the lower leg, attaching in various places along the bottom of the foot. They pull up on the plantar surface of the foot, acting as guy wires suspending the arches from above. Ineffective support of the foot through muscular weakness is evident in legs that lack shape and proportion. Abnormal thickening in the legs denotes lack of fluid flow, caused by the inefficient pumping action of toneless muscles. As effective neuromuscular patterns of action are taught to the leg muscles through integrated deep tissue therapy, diminished arches can be effectively strengthened and raised. This re-education of the foot and leg muscles results in better-coordinated action throughout the body.

The joints of the legs are meant to operate in a relay fashion, meaning that the hip, knee, and ankle should all flex together and extend together during most leg movements. Although these three joints are not all technically hinges, they can be thought of in that way when working as a unit. They should be positioned so that they are aligned directly over each other in flexion movements, with the hinge at each joint forming a horizontal platform in relation to the vertical standing body. This alignment allows the muscles of the leg to store power when the joints flex, as in a preparation to jump, and to release that power effectively when the joints extend. Deep tissue work can help to restore this balanced alignment.

MUSCULOSKELETAL ANATOMY AND FUNCTION (ESSENTIAL ANATOMY BOX 8-1)

The ankle and foot should be thought of as a unit because their function is interdependent. Structurally, they are similar to the wrist and hand and are potentially capable of many of the same movements. The foot is organized as a series of arches meant to distribute weight. The foot also acts as a springboard to push the body away from the ground and propel it through space. To accomplish these functions, the foot must be both strong and mobile. It is composed of 26 bones, 31 joints, and 20 intrinsic muscles. The bones of the foot are connected by a series of more than 100 ligaments. These ligaments reinforce the arches and limit movement at the joints so that the foot can maintain its integrity.

There are three major arches in the foot. The inner longitudinal arch is largely responsible for pushing the foot forward in locomotor movements. It is made up of the

---

ESSENTIAL ANATOMY BOX 8–1

The Foot, Leg, and Knee Routines

Muscles

Toe tendons
Insertion points of flexor
　　hallucis longus, flexor
　　hallucis brevis, and
　　abductor hallucis
Muscles of the plantar
　　surface of the foot
Muscles of the dorsal surface
　　of the foot
Ankle retinaculum
Flexor digitorum longus
Lateral leg muscles-tibialis
　　anterior, extensor hallucis
　　longus, extensor digitorum
　　longus, peroneals
Gastrocnemius
Soleus
Knee-ligaments and tendons

Bones and Landmarks

Bones of the foot—phalanges,
　　metatarsals, cuboid, navicular, talus
Tibia
Lateral malleolus
Medial malleolus
Tibial tuberosity
Fibula
Head of fibula
Patella

inner portion of the calcaneus, the talus, the navicular, the three cuneiforms, and the first three metatarsals and phalanges. The outer longitudinal arch is more weight-bearing and weight-distributing. It supports the inner arch by supplying lift and balance. It is formed by the calcaneus, cuboid, and the fourth and fifth metatarsals and phalanges. When the outer longitudinal arch is collapsed, the weight of the body is thrown too much onto the outer portion of the foot and the integrity of the balance of the lower limb is lost.

The third arch is actually a series of transverse arches crossing the foot. They are formed by the relationship of the tarsal and metatarsal bones with the surrounding muscles and ligaments. All the arches of the foot depend on strong muscular stability and action as well as ligamentous support. The majority of these muscles attach on the tibia or fibula, providing a long lever of support. The long and short plantar ligaments are crucial in maintaining the shape of the arches. They connect the bones that form the ends of the longitudinal arches, like the string of a bow, preventing them from sliding too far apart when weight is placed on the foot.

The superficial intrinsic muscles on the plantar surface of the foot are **extensor hallucis brevis, abductor hallucis, flexor digitorum brevis,** and **abductor digiti minimi** (Fig. 8-1A). The only intrinsic muscle on the dorsal surface of the foot is the extensor digitorum brevis. Overall, these muscles serve to stabilize the foot when balancing on one leg and are used in walking and running. Flexor digitorum brevis is responsible for clutching actions of the foot, where the toe joints are flexed and the person appears to be grasping the ground with the feet. This stance is indicative of tension and instability higher up in the body. Sore feet and pain when walking may indicate the presence of trigger points in the intrinsic foot muscles.

The deep intrinsic muscles consist of the **quadratus plantae** and **lumbricales, flexor hallucis brevis, adductor hallucis, flexor digiti minimi brevis,** and the **interossei.**

Their primary function is to align and stabilize the bones of the foot during propulsion. They guide and move the toes, providing a balanced pulling action on the bones so that the foot tracks forward properly with the toes not spread too far apart or overlapping each other. Restricted movement or hypermobility of the toes, as well as calluses on them, may indicate tension in the deep intrinsic muscles.

The ankle joint consists of the articulation of the tibia over the talus bone. The medial malleolus, which is a projection on the tibia, and the lateral malleolus at the lower end of the fibula form the sides of a cavity that fits over the talus, creating a pure hinge joint.

The talus articulates with the calcaneus bone below it, transferring weight to it from the tibia and forming another joint capable of inversion and eversion (the lifting and lowering of the medial side of the foot). This joint is extremely important in maintaining the integrity of the foot because the strength of the arches is largely dependent on the position of the calcaneus. When the calcaneus slides out to the side from underneath the talus, it causes the inner arch to fall and the tibia to rotate medially. In the case of an abnormally high medial arch, the calcaneus has pulled inward under the talus, decreasing the length of the foot and throwing weight to the outside of the foot. An overly high arch inhibits flexibility in the foot, causing the ankle to become looser since it has to accommodate adjustments that would normally be made by a more flexible foot.

The bones of the leg are the tibia and fibula. The tibia supports more weight than the femur yet it is smaller. The fibula attaches to the tibia via an interosseus membrane. It reinforces the tibia, giving increased elasticity and flexibility to the leg, and provides attachment points for important muscles of the lower extremity.

The following groups of muscles control movements of the foot but have their origins on various places on the leg (Fig. 8-1B). **Extensor hallucis longus** dorsiflexes the big toe and foot, while **extensor digitorum longus** flexes the other four toes. Both muscles are important in preventing the entire foot from dropping hard against the ground during walking. Night cramps of the toes are caused by spasms in these muscles.

Flexor hallucis longus plantar flexes the big toe and ankle, inverts the foot, and assists support of the medial arch. **Flexor digitorum longus** plantar flexes the four toes and ankle and also provides support for the arches. Both of these muscles provide stability when a person is standing on tiptoe.

Tibialis anterior is the strongest dorsiflexor of the foot and inverts the foot. It is highly active during running and jumping movements. Attaching on the base of the first metatarsal bone and the medial cuneiform, the tibialis anterior supports the medial arch. Overuse of this muscle is one of the primary causes of shin splints. Driving a car for long periods with the foot on the accelerator pedal held in a dorsiflexed position can also be stressful to the tibialis anterior muscle. Regular stretching of the gastrocnemius and soleus, the antagonist muscles on the back of the leg, helps to keep tibialis anterior in proper balance.

Peroneus longus and **peroneus brevis** are responsible for plantar flexion, eversion of the foot, and support of the lateral arch. They oppose tibialis anterior in their actions. The coordinated action of these muscles is crucial in preventing sideways rolling of the foot.

The **gastrocnemius** crosses the ankle and knee joints (Fig. 8-1B). When the knee is extended or slightly flexed, it is a strong plantar flexor of the ankle. This muscle also flexes and medially rotates the knee. When the knee is flexed, the gastrocnemius is too slack to be effective as an ankle flexor.

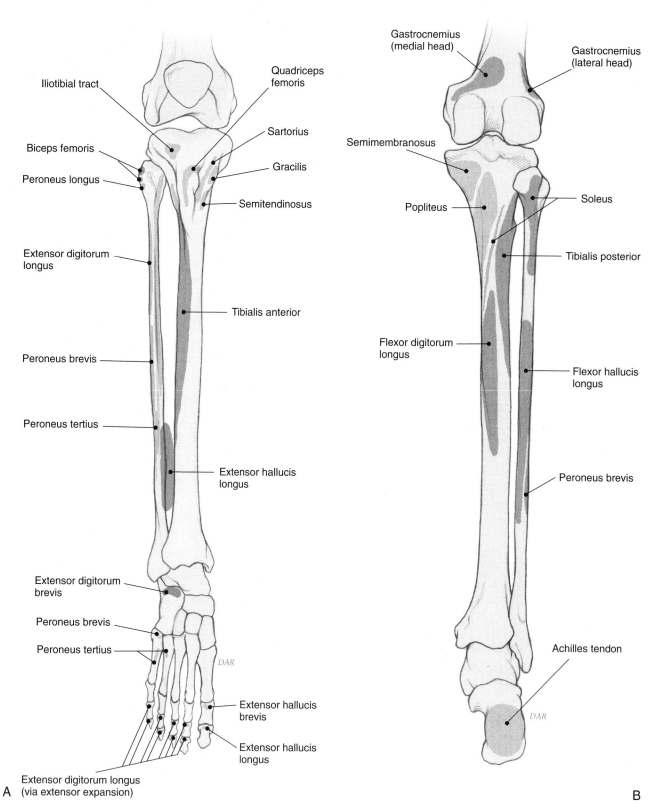

Iliotibial tract

Quadriceps femoris

Biceps femoris

Sartorius

Peroneus longus

Gracilis

Semitendinosus

Extensor digitorum longus

Tibialis anterior

Peroneus brevis

Peroneus tertius

Extensor hallucis longus

Extensor digitorum brevis

Peroneus brevis

Peroneus tertius

DAR

Extensor hallucis brevis

Extensor hallucis longus

Extensor digitorum longus (via extensor expansion)

A

Gastrocnemius (medial head)

Gastrocnemius (lateral head)

Semimembranosus

Popliteus

Soleus

Tibialis posterior

Flexor digitorum longus

Flexor hallucis longus

Peroneus brevis

Achilles tendon

DAR

B

FIGURE 8-1   (A) Muscles of leg and foot—anterior view. **(B)** Muscles of the leg—posterior view. *(continued)*

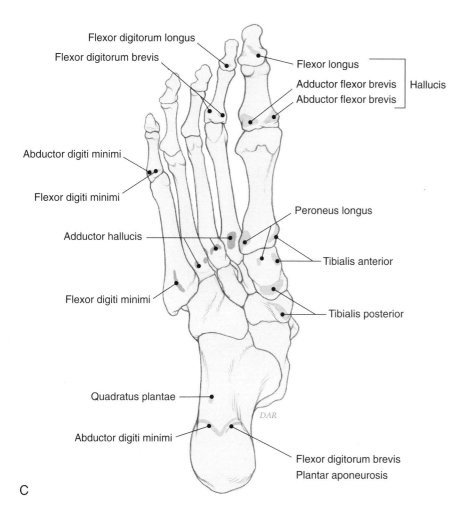

Flexor digitorum longus
Flexor digitorum brevis
Flexor longus
Adductor flexor brevis } Hallucis
Abductor flexor brevis
Abductor digiti minimi
Flexor digiti minimi
Peroneus longus
Adductor hallucis
Tibialis anterior
Flexor digiti minimi
Tibialis posterior
Quadratus plantae
Abductor digiti minimi
Flexor digitorum brevis
Plantar aponeurosis
DAR

C

FIGURE 8-1   *Continued.* (**C**) Muscles of the plantar surface of the foot.

The **soleus** is deep to the gastrocnemius. The two muscles act as a unit in their action at the ankle, merging at the Achilles tendon. The soleus attaches broadly on the tibia and fibula. Both muscles act to prevent overflexion of the knee during walking by stabilizing the ankle.

The articulation of the tibia and femur forms the knee joint. The two convex condyles of the femur fit into the two concave condyles of the tibia, allowing for flexion, extension, and slight rotation movements at the beginning of flexion, due to the uneven size of the condyles. The femur moves on the tibia with a combination of rolling and gliding movements. It is prevented from sliding off the tibia through the reinforcement of strong muscles and ligaments.

Eight ligaments reinforce the knee joint. The four primary ones are the anterior and posterior cruciate ligaments and the lateral and medial collateral ligaments. Two other ligaments, known as the menisci, are ring-shaped structures of cartilage formed at the top of tibia. They provide cushioning, even weight distribution, and shock absorption between the femur and tibia.

The patella is a small, triangular-shaped bone in front of the knee joint that is formed within the quadriceps tendon. It protects the knee and provides greater leverage for the action of the quadriceps muscle by acting as a pulley.

Twelve muscles directly affect movement at the knee. Eight of them are two-joint muscles, meaning they cross two joints; the remaining four are one-joint muscles (the popliteal and three of the quadricep muscles). Six of the two-joint muscles affect the movements of the femoral and knee joints. They are the three hamstring muscles: the rectus femoris, sartorius, and gracilis. The other two affect movements of the knee and ankle joints. They are the gastrocnemius and the plantaris. These muscles need to be balanced and coordinated for proper function of the knee to occur. They should be examined in conjunction with the muscles controlling the arches of the foot to assure stress-free movements of the knee.

CONDITIONS (INDICATIONS/CONTRAINDICATIONS BOX 8-1)

FEET AND ANKLES

1. To help a *fallen medial arch*:
   - Have the client perform exercises to build the arch (e.g., picking up marbles with the toes).
   - Release the peroneal muscles, because the foot will be overly everted.

Indications

Uneven weight placement on
   feet

Collapsed arches

Bunions

Misalignments of toes

Muscle strain

Muscle cramps

Well-healed foot surgery

Knee problems

Contraindications

Acute shin splints

Stress fracture

Broken bones

Varicose veins

Phlebitis

Spreadable rashes or fungus

---

2. A *callus* indicates too much strain or wear on that section of the foot, due to misalignment or improperly fitted shoes. Sometimes releasing the muscles that are pulling the toes or metatarsal out of position will reduce the callus.
3. *Plantar fascitis* is an inflammation of the plantar fascia, often due to overuse of the foot through walking, running, or jumping. Ice packs may be applied. Massage is contraindicated.
4. With a *sprained ankle*, ligaments will be damaged and at least partially torn. Damage can also be more severe. Apply ice immediately. Have the ankle checked by a physician. Massage work may be indicated after the initial swelling has subsided. Range of motion assessment can indicate more specifically which ligaments have been damaged.

LEG

1. *"Shin splints"* is a vague term describing a variety of strain conditions affecting the lower leg. Any of the muscles along the lower leg that move the foot may be subject to slight tearing away from the bone when overused or fatigued, resulting in pain and inflammation. Treatment consists of rest, ice application, and mild massage to bring blood to the area. Shin splints left untreated may result in stress fractures to the tibia.
2. *Achilles tendinitis* is an inflammatory condition brought about by overuse of the gastrocnemius and soleus muscles. Rest and ice are the appropriate treatment. Shortness of the gastrocnemius muscle is a common cause of strain in the Achilles tendon. Regular massage and stretching of this muscle is an excellent preventive measure (see page 137).
3. *Muscle cramps* occur frequently in the gastrocnemius muscles. To relieve cramping, stretch the muscle by

dorsiflexing the foot and holding it for at least 30 seconds. If the cramp does not subside, rest and ice are appropriate treatment.

KNEES

1. *Pain around the knee* may be caused by poor alignment of the leg. Pain on the medial side can be an indication of shearing actions. Pain in the patellar ligament below the knee can be caused by overly deep forward lunging actions or hyperextension of the knee, which is often accompanied by pain in the ligaments at the back of the knee.
2. *Chondromalacia* is a softening or roughening of the underside of the patella that can be caused by a blow to the knee or by poor muscle tone around the knee. It is accompanied by a grinding or creaking sound when the knee is flexed. Strengthening the quadriceps muscles is recommended.

THE MIND/BODY CONNECTION

The feet and ankles support and move the entire body. They are also our physical connection to the ground beneath us. Any form of imbalance or distortion in this area may be reflected as a sense of insecurity. How can we take a strong stance in life or move with grace and fluidity if we are unsure of our self at our foundation? A person who takes solid steps, being trusting of firm support underneath his or her feet, exudes a sense of confidence. Such persons know their places and stand their ground.

A close examination of the feet not only reveals structural imbalances higher up in the body, but also provides a map of how an individual might be compensating for feelings of insecurity. The way the feet relate to the earth mirrors the way the individual relates to the issues of contact and grounding. For example, a person with flat feet is making a fuller contact with the ground. Such a person may need the feeling of knowing that he or she is supported or held up by external influences. Someone with extremely high arches is making minimal contact with the earth. That person may experience a sense of disconnection with the ground or the kind of diminished mental clarity associated with a lack of grounding.

The ankle joints are essential for moving the feet. They express, as do all joints, the ability to adapt and change direction. Inflexible ankles prevent the feet from pointing in various directions and stepping on different paths, limiting the number of choices a person may feel he or she is able to make in life. Ankles that are weak and buckle under prevent individuals from feeling that they can stand up fully and carry their own weight.

The knees are important joints for weight support and transfer. They tie in with a wide variety of emotions. We tend to collapse and shake at our knees in response to a number of emotional stimuli. Fear can cause a person to feel weak in the knees, as can powerful joy and excitement.

When the knees, ankles, and feet are aligned through the vertical axis, with the feet pointing straight forward, energy is able to flow freely through the lower extremity. The feet relate to the root chakra, dealing with issues of survival and sustenance of the physical body. Interpretations of body stances are subjective, with many possible nuances of meaning, and should only be used as indicators, not as blanket categorizations of personality or behavior.

POSTURAL EVALUATION (TABLES 8-1 AND 8-2)

1. Check the alignment of the legs.
   - How does the line of gravity flow from the knee to the foot?
   - What is the shape of the legs: straight, bowed, knock-kneed?
2. Observe where the body's weight is concentrated on the feet. Is it forward, back, medial, or lateral?
3. Compare the directions in which the right and left feet are facing.
4. Observe the arches.
   - Are they high?
   - Are they collapsed?
5. Describe the shape and configuration of the toes.
   - Squeezed together.
   - Spread apart.
   - Curled under.
   - Does the big toe pull inward?
6. Check for bunions, calluses, and blisters on the feet. They indicate stress points on the feet.
7. Observe imbalance and/or weakness in the ankles. Compare the right and left ankles.
   Are the ankle joints on the same horizontal plane?
8. Look at the shape of the lower legs.
   - Are the muscles toned?
   - Is there swelling?
9. Describe the positioning of the knees.
   - Are they locked or hyperextended?
   - Are they flexed?
   - Are the patellae drawn up?
   - Are there bulges on the medial side of the knees, indicating a bracing of the soft tissues against gravity?
10. Examine the shape and muscle tone of the posterior legs.
    - What is the muscular condition of the calves? Are they large, underdeveloped, of equal size and shape on both sides? Are there differences between the right and left legs?
    - Are the Achilles tendons on both legs vertical or is one or both pulling to the side?

TABLE 8–1 Body Reading for the Feet	
Conditions	**Muscles that May Be Shortened**
Pigeon-toed—legs rotate medially, feet turn in	Adductors Gluteus medius and minimus Tensor fascia latae
Duck feet—legs rotate laterally, feet turn out	Gluteus maximus Iliopsoas Piriformis, deep lateral rotators
Problem feet—high insteps, fallen arches, hammer toes, and others	Deviations in the feet are often due to misalignment at the knee and hip; working the foot muscles may help to reshape the foot

TABLE 8–2   Range of Motion (ROM) for the Knee and Ankle

Action	Muscles
Knee	
Flexion (ROM 135°)	Biceps femoris
	Semitendinosus
	Semimembranosus
	Sartorius
	Gracilis
	Gastrocnemius
	Plantaris
	Popliteus
Extension (ROM 0°)	Quadriceps
	Tensor fascia latae
Internal rotation (ROM 10°)	Semitendinosus
	Semimembranosus
	Popliteus
	Gracilis
	Sartorius
External rotation (ROM 10°)	Biceps femoris
Ankle	
Dorsiflexion (ROM 10°)	Tibialis anterior
	External digitorum longus
	Peroneus tertius
	Extensor hallucis longus
Plantar flexion (ROM 65°)	Gastrocnemius
	Soleus
	Plantaris
	Peroneus longus
	Peroneus brevis
	Tibialis posterior
	Flexor hallucis longus
Inversion of the foot (ROM 5°)	Tibialis anterior
	Tibialis posterior
Eversion of the foot (ROM 5°)	Peroneus tertius
	Peroneus longus
	Peroneus brevis

EXERCISES AND SELF-TREATMENT

FEET AND ANKLES

Position

Lie down on your back with both knees flexed. Both feet are on the floor and parallel to each other. Bring the right knee to the chest. Place both hands around the knee to stabilize it.

1. *Foot circles.* Rotate the foot slowly in a full circle, as if tracing the face of a clock. Inhale during the first half the circle; exhale while completing the circle. Repeat the movement three times in each direction. (Alternately stretches and strengthens all the muscles that move the ankle joints.)

2. *Flexing.* Begin the exercise with the right foot fully flexed. Slowly, with resistance, point the foot, articulating each joint. Reverse the motion, bringing the foot back to full dorsiflexion. Repeat the movement two more times. (Alternately stretches and strengthens the intrinsic muscles of the foot and the plantar and dorsiflexor muscles of the ankle.)

3. *Toe clutching.* Begin with the foot dorsiflexed. Imagine a pencil placed behind the toes. On exhala-

tion, imagine squeezing the pencil with the toes, making a fist with the foot. Inhaling, release the flexion of the toes. Repeat the movement three times. (Alternately stretches and strengthens the flexors and extensors of the toes.)
4. Repeat the above three exercises on the left side.

CALF MUSCLES

Position

Stack two telephone books against the base of a wall. Stand facing the wall, with the balls of your feet on the edge of the telephone books. Put your hands against the wall for support.

1. *Toe raises.* Slowly raise up onto the balls of the feet. Hold for three counts. Lower your feet until the heels are parallel to the top of the telephone books. Repeat the toe raise several times. (Strengthens the gastrocnemius, soleus, tibialis posterior, peroneus longus and brevis, flexor hallucis longus.)
2. *Calf stretch.* Slowly lower your heels toward the floor, until you feel a stretch in the calf muscles. Hold the stretch for a minimum of 20 seconds. (Stretches gastrocnemius, soleus, tibialis posterior, and other plantar flexor muscles.)

FOOT, LEG, AND KNEE ROUTINE

OBJECTIVES

■ To balance the muscles that control the foot so that weight placement and walking patterns can be improved.
■ To relieve stress and uneven pulls on the muscles of the foot so that the formation of bunions, calluses, and other manifestations of foot dysfunction are minimized.
■ To balance muscular action around the knee, allowing the knee to track properly, thus eliminating strain on the soft tissue components of the joint.
■ To help relieve painful conditions that manifest in the muscles of the leg, such as spasms, shin splints, and trigger points.

ENERGY

Position

The client is lying supine on the table. A bolster under the knees is optional.
The therapist is standing at the foot of the table.

Polarity

Hold the toes of each foot between the thumb and index finger for 10 seconds each, beginning with the fifth toe and ending with the big toe. According to polarity theory, the tip of each toe is the culmination point of a vertical line of force that runs through the body from head to toe. These energy currents stimulate proper physiologic and psychological functioning. Moving from the fifth toe to the big toe, the energy currents are labeled earth, water, fire, air, and ether, in accordance with ayurvedic terminology. Holding each toe assists in clearing any blockages along these five energetic pathways.

Shiatsu

1. Compress the leg with both hands, from the knee to the ankle. This stimulates the flow of qi through the channels that flow through the leg. The yang channels on the outside of the leg are the gallbladder and stomach. The yin channels on the inside portion of the leg are the spleen, liver, and kidney.
2. Squeeze down the sides of the foot to the toes (Fig. 8-2).

SWEDISH/CROSS FIBER

1. Alternately apply effleurage strokes down the dorsal and plantar surfaces of the foot.
2. Perform knuckle kneading on the plantar surface of the foot.
3. Perform thumb gliding on the dorsal surface of the foot.
4. Perform effleurage and draining strokes from the ankle to the knee.

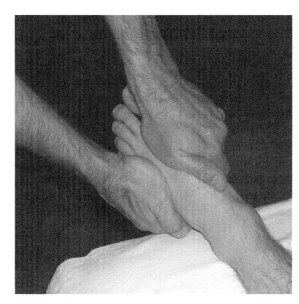

FIGURE 8-2 Shiatsu compression of the foot.

5. Reach the fingers of both hands underneath the calf, placing the fingertips between the heads of the gastrocnemius muscles. Rake outward, drawing the hands away from each other. Cover the entire calf, from several inches above the ankle to the knee.
6. Perform thumb gliding around the knee.

CONNECTIVE TISSUE

Myofascial Spreading Techniques

1. Facing the dorsal side of the client's foot from the side of the table, place the hands around the sides of the foot, with the fingertips touching at the midline of the plantar surface. Sink in with the fingers and spread from the midline to the outside edges of the foot.
2. Standing at the foot of the table, place the fingers on the dorsal surface of the foot at the base of the toes. Sink into the tissues and slowly glide toward the ankle.
3. Place the heels of the hands at the midline of the leg, above the ankle. Slowly spread the hands apart. Work in horizontal strips to the knee.

DEEP TISSUE/NMT

Sequence

1. Tendons of the toes
2. Insertion points of flexor hallucis longus, flexor hallucis brevis, and abductor hallucis
3. Muscles of the plantar surface of the foot
   First layer—abductor digiti minimi, flexor digitorum brevis, abductor hallucis
   Second layer—flexor hallucis longus, flexor digitorum longus, four lumbricals, quadratus plantae
   Third layer—flexor digiti minimi, adductor hallucis, flexor hallucis brevis
   Fourth layer—three plantar and four dorsal interossei; tendons of peroneus longus and tibialis posterior
4. Muscles of the dorsal surface of the foot
   Tendons—tibialis anterior, extensor hallucis longus, extensor digitorum longus, peroneus tertius
   Muscles—interossei, extensor hallucis brevis, extensor digitorum brevis, abductor digiti minimi
5. Retinaculum of the ankle—anterior portion
6. Medial leg muscles—flexor digitorum longus, soleus, gastrocnemius
7. Lateral leg muscles—tibialis anterior, extensor hallucis longus, extensor digitorum longus, peroneus longus, peroneus brevis, peroneus tertius, soleus
8. Retinaculum of the ankle—posterior portion
9. Gastrocnemius
10. Soleus and deep posterior leg muscles
11. Knee—ligaments and tendons

1. Tendons of the Toes

- Standing at the foot of the table, grasp the base of the proximal phalanx of the big toe, front and back, with the thumb and index finger (Fig. 8-3). Do short up-and-down strokes on the flexor and extensor tendons. Repeat on the distal phalanx.
- Repeat the above stroke on each of the other four toes, moving in sequence from the base of the second toe to the fifth toe.

2. Insertions of Flexor Hallucis Longus, Flexor Hallucis Brevis, Abductor Hallucis, and Adductor Hallucis

Flexor Hallucis Longus
The attachment point is located at the center of the base of the distal phalanx of the big toe, just above the joint, on the plantar surface of the foot.

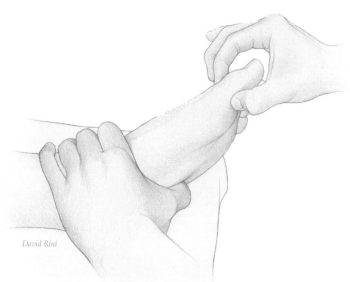
David Rini

FIGURE 8-3 Contacting the flexor and extensor tendons of the toes.

Do static compression and cross fiber friction on the attachment with the tip of your thumb or index finger.

Flexor Hallucis Brevis

The medial part inserts on the medial side of the base of the proximal phalanx of the hallux. The lateral part inserts on the lateral side of the base of the proximal phalanx of the hallux.

Abductor Hallucis

Inserts on the medial side of the base of the proximal phalanx of the hallux.

Adductor Hallucis

Inserts on the lateral side of the base of the proximal phalanx of the hallux.

To contact these attachments, hold the base of the big toe on both sides between your thumb and index finger. Feel for the tender spots on either side of the toe. Apply static compression and cross fiber friction on tender areas.

3. Muscles of the Plantar Surface of the Foot

Position

The therapist sits at the foot of the table, with the non-working hand holding the client's foot around the toes, maintaining a dorsiflexed position.

Flexor Hallucis Brevis

Origin: Medial portion of cuboid bone, lateral cuneiform bone.
Insertion: Base of proximal phalanx of hallux on the medial and lateral sides.
Action: Flexes proximal phalanx of the hallux.

Abductor Hallucis

Origin: Tuberosity of calcaneus, flexor retinaculum, plantar aponeurosis.
Insertion: Medial side of base of proximal phalanx of hallux.
Action: Abduction of hallux.

Trigger points tend to collect in the flexor hallucis brevis and abductor hallucis, muscles that insert at the medial side of the base of the big toe. The referred pain zone for flexor hallucis brevis is the region of the head of the first metatarsal and perhaps into the big toe. Trigger point pain from abductor hallucis can run across the ball of the foot. Check carefully along the toe tendons also.

- Using a **soft fist,** stroke down the plantar surface of the foot from the base of the toes to the heel (Fig. 8-4).
- Lumbricales muscles: to reach the muscles, stroke along the sides of each of the toe muscle tendons with the knuckle of the index finger or the thumb, from the base of the toes to the heel (Fig. 8-5). Maintain static compression on tender spots.

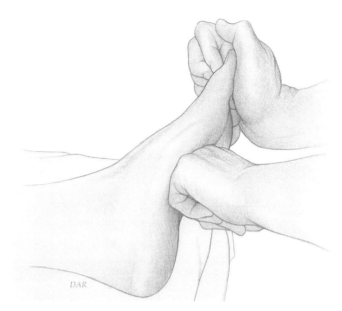

FIGURE 8-4 Deep tissue stroke on the muscles of the plantar surface of the foot.

4. Muscles of the Dorsal Surface of the Foot

Extensor Digitorum Brevis

Origin: Anterior and lateral surfaces of calcaneus, lateral talocalcaneal ligament, extensor retinaculum.
Insertion: Base of proximal phalanx of hallux, joins lateral sides of tendons of extensor digitorum longus on toes 2, 3, and 4.
Action: Extends the hallux (big toe) and toes 2, 3, and 4.

To check for trigger points, feel for tenderness in the extensor digitorum brevis muscle, near the ankle crease.

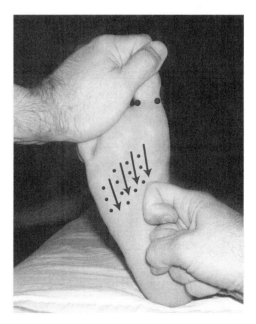

FIGURE 8-5 Stroking the lumbricales muscles between the toe tendons.

Pain from trigger points can radiate over the entire dorsal surface but will be most pronounced near the ankle.

Extensor Digitorum Brevis
With the knuckle of the index finger or the thumb, stroke along the sides of the toe tendons from the base of the toes to the ankle (Fig. 8-6).

5. Retinaculum of the Ankle—Anterior Portion
Place both thumbs at the midline of the ankle joint. Simultaneously move the thumbs in short up-and-down strokes, sliding the retinaculum over the tendon sheaths. Separating the thumbs slightly, repeat the stroke (Fig. 8-7). Continue to the medial and lateral malleoli.

6. Medial Leg Muscles (Flexor Digitorum Longus, Soleus, Gastrocnemius)

Position
Stand at the side of the table, placing the fingers of both hands along the medial border of the tibia, behind the medial malleolus.

- Perform circular friction strokes with the fingertips on the muscles medial to the edge of the tibia bone. Work from the medial malleolus to the knee.
- Perform short up-and-down and side-to-side strokes with the fingertips on the borders of the muscles just medial to the edge of the tibia, from the medial malleolus to the knee (Fig. 8-8).

7. Lateral Leg Muscles (Tibialis Anterior, Extensor Hallucis Longus, Extensor Digitorum Longus, Peroneus Longus, Peroneus Brevis, Peroneus Tertius, Soleus)

Tibialis Anterior
Origin: Lateral condyle and proximal two-thirds of lateral surface of tibia, interosseus membrane.

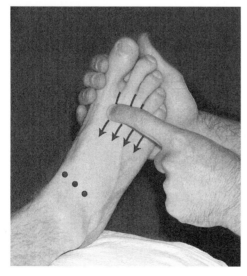

FIGURE 8-6 Direction of deep tissue stroke on extensor digitorum brevis.

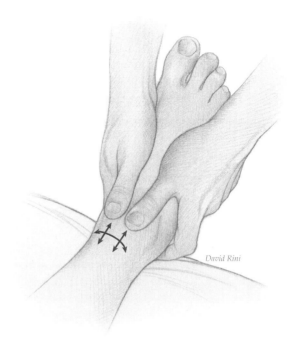

FIGURE 8-7 Directions of strokes on the retinaculum of the ankle.

Insertion: First medial cuneiform on medial and plantar surfaces, base of first metatarsal.
Action: Dorsiflexion of ankle at talocrural joint; inversion (supination) of foot at subtalar and midtarsal joints.

Trigger points are most often found in the upper third of the tibialis anterior muscle. The referred pain zone will be on the front of the ankle toward the medial side and over the entire big toe (hallux).

Note—It may be easier to work on the tibialis anterior muscle with the client in a supine position.

Peroneus Longus
Origin: Head and upper two-thirds of lateral shaft of the fibula.
Insertion: Lateral plantar side of base of first metatarsal, lateral plantar side of first cuneiform.
Action: Eversion of foot, assists plantar flexion of ankle, support of transverse arch.

Check the fibers of peroneus longus approximately 1 inch below the head of the fibula. The trigger point referral zone is around the lateral malleolus, extending along the lateral side of the foot.

Peroneus Brevis
Origin: Distal two-thirds of lateral surface of shaft of the fibula.
Insertion: Tuberosity on lateral surface of fifth metatarsal.
Action: Eversion of foot, assists plantar flexion of ankle.

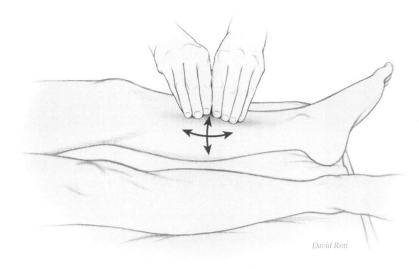

David Rini

FIGURE 8-8 Directions of deep tissue strokes on the medial leg muscles.

Peroneus Tertius
Origin: Distal one-third of medial surface of fibula.
Insertion: Dorsal surface of base of fifth metatarsal.
Action: Dorsiflexion of ankle, assists foot eversion.

- Trace the lateral side of the lateral malleolus with the knuckle or thumb to contact the tendons of the peroneal muscles. Perform the short up-and-down strokes on the tendons.
- Tibialis anterior: perform an elongation stroke with the elbow lateral to the shaft of the tibia from the ankle to the lateral condyle of the tibia (Fig. 8-9).

Position
The client is turned onto his or her side so that the leg to be worked on is uppermost. The top leg is flexed 90° at the hip and knee. A bolster is placed under the leg so that the hip does not roll forward.

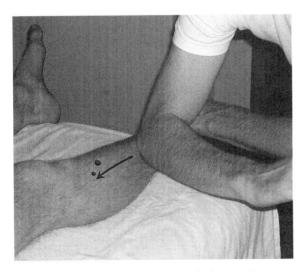

FIGURE 8-9 Elongation stroke on the tibialis anterior.

- Peroneal muscles: perform elongation strokes with the elbow from the lateral malleolus to the head of the fibula (Fig. 8-10).
- Using the elbow, separate the lateral leg muscles by stroking along their borders, from the ankle to the knee.
- A cross-fiber motion with the elbow may be used to locate trigger points.

The Posterior Leg

Position
The client is placed in the prone position; a bolster is placed under the ankle, if required.

The therapist is standing at the side of the table next to the client's foot.

The therapist warms up the posterior leg muscles as described above for the anterior leg.

8. Retinaculum of the Ankle—Posterior Portion
Place the thumbs on either side of the Achilles tendon. Do short up-and-down strokes on the retinaculum, sliding it over the underlying tendons. Separating the thumbs slightly, repeat the stroke. Continue to repeat the stroke, widening the distance between the thumbs, to the lateral and medial malleoli.

9. Gastrocnemius
Origin: Lateral head—lateral epicondyle and posterior surface of shaft of femur above the condyle. **Medial head**—popliteal surface of femur above the medial condyle.
Insertion: Middle posterior surface of calcaneus via tendo calcaneus.
Action: Plantar flexion of foot, assists in knee flexion.

Clusters of trigger points may form symmetrically in the upper quadrant of the gastrocnemius, in the medial and lateral heads. The referred pain zone is for the most

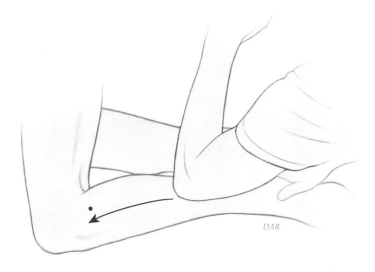

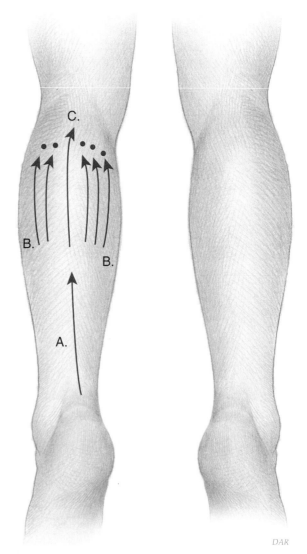

FIGURE 8-10 Elongation stroke on the peroneal muscles.

part local, radiating in the upper portion of the muscle and over the knee joint. A trigger point found just above the midline of the medial head of the muscle refers pain primarily to the instep of the foot and along the back of the calf on the medial side.

- Perform an elongation stroke using the forearm or knuckles, from the calcaneus to mid-calf region (A in Fig. 8-11).
- Reposition the forearm or knuckles directly over the lateral head of the gastrocnemius. Continue the elongation stroke to the knee. Repeat on the medial head (B in Fig. 8-11).

 Never stroke over the center of the back of the knee (popliteal fossa). Stay on the muscle by stroking on the side of the knee, maintaining your pressure on the muscle fibers of the gastrocnemius.

- Perform an elongation stroke with the thumbs up the midline of the posterior leg to separate the heads of the gastrocnemius (C in Fig. 8-11).
- Palpate trigger points in the bellies of the muscle using short up-and-down and side-to-side strokes with the thumbs. Treat any that are found.

10. Soleus and Deep Posterior Muscles

Soleus
Origin: Middle third of medial side of shaft of tibia, proximal third of shaft on posterior surface and head of fibula, fibrous arch between tibia and fibula.
Insertion: Posterior surface of calcaneus via tendo calcaneus (along with gastrocnemius).
Action: Plantar flexion of foot. Strong stabilizer of the body in standing position, prevents falling forward.

FIGURE 8-11 Sequence of strokes on the gastrocnemius.

The best way to examine the soleus is to disengage the gastrocnemius by flexing the client's leg 90°. The most frequent trigger point that forms in the soleus is found on the medial side, just above the Achilles tendon. It refers pain into the Achilles tendon and heel primarily, but may also radiate up into the medial side of the soleus.

■ Place thumbs or fingertips on both sides of the Achilles tendon. Working in small sections, apply up-and-down strokes lateral to the gastrocnemius muscle, from the ankle to the knee. Seek out areas of tightness and sensitivity to treat in the deeper layers of muscles.
■ Trigger points in the soleus muscle may be palpated by pressing deeply through the gastrocnemius.

11. The Knee

Position

The client is placed in a supine position, with a bolster under the knee.

The therapist is standing at the side of the table next to the client's knee.

Static compression as well as up-and-down and side-to-side strokes are used on the following attachment points (Fig. 8-12):

Pes anserinus (insertion point of semitendinosus, sartorius, and gracilis)—on the head of the tibia, medial to the patella.

Biceps femoris and peroneus longus—on the head of the fibula on the lateral side of the leg.

Quadriceps femoris—on the center of the head of the tibia, slightly superior to the tuberosity.

Patellar ligament—place the thumbs just above the tuberosity of the tibia. Do short up-and-down and side-to-side strokes on the ligament to the inferior border of the patella.

Medial and lateral patellar retinaculum—place the thumbs on either side of the patellar ligament. Move up-and-down and side-to-side, sliding the retinaculum. Pause at tender points.

Stretches

1. Standing at the foot of the table, grasp the toes of the client's foot with one hand while the other hand holds the foot at the heel. Flex and extend the toes several times.
2. Dorsiflex the foot and hold for several seconds.
3. Plantar-flex the foot and hold for several seconds.

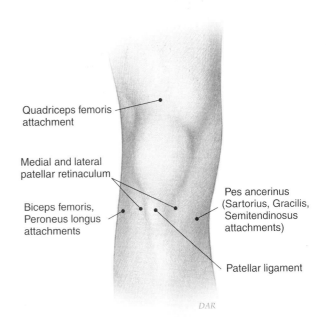

FIGURE 8-12 Attachment points at the knee.

(Stretches 2 and 3 above may be performed with the client lying in the supine or prone position, with the leg flexed 90° at the knee.)

4. Sandwich the foot between the palms. Invert the foot and hold for a few seconds. Evert the foot and hold for a few seconds.

Accessory Work

1. Hand and forearm massage complement this session well because these areas correspond reflexively to the foot and leg.
2. Neck and cranial massage will help to balance the upper pole of the body after this work.

Closing

Sitting at the head of the table, lightly cup the client's head in both your hands and hold for at least 30 seconds, allowing the client to relax and assimilate the effects of the session.

REFERENCE

1. Rolf IP. Rolfing: the integration of human structures. New York: Harper and Row, 1977: 58–60.

Stabilizing the Core

This chapter focuses primarily on re-establishing balanced action of the muscles that act on the pelvis. These include many of the thigh muscles as well as the abdominal and pelvic muscles. The thigh/hip and abdominal/pelvic regions are discussed separately to clarify anatomic and functional distinctions. However, these areas are integrated within the routines to promote coordination of all the muscles affecting pelvic placement and movement.

The four routines presented in this chapter should be viewed as a progressive unit. They should be performed in the prescribed order to achieve maximum results and prevent imbalance or trauma to the pelvic region. The deeply-lying psoas and iliacus muscles should never be massaged until the surface abdominal muscles and thigh muscles have been released. Premature work on the iliopsoas can seriously disrupt the integrity of the pelvic core.

The four sessions should be scheduled at close intervals, with no more than 2 weeks between each one, so that the results from the previous session can effectively be carried over to the next. The therapist should teach the client the exercises described in the lessons to stretch the muscles worked on so that the client may better integrate the muscular release and increased core awareness achieved within the sessions.

The order of the routines is as follows:

1. The posterior thigh muscles and hip muscles.
2. The abdominal muscles, including their attachments on the ribcage and pelvis.
3. The lateral and medial thigh muscles and massage to the intestines.
4. The anterior thigh muscles and hip flexors, including the rectus femoris and iliopsoas.

THE THIGH AND HIP

INTRODUCTION

The thigh consists of the femur, which is the longest and strongest bone in the body, and the muscles attached to it. The hip is the articulation of the femur with the pelvis. It is a ball-and-socket joint capable of a broad range of movements, including flexion and extension, abduction and adduction, rotation, and circumduction. The thigh and hip are active in balancing the body in standing and in initiating movement of the lower limb. The muscles at the front of the thigh, the quadriceps, are among the most powerful in the body. They are balanced by groups of muscles on the sides and back of the thigh.

A total of 22 muscles are involved in moving the femur at both of its joints. Twenty-one of these muscles have their origin at various places on the pelvis. In a standing position the legs are fixed in their position over the feet. Therefore, when the thigh muscles are shortened they tend to pull from their attachment on the pelvis, moving it out of position. One of the goals of deep tissue work on the thigh muscles is to balance their action so that the pelvis can sit freely over the heads of the femurs without being chronically pulled into a distorted alignment.

The hip joint is reinforced by strong ligaments and muscles. Because of its ball-and-socket design the hip joint is capable of rotary and circular movements. However, in walking and running its movement is limited by the hinge design of the knee and ankle beneath it, which are capable of flexion and extension movements only. The femur must meet the challenge of absorbing and transferring a large number of stresses coming from various angles at both its ends. Much stress is therefore placed on the knee. The knee must process the forces coming to it from the weight of the body above and the movements of the hip. It must also be able to absorb the shock from the impact of weight rising up to it from the ground below in walking and running movements.

In proper alignment of the thigh, a vertical axis passes from the center of the hip joint at the front of the thigh to the center of the knee joint. This axis is distorted in both knock-kneed and bow-legged conditions, adding additional stress to the joints of the legs. The deep tissue ther-

---

ESSENTIAL ANATOMY BOX 9–1

The Thigh and Hip Routines

Muscles

Quadriceps: rectus femoris, vastus lateralis, medialis, and intermedius

Adductors: adductor brevis, longus, and magnus, gracilis, pectineus

Hamstrings: biceps femoris, semimembranosus, semitendinosus

Lateral rotators: piriformis, obturator internus, gemellus superior, gemellus inferior, obturator externus, quadratus femoris

Gluteus maximus, medius, minimus

Tensor fascia latae and iliotibial band

Sartorius

Bones and Landmarks

Anterior superior iliac spine (ASIS)

Anterior inferior iliac spine (AIIS)

Sacrum

Coccyx

Ischial tuberosity

Femur

Greater trochanter

Lesser trochanter

Patella

Tibia

Tibial tuberosity

Fibula

Head of fibula

apist should be aware of this vertical axis when working on the thigh muscles and attempt to re-establish it by releasing uneven pulls in the musculature of the thigh.

MUSCULOSKELETAL ANATOMY AND FUNCTION (ESSENTIAL ANATOMY BOX 9-1 AND FIG. 9-1A AND B)

The proximal end of the femur consists of a rounded head, a neck, and two projections, called the greater and lesser trochanter. The head fits into a round cavity in the pelvis called the acetabulum, formed by the junction of the ilium, pubis, and ischium. The entire circumference of the acetabulum is coated by a ring of cartilage called the labrum. This ring holds onto the head of the femur, creating a snug fit for it in the hip joint. Extending from the labrum is a thick sleeve, or joint capsule, that encases the neck of the femur, reinforcing and protecting the joint.

Seven ligaments surround the hip joint, giving it additional strength and support. The strongest of these is the iliofemoral or Y ligament. It attaches in front of the hip joint, at the anterior inferior iliac spine (AIIS), and in the space on the femur between the two trochanters. The ischiofemoral ligament is situated at the back of the joint, attaching to the ischium below the acetabulum, and to the posterior femoral neck. These ligaments help hold the head of the femur firmly in the hip socket during movements of the thigh.

The neck of the femur extends diagonally upward from the shaft of the bone. Its design keeps the thigh clear of the pelvis, allowing for greater mobility of the pelvis over the legs. The disadvantage of the shape of the neck is that it is in the form of a bent lever, subjecting it to greater stress than a straight column. It is potentially the weakest point on the thigh. Many older people break their leg at the neck of the femur.

The greater trochanter is the site of attachment for many muscles that initiate movements of the thigh. The six lateral rotators as well as the **gluteus medius and minimus** (the medial rotators) have their insertion there. These two sets of muscles oppose each other in rotation of the femur. They must all be in balance to allow the full range of movements of the head of the femur in the acetabulum. Muscular imbalance pulls the head of the femur out of position slightly and over time may result in arthritis of the hip joint. Movement restriction at the hip often has a relay effect, creating stress and imbalance at the knee and sometimes the ankle as well.

The muscles in front of the thigh, the flexors, move the leg forward in locomotor movements (Fig. 9-1C and D). The primary hip flexors are the **iliopsoas** and the **rectus femoris**. The rectus femoris is also active in knee exten-

sion. Secondary flexors are the **sartorius** and **tensor fascia lata**. Of all these muscles, the iliopsoas is most important. Due to its location at the body's core, it possesses the greatest power and leverage. It should be the foremost initiator of hip flexion. In a balanced body, walking motions are not initiated by the legs, but in the trunk. The movement is then transferred to the legs by means of the psoas. The psoas muscle does not attach to the pelvis, but to the anterior portion of the lumbar spine. Its insertion is on the lesser trochanter on the inner surface of the femur.

The psoas and rectus femoris muscles need to be in balance with each other for a smooth, coordinated walking action to occur. Often the rectus femoris takes over hip flexion, while the psoas becomes shortened and weak, which tends to increase the lumbar curve and tips the ribcage downward and forward. This causes misalignment in the body segments, with an inevitable breakdown in full-body movement integration.

When the psoas is functioning properly in hip flexion, the upper and lower body are coordinated around the lumbar spine. As a result of this integration, the sides of the pelvis will swing with each step, rather than being held rigid by tight, inhibited muscles. In walking, the knees will swing forward and back, and the feet will roll like the base of a rocking chair, with weight moving from heels to toes. This connected chain of movement through the body creates a gentle undulation of the spine, which helps enhance physiologic processes through the increased pumping of fluids through the trunk, including the cerebrospinal fluid that flows through the spinal cord.

The opposing muscles to the hip flexors are the hip extensors, which include the three hamstrings and the **gluteus maximus**. The hamstrings are two-joint muscles originating at the ischial tuberosity and inserting on the tibia. They also serve as knee flexors. Their movement is restricted by the presence of the iliofemoral ligament in the front of the hip, limiting pure extension to about 45°.

The primary hip abductors are the gluteus medius and minimus, with the tensor fascia lata assisting in abduction when the hip is flexed. The most important function of the tensor fascia lata is to maintain tension in the **iliotibial band**. This band of fascia, located on the outside of the thigh, assists in absorbing tensile or stretching stresses acting on the femur. Bones are designed to absorb compression, or shortening stresses better than tension, or lengthening stresses, which are absorbed by the muscles and fascia. Therefore, this additional support is crucial in strengthening the thigh.

The hip adductor muscles are the **pectineus, adductor brevis, adductor longus, adductor magnus,** and the **gracilis**. The gracilis is the only two-joint muscle of this group, inserting on the medial surface of the shaft of the tibia.

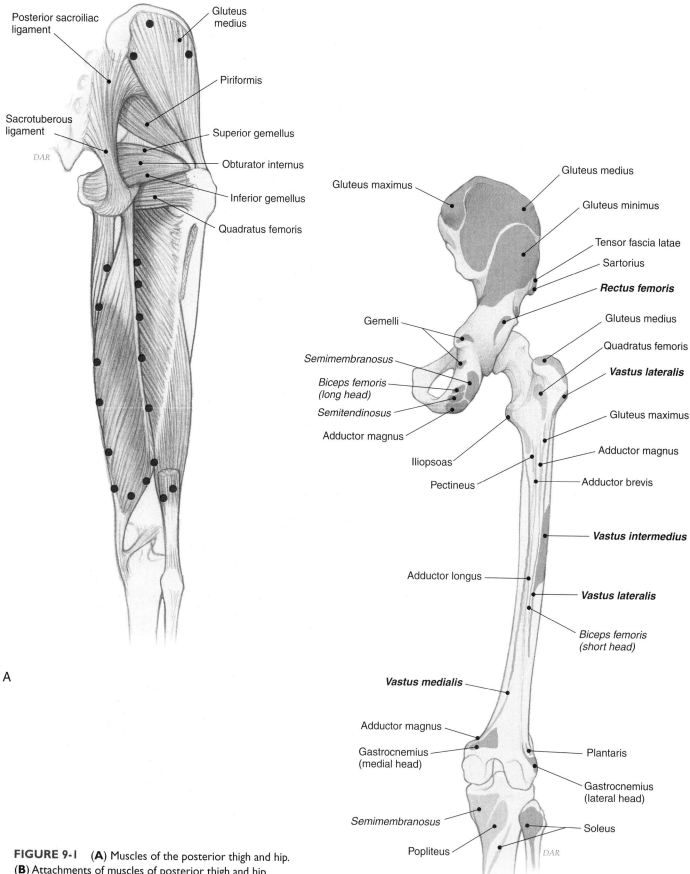

FIGURE 9-1 **(A)** Muscles of the posterior thigh and hip. **(B)** Attachments of muscles of posterior thigh and hip. *(continued)*

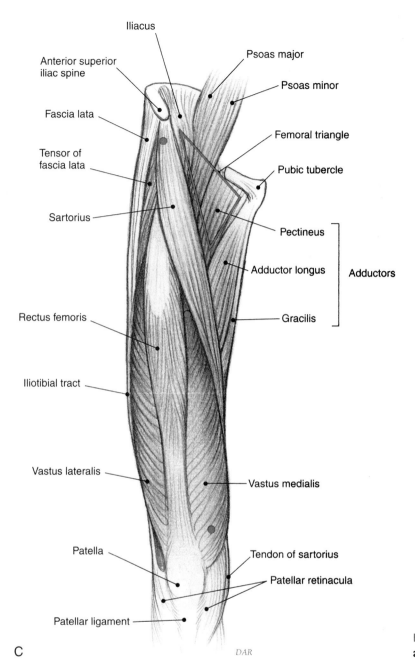

Iliacus

Anterior superior
iliac spine

Psoas major

Psoas minor

Fascia lata

Femoral triangle

Tensor of
fascia lata

Pubic tubercle

Sartorius

Pectineus

Adductor longus   Adductors

Rectus femoris

Gracilis

Iliotibial tract

Vastus lateralis

Vastus medialis

Patella

Tendon of sartorius

Patellar retinacula

Patellar ligament

C

DAR

FIGURE 9-1   *Continued.* **(C)** Muscles of the thigh—
anterior view. *(continued)*

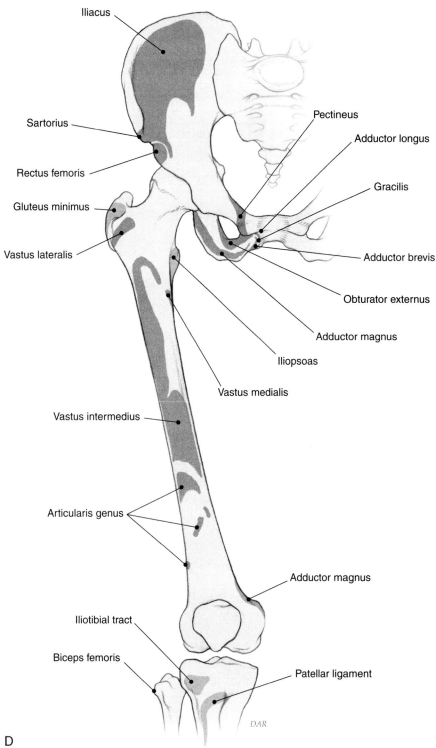

D

FIGURE 9-1 *Continued.* (**D**) Muscle attachments on the thigh and pelvis.

Indications	Contraindications	
		INDICATIONS/ CONTRAINDICATIONS BOX 9-1
Fatigue	Varicose veins	
Low back pain	Broken bones	
Hip pain	Acute injury	
Leg pain	Recent trauma	*Conditions Affecting Massage of the Thigh and Hip*
Pelvic misalignment	Severe bruises	
Cellulite	Phlebitis	
Muscle strain	Rashes	
Muscle cramps	Burns	
Poor circulation		
Polio and similar conditions		
Amputation		
Sciatica		

CONDITIONS (INDICATIONS/ CONTRAINDICATIONS BOX 9-1)

1. *Muscle strains* in thigh muscles are common. Rest and appropriately applied massage techniques are often adequate treatment.
2. *Varicose veins* result from swelling of the veins due to a breakdown of the one-way valves that prevent venous blood from flowing downward instead of toward the heart. The condition is caused by a weakening of the vein walls, which allows them to stretch and pull the valves open.

   There seems to be a genetic component in the tendency to develop varicose veins. Pregnancy can often trigger them or exacerbate the condition. Certain dietary supplements may help to strengthen the vein walls. The client should consult a physician for guidance in this area. The best home care treatment is elevation of the legs for a period everyday, to assist the flow of blood out of the legs. Deep tissue massage is contraindicated.

THE MIND/BODY CONNECTION

Like the leg and foot, the thigh is involved in moving the body. The muscles of the thigh, being closer to the core of the body, are more involved in initiating movement. The lower portion of the leg mirrors how we handle ourselves once we have completed our movement and planted our feet.

The thighs have been called the prime movers of the body. Observing their shape and tone indicates how a person moves through life. The quadriceps are thick, fiber-dense muscles. They are powerful, potentially able to lift more weight than any other muscle group. The hamstring muscles, when chronically contracted, pull the ischial tuberosities of the pelvis downward, restricting pelvic movement and putting strain on the back of the knees.

These two muscle groups must be well-coordinated to effectively orchestrate the movements of flexion and extension at the knee joint and anterior and posterior tipping of the pelvis. The hamstrings are often weak in relation to the quadriceps, allowing them to pull too strongly on the front of the knee, causing hyperextension of the joint.

Holding onto the adductor muscles often denotes a shielding or protective stance. Squeezing the inner thighs blocks access to the pelvic region. Constriction of the outer thigh often accompanies contraction of the gluteal muscles. These muscles tighten in an effort to contain feelings and sensations.

As the hip and thigh are released through deep tissue sessions, a client may experience a renewed surge to move ahead with life. Reconnecting with the ground gives a sense of sustenance and a feeling of belonging here on the earth. This, coupled with tapping into the vast reserve of personal power we all contain, as represented by the thighs, is powerful motivation to create positive changes in one's life.

POSTURAL EVALUATION

1. Check the overall alignment of the anterior thigh.
   - Does the line of gravity appear to fall in a straight line between the center of the hip joint in the front of the thigh and the center of the knee?
   - If not, how does it deviate?

2. Observe the shape and muscular tone of the thighs.
   - What is the degree of muscular development? Bound, flaccid, or well-toned?
   - Do the muscles appear to be pulling in any particular direction?
   - Note any differences between the right and left thigh.

3. In what direction(s) are the thigh muscles pulling the pelvis? Which muscles are involved?
4. Check the alignment of the back of the thighs.
   - Where does the line of gravity fall through the back of the thighs?
   - Is the gluteal line at the base of the buttocks horizontal?

TABLE 9–1   Range of Motion for the Hip

Action	Muscles
Flexion (knee extended) (ROM 90°)	Psoas major
	Sartorius
	Pectineus
	Adductor longus
	Adductor brevis
	Adductor magnus (ant.)
	Sartorius
	Rectus femoris
Extension (ROM 45°)	Gluteus maximus
	Biceps femoris (long head)
	Semitendinosus
	Semimembranosus
	Adductor magnus
	Gracilis
	Pectineus
Abduction (ROM 45°)	Gluteus medius
	Gluteus minimus
	Iliopsoas
	Tensor fascia latae
	Sartorius
Adduction (ROM 25°)	Adductor brevis
	Adductor longus
	Adductor magnus
	Gracilis
	Pectineus
Internal rotation (sitting) (ROM 35°)	Gluteus medius
	Gluteus minimus
	Tensor fascia latae
	Pectineus
	Adductor-longus, brevis, magnus
External rotation (sitting) (ROM 40°)	Piriformis
	Gemellus superior
	Obturator internus
	Gemellus inferior
	Obturator externus
	Quadratus femoris
	Gluteus maximus

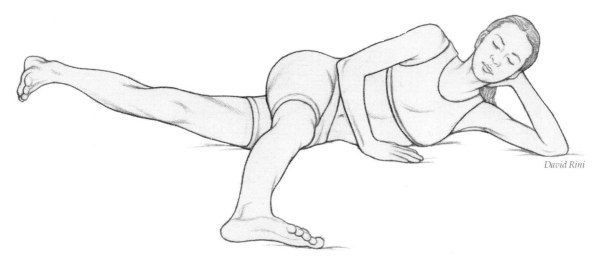

David Rini

FIGURE 9-2   Inner thigh lift.

5. Observe the muscles of the posterior thigh and hip region (Table 9-1).
   - What is the muscular condition of the back of the thigh? Well-toned, weak, or contracted?
   - What is the shape and tone of the gluteal region? Tight, loose, squeezed, overdeveloped, or underdeveloped?
   - Are the tendons of the hamstrings prominent at the back of the knees? Do they appear even on the right and left legs?
   - Do the hamstrings appear to be pulling the pelvis downward?
   - Does the degree of muscularity match that of the front of the thighs?

EXERCISES AND SELF-TREATMENT

ADDUCTORS

1. Inner Thigh Lift (Strengthens Adductors)

Preparation
Lie on your right side. The right leg is fully extended along the floor, under you. The left leg is extended straight in front at hip level. Place your left hand on the floor in front of your chest for support. Hold your head in your right hand (Fig. 9-2).

Execution
Exhaling, lift the right leg straight up, keeping the instep parallel to the floor. Think of squeezing the right inner thigh against the left inner thigh. Inhale as you lower the

leg. Repeat several times. Reverse the position to do the left side.

2. Inner Thigh Stretch (Stretches Adductors)

Preparation
Lying on your back, bring the soles of your feet together in front of you, close to your pelvis. Wrapping your hands around the outside edges of the feet, turn the knees outward (Fig. 9-3).

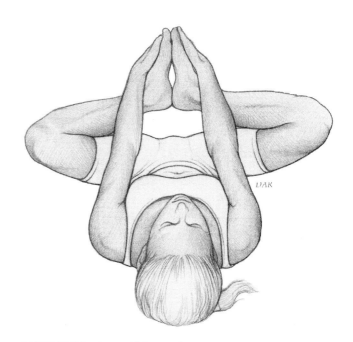

DAK

FIGURE 9-3   Inner thigh stretch.

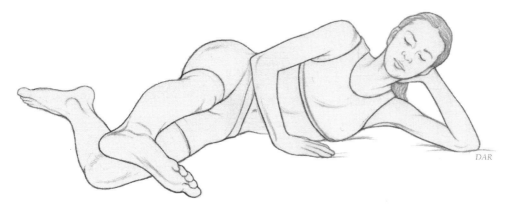

FIGURE 9-4 Outer thigh lift.

Execution

Exhaling, draw the heels toward you as you continue to turn the knees out until you feel a stretch in the adductor muscles. Hold for a minimum of 20 seconds.

ABDUCTORS

1. Outer Thigh Lift (Strengthens Gluteus Medius, Gluteus Minimus, Tensor Fascia Latae)

Preparation

The starting position is the same as for the inner thigh lift above, except that the bottom leg is flexed instead of straight. Medially rotate the leg extended in front of you at hip level so that the toes are pointing downward about 45° (Fig. 9-4).

Execution

Exhaling, lift the leg extended in front of you straight up in the air approximately 2 feet. Hold for a moment, then lower the leg as you inhale until the side of the big toe touches the floor. Repeat several more times. Reverse your body position to do the exercise on the other side.

2. Outer Thigh Stretch (Stretches Gluteus Medius, Gluteus Minimus, Tensor Fascia Latae, Piriformis).

Preparation

Lie on your back with both legs extended and your arms out to your sides at shoulder level. Circle the right leg along the floor to the left side, bringing it in the direction of your left shoulder.

Execution

Reach down and take hold of the right ankle with your left hand. Slowly bring the leg toward your left shoulder

until you feel a stretch in the outer thigh and hip of the right leg. Hold for 30 seconds. Repeat the stretch for the left leg.

QUADRICEPS

1. Quadricep Strengthener (Strengthens Vastus Lateralis, Vastus Medialis, Vastus Intermedius, Rectus Femoris)

Preparation

Sit up tall with the legs extended in front of you. Keeping the right leg extended and the right foot strongly flexed, slide the left thigh toward your chest, keeping the foot on the floor. Hold the left knee with both hands (Fig. 9-5).

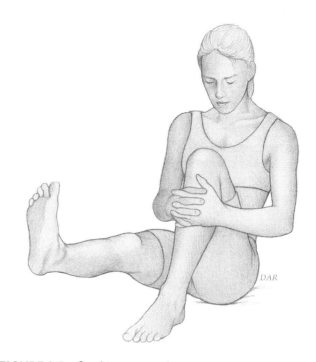

FIGURE 9-5 Quadriceps strengthener.

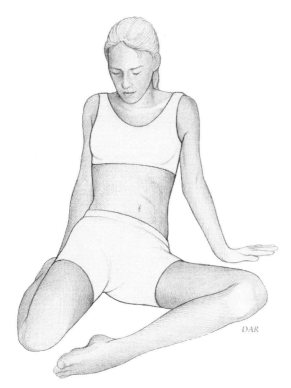

FIGURE 9-6 Quadriceps stretch.

Execution

Exhaling, lift the right leg straight up off the ground a few inches while pulling up on the patella. Hold for a few seconds. Inhaling, lower the leg to the floor. Adjust the position of your back, making sure it is straight, and repeat the leg lift a few more times. Reverse your position and repeat on the left side.

2. Quadricep Stretch (Stretches Vastus Lateralis, Vastus Medialis, Vastus Intermedius, Rectus Femoris)

Preparation

To stretch your right thigh, lie on your left side. Place your head in your left hand. Flex both legs.

Execution

Lift your right leg, bringing the thigh toward the chest. Reach down and take hold of the top of the right ankle with your right hand. Slowly draw the thigh back until you feel a stretch in the center of your right thigh (Fig. 9-6). Hold for 20 seconds. Reverse the body position and stretch the left thigh.

HAMSTRINGS

1. Hamstring Strengthener (Strengthens Biceps Femoris, Semitendinosus, Semimembranosus)

Preparation

Lie face down on the floor, turning your head to one side. Flex your right leg at the knee. Place your left foot behind the right ankle (Fig. 9-7).

Execution

Try to draw the right heel toward your hip as you resist the movement by pressing against the right ankle with your left leg. Flex the right leg toward the hip several times, with resistance. Then hold an isometric contraction of the right hamstring muscles for up to 30 seconds.

2. Hamstring Stretch (Stretches Biceps Femoris, Semitendinosus, Semimembranosus)

Preparation

Have a belt or tie handy. Lie on the floor on your back, with the left knee flexed and the left foot placed on the floor. Bringing your right thigh to your chest, loop the belt around the ball of the foot.

Execution

Exhaling, slowly extend the right leg toward the ceiling. Push upward with the heel as you flex the foot by pulling down on the sides of the belt (Fig. 9-8). Hold for 30 seconds.

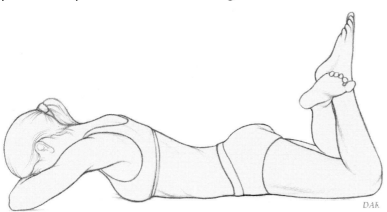

FIGURE 9-7 Hamstring strengthener.

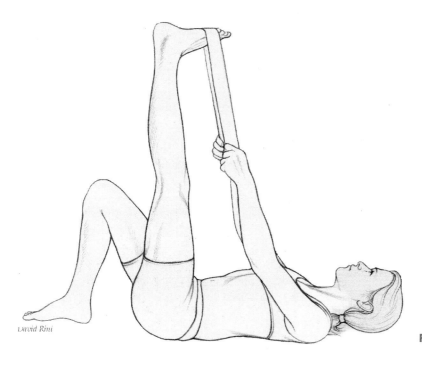

David Rini

FIGURE 9-8   Stretching the hamstrings using a belt.

HIPS

1. Gluteal Strengthener (Strengthens Gluteus Maximus)

Preparation
Position yourself on your forearms and knees, with the right leg extended straight back and turned out, so that the big toe is touching the floor.

Execution
Exhaling, lift the right leg straight up until you feel the gluteus maximus tighten (Fig. 9-9). Do not arch your back.

Lower the right leg and repeat several more times. Reverse the leg position and repeat the lifts with the left leg.

2. Gluteal Stretch (Stretches Gluteus Maximus, Piriformis)

Preparation
Sit cross-legged with the right heel placed in front of the left. Leaning forward slightly from the hip joints, place both hands on the floor in front of the legs.

Execution
Exhaling, slide the hands forward, slowly folding the trunk toward the floor until you feel a stretch in the back

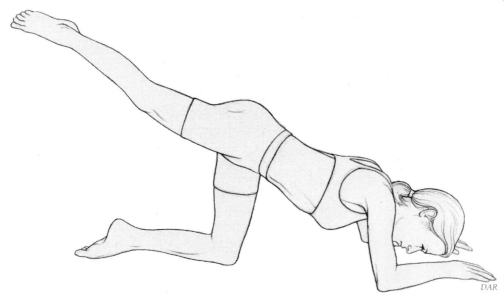

DAR

FIGURE 9-9   Gluteal strengthener.

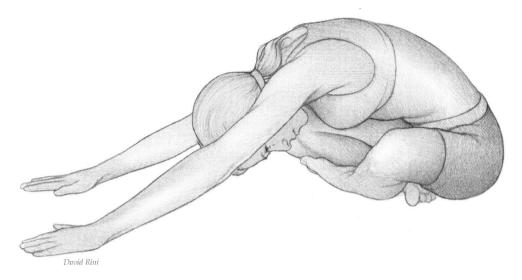

David Rini

FIGURE 9-10   Position to stretch the gluteal and piriformis muscles.

of the right hip (Fig. 9-10). Make sure both hips are touching the floor. Hold the stretch for 30 seconds. Repeat, with the left foot in front to stretch the left hip.

3. Hip Release

Preparation

Lying on the floor on your back, flex both knees, keeping the soles of the feet on the floor.

Execution

Bring your right thigh to your chest, placing both hands around the knee. Circle the thigh slowly as you imagine breathing into the right hip joint. Keep the thigh muscles totally relaxed. Let your arms guide the movement. Circle a few times in the other direction. Repeat the hip circles with the left leg.

POSTERIOR THIGH AND HIP ROUTINE

OBJECTIVES

- To release restriction in the hamstring muscles and their attachments, which can contribute to low back problems and pelvic distortion.
- To open up the gluteal muscles, often a major site of stored tension.
- To release the deep lateral rotators, which helps to improve the walking pattern.
- To reduce sciatic pain generated by a tight piriformis muscle.
- To help heal injuries in the sacral ligaments, an overlooked contributor to low back pain.

- To bring balance to the soft tissues acting on the sacrum, allowing it to find its natural position. This brings greater ease throughout the body, as the upper and lower halves balance around the sacrum.

ENERGY

Position

The client is lying prone on the table. A bolster may be placed under the ankles.

The therapist is standing on the left side of the table facing the client's back.

Polarity

Sacral Rock

1. The left hand contacts the C7–T1 area of the upper back. The palm of the right hand contacts the sacrum. Gently rock the sacrum with the right hand while the left hand stabilizes the upper back. Continue for at least 30 seconds.

   This procedure helps to mobilize the lumbar vertebrae by freeing constrictions around the joints as well as relaxing the muscles of the pelvis. It also helps the client to experience a feeling of continuity throughout the length of the spinal column

2. The therapist's left hand (negative pole) contacts the client's sacrum (positive pole). The right hand (positive pole) rests on the back of the client's left knee (negative pole).

   a. Rock the sacrum with the left hand.

   b. Place the right hand (positive pole) on the right knee (negative pole), continuing to rock the sacrum.

This polarity procedure integrates the pelvis with the thighs.

Shiatsu

1. Compress the back of the left thigh with both hands, from the hip to the knee. Repeat on the other leg. This Shiatsu move stimulates qi flow through the bladder channel, which runs down the back of the leg.
2. Roll both fists across the muscles in the gluteal area. The bladder and gallbladder channels run through the back of the pelvis.

SWEDISH/CROSS FIBER

1. Perform effleurage strokes on the posterior thigh and gluteal area.
2. Perform pétrissage strokes on the posterior thigh and gluteal area.
3. Perform friction strokes on the posterior thigh and gluteal area.
4. Apply cross fiber strokes across the hamstrings and gluteal muscles using the broad side of the thumb and/or the heel of the hand.

CONNECTIVE TISSUE

Myofascial Spreading Techniques

1. Starting at the midline of the posterior thigh, spread outward, using the heels of both hands. Work in horizontal strips from the knee to the hip.
2. Spread the gluteal muscles using the heels of the hand and/or fingertips.

DEEP TISSUE/NMT

Sequence

1. Hamstrings—bellies and attachments.
2. Gluteus maximus, medius, and minimus.
3. Lateral rotators—piriformis, obturator internus, obturator externus, gemellus superior, gemellus inferior, and quadratus femoris.
4. Sacral ligaments—sacrotuberous, posterior sacroiliac

1. Hamstrings

Biceps Femoris
Origin: Long head—ischial tuberosity (inferior and medial aspects, sharing same tendon as semitendinosus), sacrotuberous ligament. **Short head**—entire length of lateral lip of linea aspera on femur, proximal two-thirds of lateral supracondylar ridge, lateral intermuscular septum.

Insertion: Lateral aspect of head of fibula, lateral condyle of tibia.
Action: Knee flexion, knee external rotation. **Long head**—hip extension.

Semitendinosus
Origin: Ischial tuberosity (inferior medial aspect).
Insertion: Shaft of tibia on proximal medial side.
Action: Knee flexion, knee internal rotation, hip extension; assists hip internal rotation.

Semimembranosus
Origin: Ischial tuberosity (superior and lateral aspects).
Insertion: Medial condyle of tibia on posterior medial aspect, lateral condyle of femur (posterior aspect via fibrous expansion, forming part of oblique popliteal ligament).
Action: Knee flexion, knee internal rotation, hip extension; assists hip internal rotation.

Trigger points tend to cluster in the distal portion of all three hamstring muscles above the knee. Checking along the borders of the muscles will often reveal trigger points. Referral patterns can be up to the gluteal area, around the ischial tuberosity, and around the back of the knee.

Position
The client is lying prone on the table. A bolster may be placed under the ankles.

The therapist is standing at the side of the table next to the client's knees.

- Flexing the client's knee, follow the tendons of the hamstrings across the knee joint to their insertions on the leg and apply static compression and cross fiber techniques with your thumbs or fingers (Fig. 9-11).
- Perform an elongation stroke with your forearm from the knee to the ischial tuberosity. Repeat, covering each of the three hamstring muscles.
- Separate the three hamstring muscles by using the elbow. Follow the tendon of each muscle from the knee to find its border on the posterior thigh. Stroke from the knee to the ischial tuberosity along the edge of each muscle.
- Apply short cross fiber strokes with your thumb or knuckle to the origins of the hamstrings at the ischial tuberosity.

2. Gluteus Maximus, Medius, and Minimus

Gluteus Maximus
Origin: Posterior gluteal line and crest of ilium, posterior surface of sacrum and coccyx, aponeurosis of erector spinae, sacrotuberous ligament.
Insertion: Iliotibial band of fascia lata, gluteal tuberosity of femur.

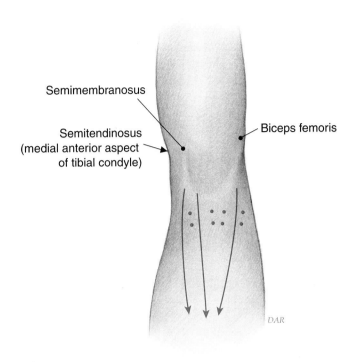

Semimembranosus

Semitendinosus
(medial anterior aspect
of tibial condyle)

Biceps femoris

FIGURE 9-11 Origin of hamstrings and direction of deep tissue strokes.

Action: Hip extension, lateral hip rotation, extension of trunk when insertion is fixed. **Upper fibers**—hip abduction. **Lower fibers**—hip adduction.

The most common trigger point in gluteus maximus is found in the fibers slightly above the ischial tuberosity. The referred pain zone can be over the entire gluteal region. Another trigger point can be located in the fibers next to the lower portion of the sacrum. Activity here can refer pain along the gluteal line at the base of the muscle. A third trigger point has been found in the most medial and inferior fibers of the muscle, near the coccyx. It refers pain to the coccyx, so that when active, people often mistakenly think they have a problem with the coccyx.

- Standing at the side of the table next to the client's pelvis, perform elongation strokes with the forearm, fist, or heel of hand, in strips, from the ilium and sacrum to the greater trochanter (Fig. 9-12).
- Taut bands may be palpated by rolling across the fibers of the muscle with the fingertips or elbow. Treat trigger points as they are found.

Gluteus Medius

Origin: Outer surface of ilium inferior to iliac crest.
Insertion: Oblique ridge on lateral surface of greater trochanter of femur.
Action: Hip abduction. **Anterior fibers**—medial rotation of hip. **Posterior fibers**—lateral rotation of hip. The

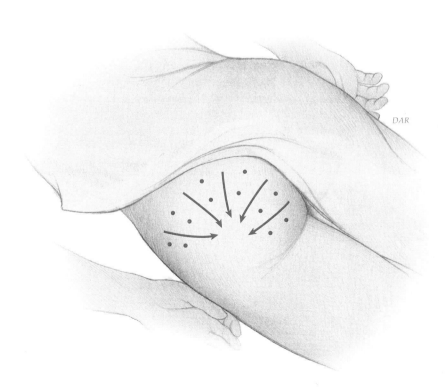

FIGURE 9-12 Direction of deep tissue strokes on gluteal muscles.

action of gluteus medius prevents the pelvis from sliding laterally and tilting during the walking motion.

The three most common trigger points in gluteus medius are located along the iliac crest, each in one of the three portions of the muscle. The first trigger point is found along the underside of the crest, near the sacroiliac joint. The pain pattern is along the iliac crest and over the sacroiliac joint and sacrum. The second trigger point is at the center point of the iliac crest, dividing it in two equal portions, front and back, and just below the lip. It refers pain to the middle of the gluteal region and sometimes down the outside of the thigh. The third point is much less common than the other two. It is found near the anterior superior iliac spine, again just below the lip of the iliac crest. Pain is referred along the iliac crest to the lower lumbar region and the sacrum.

Gluteus Minimus
Origin: Outer surface of ilium between the middle and inferior gluteal lines.
Insertion: Anterior border of greater trochanter of femur.
Action: Hip abduction, medial rotation of hip.

Trigger point pain from gluteus minimus is characteristically deep and quite severe. It projects down the leg more so than referred pain from the other gluteal muscles. There are two portions of the muscle. Trigger points in the anterior portion lie along the fibers vertically in a line to the greater trochanter. They refer pain to the lower buttock region and along the side of the thigh, sometimes all the way down to the ankle. Trigger points in the posterior portion accumulate in a fan-shaped pattern across the muscle near its origin on the ilium. The pain pattern will cover the buttock and run down the back of the thigh, over the knee to the posterior calf region.

- Perform elongation strokes with the forearm, elbow, or fist, in strips, from the lateral portion of the iliac crest to the upper portion of the femur just below the greater trochanter.
- Taut bands may be palpated by rolling across the fibers of the muscle with the fingertips or elbow. Treat trigger points as they are found.

3. Lateral Rotators (Piriformis, Obturator Internus, Gemellus Superior, Gemellus Inferior, Obturator Externus, Quadratus Femoris)

Piriformis
Origin: Anterior surface of sacrum, sacrotuberous ligament.
Insertion: Superior border of medial aspect of greater trochanter of femur.
Action: Lateral rotation of hip.

Obturator Internus
Origin: Margin of obturator foramen on pelvis, ramus of ischium, inferior ramus of pubis, pelvic surface of obturator membrane.

Insertion: Medial surface of greater trochanter of femur.
Action: Lateral rotation of hip.

Gemellus Superior
Origin: Gluteal surface of ischial spine.
Insertion: Superior border of greater trochanter.
Action: Lateral rotation of hip.

Gemellus Inferior
Origin: Superior surface of ischial tuberosity.
Insertion: Superior border of greater trochanter.
Action: Lateral rotation of hip.

Obturator Externus
Origin: Medial margin of obturator foramen formed by rami of pubis and ischium.
Insertion: Trochanteric fossa of femur.
Action: Lateral rotation of hip.

Quadratus Femoris
Origin: Lateral border of ischial tuberosity.
Insertion: Quadrate tubercle on posterior aspect of femur.
Action: Lateral rotation of hip.

- Apply short side-to-side strokes with the elbow or thumbs next to the border of the sacrum to contact the medial portion of the piriformis near its origin on the anterior sacrum (A in Fig. 9-13).
- Perform an elongation stroke with the elbow, fist, or heel of the hand, from the border of the sacrum to the greater trochanter, following the length of the piriformis from origin to insertion (B in Fig. 9-13).

 Be careful doing this move as the piriformis covers the sciatic notch, where the sciatic nerve surfaces from the pelvis. Pressure on the sciatic nerve causes a shooting pain down the posterior thigh and should be avoided.

- Roll across the fibers of the lateral rotator muscles with the fingertips or elbow, from the border of the sacrum to the greater trochanter. Treat trigger points as they are found.
- Apply static compression and cross fiber strokes against the insertion points of the muscles on the greater trochanter, using the elbow or thumbs (C in Fig. 9-13).

4. Sacral Ligaments

Sacrotuberous Ligament
- Palpate the lateral edge of the sacrum just above the coccyx. Palpate the ischial tuberosity on the same side of the pelvis. The ligament runs between these two locations (Fig. 9-14).

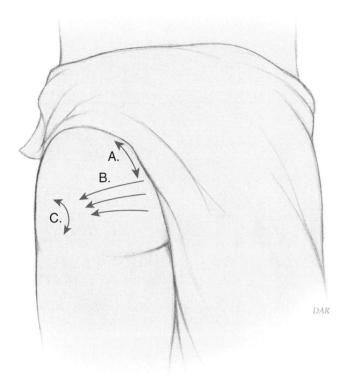

FIGURE 9-13 Directions of strokes on the lateral rotator muscles.

- Starting just lateral to the sacral edge, slide both thumbs under the gluteal muscles, then press up in a superior direction until you feel a dense, taut band of tissue.

Move the thumbs slowly side to side along the ligament, checking for tenderness. Hold painful areas with static compression for 8 to 12 seconds.

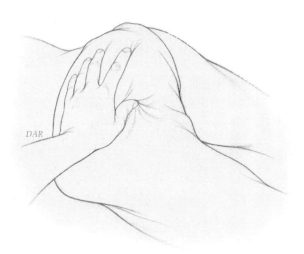

FIGURE 9-14 Contacting the sacrotuberous ligament.

Posterior Sacroiliac Ligament

Injuries to this ligament will project pain across the low back and perhaps into the groin, thigh, and leg on the injured side.

- Locate the posterior superior iliac spine with your thumbs. Press in and up on the underside of it with the thumb pads (Fig. 9-15). Perform short cross fiber strokes against the edge of the bone.
- With your fingertips, do short up-and-down and side-to-side strokes on the sacrum, covering the entire surface.

Stretches

Position

The client is lying supine, with the leg to be stretched extended along the table and the other leg flexed, with the sole of the foot against the table.

The therapist stands at the side of the table near the client's foot.

1. *Hamstrings*—using your inside hand, hold the client's foot behind the heel and lift the straight leg off the table. You may place the client's leg against your shoulder for additional support. Your other hand is placed on the client's anterior thigh. Stretch the leg by pressing forward and upward on the heel. Press against the anterior thigh with your other hand or forearm to encourage the knee to straighten (Fig. 9-16).
2. *Gluteus maximus*—the client's knee is brought to his or her chest. The client and therapist both place their hands over the knee. As the client draws the knee toward his or her chest, lean forward to apply additional impetus to the stretch (Fig. 9-17).
3. *Gluteus medius and minimus*—holding the client's ankle, bring the client's straight leg across his or her body to an adducted position. Rotating the leg laterally so that the toes and knee are facing upward, press the leg downward in the direction of the table until a stretch is felt in the gluteals (Fig. 9-18).
4. *Lateral rotators*—the leg of the side to be stretched is flexed at the knee and hip. The other leg is also flexed at the knee and hip, with the sole of the foot against the table. Holding the client's knee and ankle, turn the knee out and place the client's foot against the thigh of the client's other leg. As the foot rests there, take hold of the knee and ankle of the supporting leg and bring it toward the client's chest, sandwiching the foot of the stretched side between the client's chest and shoulder. Continue to bring the thigh toward the chest until a stretch is felt in the lateral rotator muscles (Fig. 9-19).

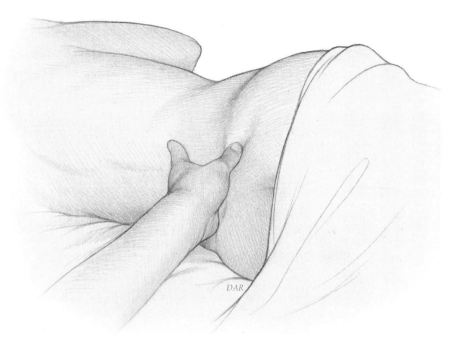

FIGURE 9-15   Contacting the posterior sacroiliac ligament.

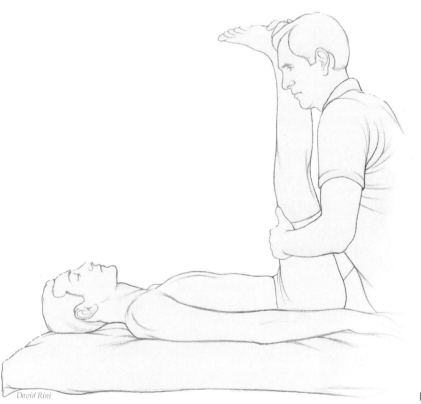

FIGURE 9-16   Hamstring stretch.

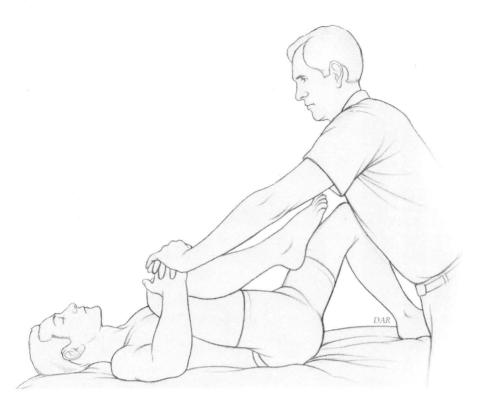

FIGURE 9-17   Gluteus maximus stretch.

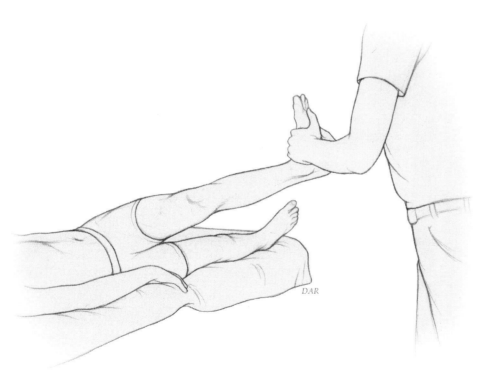

FIGURE 9-18   Stretch for gluteus medius and minimus.

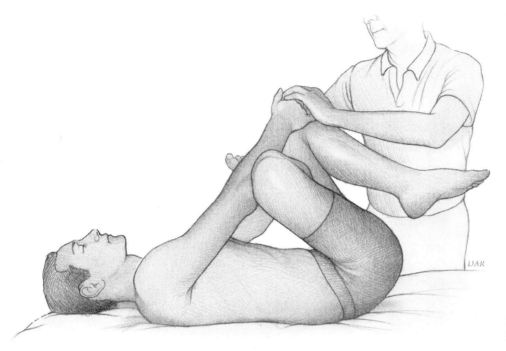

FIGURE 9-19 Stretch for the lateral rotators.

Accessory Work

1. This session is complemented with work on the rectus abdominus muscle, which, when shortened, contributes to posterior pelvic tilt along with shortened hamstrings.
2. Polarity balancing of the cranium and feet reinforces the release work that was done with the sacrum in this session.

Closing

- Sitting at the head of the table, lightly cup the client's head in both your hands and hold for at least 30 seconds, allowing the client to relax and assimilate the effects of the session.
- Move to the foot of the table. Lightly cup the client's heels with your hands. Hold for at least 30 seconds. Remove your hands slowly to complete the session.

THE PELVIS AND ABDOMEN

INTRODUCTION

The pelvis forms the body's core. Functionally, it is analogous to the hub of a wheel, with the spine and limbs acting as spokes radiating from it. The pelvis serves four main purposes:

1. It houses and protects the vital organs.
2. It provides attachment sites for the muscles that control the trunk, legs, and arms.
3. It absorbs and distributes the shock that is transferred up the lower limbs in movement activities like walking.
4. It transfers the weight of the upper body to the legs and feet.

The pelvic bones create a series of arches and curves that when joined together form a bowl. This shape allows weight to be easily moved around and through the pelvis without jarring the bowl's contents. The pelvis is a highly mobile structure, able to alter its position to accommodate weight shifts brought about by the movement of body segments above and below it. The pelvis moves freely between the spine and the heads of the femora with its position mostly determined by muscular action.

The muscles of the thigh and trunk that attach to the pelvis must be balanced for correct pelvic alignment. Chronic shortness in any of these muscles creates compensatory tightening in other muscles, ligaments, and fascia, leading to stress and dysfunction in the hips and low back. Releasing chronic muscular tension patterns in the pelvis is a primary concern of the deep tissue therapist. The body as a whole cannot become integrated until the process of relaxing the core is initiated.

The primary pelvic muscle group is the iliopsoas. The psoas is the major integration muscle for the entire body.

It connects the spine to the thigh and contributes to determining the pelvis' position. When the psoas is functioning properly, the body's movements come under the control of the core, giving increased power, grace, and stamina.

The area of the trunk joining the pelvis and ribcage is known as the abdomen. The entire region is wrapped in muscles and fascial sheaths. The muscles of the abdomen are responsible for the movements of forward and lateral flexion as well as rotation of the trunk. These muscles attach along the ribs and the pelvic rim. They provide support and protection for the abdominal organs. The deepest muscle of the abdomen is the quadratus lumborum. It forms the back of the abdominal wall and contributes to extension and lateral flexion of the spine. The abdominal muscles work in conjunction with the back muscles to maintain pelvic alignment from above.

Correct alignment of the pelvis is crucial for maintaining the health and vitality of the abdominal organs. Poor posture compresses the organs and diminishes their efficiency. Sluggish or irregular function of the intestines is a major problem affecting a high percentage of the population. The factors contributing to intestinal dysfunction include poor diet, lack of exercise, inadequate intake of water, and lack of tone and balance of the abdominal muscles. Proper intestinal activity is encouraged by deep tissue massage.

MUSCULOSKELETAL ANATOMY AND FUNCTION (ESSENTIAL ANATOMY BOXES 9-2 AND 9-3)

The pelvis is made up of three pairs of bones: the ilia, the ischia, and the pubic bones. The ilium bones brace the sacrum, which is situated in the center of the back of the pelvis. The articulation of the ilium and sacrum is called the sacroiliac joint. The ilia flare in the back in a fan shape. They taper as they curve around to the front, fusing with the pubic bones. The pubic bones join in the front of the pelvis at the pubic symphysis, a moveable joint with a disc between the two bones. The ilia and pubic bones join with the ischia. The acetabulum is a cavity formed where the three pelvic bones join. It consists of equal portions of the ilium, pubic bone, and ischium. This arrangement allows equal forces from all three bones in the pelvis to pass to the hip joint.

The sacrum is the keystone for the human skeleton. Weight from the upper body accumulates at the sacrum. It then passes from the sacroiliac joints across the ilia to the hip joints and, when a person is standing, from there to the heads of the femora. In a seated position, the weight is transferred to the ischial tuberosities, which are ring-shaped projections at the base of the ischia. This balanced weight transfer depends on soft tissue interaction to keep the joints aligned. The sacrum is subject to a variety of displacements, including slight rotation and posterior deviation, but by far the most common aberration is anterior displacement.

Weight pressing on the sacrum tends to shift the upper portion forward, causing it to become displaced below the fifth lumbar vertebra. This tendency is counteracted by strong ligaments that wrap the sacrum and prevent it from sliding. The attachment of the **piriformis** muscle to the front side of the sacrum also contributes to its stability. When the sacrum shifts, it causes irritation and pain in the sacroiliac joints and disrupts the sequence of weight transfer through the lower body. The piriformis muscles

Muscles	Bones and Landmarks	
Rectus abdominus	Costal cartilage	**ESSENTIAL ANATOMY BOX 9–2**
External obliques	Ilium	
Internal obliques	Anterior superior iliac spine (ASIS)	
Transverse abdominus	Pubic bone	
	Inguinal ligament	
	Small intestine	
	Areas of the colon: Ascending, transverse, descending	*The Abdominal Routines*
	Ileocecal valve	
	Appendix	
	Hepatic and splenic flexures	
	Sigmoid colon and rectum	
	Aorta	

Muscles	Bones and Landmarks
Psoas major and minor	Ilium
Iliacus	Iliac crest
Rectus abdominus	Ischium
Obliques-external and	Pubic symphysis
internal	Sacrum
Gluteus maximus, medius,	Sacroiliac joint
and minimus	Lesser trochanter of the femur
Inguinal ligament	

become contracted as they attempt to stabilize the sacrum and pass this tightness to the other lateral rotator muscles. During massage work, the therapist should never press down hard on a client's sacrum, as this causes it to slide anteriorly, creating the problems described above.

The base of the pelvis is a diaphragm composed of muscles and ligaments, known as the pelvic floor. The principle muscle is the levator ani, which operates like a sling supporting the pelvic organs above it. It attaches to the inner surfaces of the pubic bones and ischia in the front, then runs posteriorly, around the genitals and anus, to attach in the back to the coccyx. The fascia that wraps this muscle is a continuation of the fascia of the inner thigh muscles, thus creating an essential bond between the pelvis and inner thigh. The degree of tightness in the inner thighs affects the condition of the internal pelvic structures. When the pelvic floor is constricted, it pulls the bones of the pelvic bowl closer together, creating compression and restriction of function in the pelvic region. For women, childbirth is much easier when the pelvic floor is able to relax. Impact injuries to the coccyx have a major effect on the tone of the levator ani muscle.

The iliopsoas is made up of three muscles, **iliacus, psoas major**, and **psoas minor**, each having a slightly different purpose (Fig. 9-20). The psoas major muscle attaches to the bodies of the 12th thoracic vertebra and the 5 lumbar vertebrae. It passes over the pelvis, like a sling, and inserts on the lesser trochanter on the inside of the femur.

When the hip joints are stable, the psoas major flexes the trunk on the legs, as in the action of a sit-up. In this capacity the psoas works in conjunction with the rectus abdominis muscle. Flexion of the spine should be initiated by the psoas since it is positioned closer to the spine. It is then reinforced by the action of the abdominal muscles. In disorganized movement patterns, the rectus abdominus muscle does most of the work while the psoas remains inactive.

The range of influence of the psoas major muscle is

extensive. The origin of the psoas on the 12 thoracic vertebra is very close to the attachments of the crura of the diaphragm. Inadequate functioning of the psoas can influence the position and action of the diaphragm, thus affect-

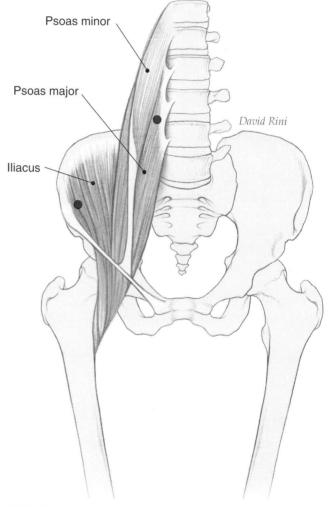

David Rini

FIGURE 9-20   The iliopsoas group.

ing respiration. The psoas also affects autonomic function in that the lumbar plexus passes through it. The nerves of this plexus control the abdominal viscera. Therefore, the general health and well-being of the body is tied to the condition of the psoas.

The psoas minor has its origin at the 12th thoracic vertebra and inserts on the ilium bone. It connects the spine with the pelvis and assists in flexion of the trunk and lumbar spine.

The iliacus muscle originates on the iliac crest and the anterior surface the ilium. It joins the psoas major in its insertion on the lesser trochanter of the femur. The iliacus connects the pelvis with the legs, giving increased power to hip flexion movements, like running and kicking. These three muscles, acting as a group, provide force and stability to the body's central core.

The muscles of the abdomen are the **rectus abdominus**, the **external obliques, internal obliques,** and the **transverse abdominus**. In addition to providing support for the abdominal contents, they are important accessory breathing muscles. As they collectively contract during exhalation, they push the diaphragm back up into position for inhalation.

The rectus abdominus forms the most superficial layer of the abdominal wall and connects the ribcage to the pelvis at the pubic bone. When it contracts, it draws the base of the pelvis upward, causing the top of the pelvis to tip posteriorly. In this action, it is the antagonist to the psoas major when a person is standing. In the standing position, when the psoas major contracts, it pulls the lumbar spine forward, causing the top of the pelvis to tilt anteriorly. The balancing action of the rectus abdominus and psoas muscles as an agonist–antagonist pair is essential for proper alignment and coordinated movement of the body as a whole.

The external obliques, acting together, also flex the spine. Unilaterally, they laterally flex the trunk and cause rotation to the opposite side. The fibers of the external obliques angle toward the midline, matching the direction of the external intercostal muscles.

The internal obliques duplicate the actions of the external obliques, except that when acting unilaterally they rotate the trunk to the same side (i.e., the right internal oblique rotates the trunk to the right, and the left internal oblique rotates the trunk to the left). The fibers of the internal obliques angle away from the midline, matching the direction of the internal intercostal muscles.

The transverse abdominus is the deepest of these three muscles. Its fibers run in a horizontal direction. It acts to compress the abdominal contents. Its strong contraction causes regurgitation.

The **quadratus lumborum** forms the posterior wall of the abdomen. It is situated behind the psoas muscle. The quadratus lumborum consists of three sections, which have their origin on the inner lip of the iliac crest and the iliolumbar ligaments. The insertions are on the lower border of the 12th rib and the transverse processes of the first 4 lumbar vertebrae. The muscle is wrapped in thoracolumbar fascia.

The quadratus lumborum is a strong stabilizer of the lumbar spine. It prevents excessive lateral bending to the opposite side. Acting bilaterally, the quadratus lumborum extends the spine. When overly contracted, it contributes to increased lordosis. Unilaterally, the muscle assists in lateral flexion to the same side. The quadratus lumborum is known as "the hip hiker." In a standing position, if the upper border of one of the iliac crests is higher than the upper border of the other, the quadratus lumborum on that side will be shortened.

CONDITIONS (INDICATIONS/ CONTRAINDICATIONS BOXES 9-2 AND 9-3)

1. *Anterior pelvic tilt* is a forward tipping of the ilium that creates an increased lumbar curve and often a protrusion of the abdomen. If the pelvis is visualized

Indications	Contraindications	INDICATIONS/ CONTRAINDICATIONS BOX 9-2
Constipation	Diverticulitis	
Low back pain	Severe hypertension	
Colitis	Pregnancy	
Distended belly	Severe illness	
Poor digestion	Recent surgery	*Conditions Affecting Abdominal Massage*
Gas	Skin rash	
Stomach ache	Recent heavy meal	
Menstrual cramps	Ulcer	

as a bowl filled with water, the water would be spilling in front of the person. The iliopsoas and rectus femoris on both sides will be shortened, causing compression of the vertebral discs and strain on the soft tissues of the lower back.

2. *Posterior pelvic tilt* is a backward tipping of the ilium. It causes the buttocks to appear tucked under. It is often accompanied by contraction in the gluteal muscles, a tight rectus abdominus, and shortened hamstrings. The erector spinae muscles will be pulled downward and the lumbar curve will be diminished, which will affect the transfer of weight through the spine.

3. *"Short leg"* is a general term, describing a lateral tilt of the pelvis, presumably because one leg is shorter than the other, causing the pelvis to lean toward the short side. In most cases, however, the unevenness of the pelvis is due to spinal curves or twists. The shortened side is often indicative of a tight psoas and quadratus lumborum muscle.

   Differences in length between the right and left psoas can also lead to pelvic rotation. The pelvis will be pulled forward and down on the side of the shortened psoas.

4. *Sciatica* is an irritation or inflammation of the sciatic nerve, which exits the spinal cord at L4–S3 and runs down the back of the leg. Compression and/or misalignment of the lumbar spine and sacrum can be responsible for the condition. In this case, the pathway of pain usually extends down the back of the leg, sometimes to the ankle.

   In some cases, the source of irritation is at the site of the piriformis muscle at the back of the hip, which the sciatic nerve passes under. (In some people, the sciatic nerve passes *through* the piriformis.) If tightness in the piriformis is the source of the irritation, the pain is usually localized at the hip and back of the thigh.

5. *Psoas strain.* The psoas muscle is difficult to pull but may become strained from extreme stretching motions of the trunk and groin, as in a jump initiated from a crouched position. This kind of injury is common in basketball players reaching for the hoop and in volleyball players. To test for psoas impairment, have the client sit on the edge of the table, with the feet hanging toward the floor. Place your hand on the thigh of the side you are checking. Have the client try to lift the thigh as you resist. If the psoas is injured, the client will experience pain in the groin area.

6. *Premenstrual syndrome and menstrual cramps.* Premenstrual syndrome occurs several days before menstruation. It can induce irritability, mood changes, pain in the pelvic region, headache, and water retention, among other symptoms. A hormonal factor is suspected in premenstrual syndrome. Deep tissue massage has been shown to have a beneficial effect on both of these conditions.[1] The relaxation of the pelvic muscles helps to diminish tension and takes pressure off the abdominal organs.

7. *Pelvic inflammatory disease* is caused by a bacterial infection, which can involve the vagina, uterus, fallopian tubes, and broad ligaments. It is a painful condition that requires medical treatment and is contraindicated for massage therapy.

8. *Abuse issues.* It is not uncommon for both male and female clients to have experienced sexual abuse, either as children or adults. As a result, they may be afraid of having the pelvic area touched. This work can be sensitive for anyone to receive, because of the societal taboos imposed on the pelvic region due to our attitudes about sex and the eliminative functions. As a therapist, always approach this work sensitively, respecting the client's limitations. It may take time for the client to fully come to terms with all the issues lodged in the pelvic area. Be patient and nurturing, allowing healing to unfold at its own pace.

   Abdominal massage should be introduced slowly to a client with a history of abuse or with concerns about having the abdominal area touched. It may take several sessions before the client is comfortable with having that area worked on. Initial contact with the abdomen may consist of gentle contact; simply holding the hands there while the client relaxes. Keeping the abdomen covered with a drape while touching it often adds to the client's sense of safety. This contact may be included in several sessions before full abdominal massage is attempted. Abdominal work should never be performed without the client's willingness and permission.

9. *Constipation.* The backup of waste matter in the intestinal tract is one of the major causes of toxic buildup in the body, which allows disease conditions to develop.[2] Several factors contribute to constipation, including poor diet, lack of abdominal tone, and inadequate intake of water. Deep tissue massage is very helpful in breaking down impacted fecal matter that is adhered to the intestinal walls so that it may move through the colon and be eliminated properly.

10. *Ileocecal valve dysfunction.* The ileocecal is a one-way valve located at the junction of the small intestine and the large intestine. This valve prevents the back-up of feces from the colon into the sterile environment of the small intestine. When this valve becomes weakened and breaks down, the waste material can enter the small intestine, creating a toxic environment that eventually makes its way to other organs via the bloodstream.[3] Lack of abdominal tone and support around the valve when eliminating is one of the primary causes of its weakening. Learning to eliminate from a squatting position is beneficial for maintaining the integrity of the ileocecal valve.

11. *Diverticulitis* is an inflammatory condition of the colon. Diverticula are tiny pouches in the colon wall filled with fecal matter. They are created by pressure from straining to push feces through the colon. When these sacs of waste material become inflamed they cause pain. This condition is a contraindication to massage work.

12. *Colitis* is an inflammation of the colon. Although its cause is unknown, episodes can be exacerbated by psychological factors, such as stress, worry, and anxiety. It is often accompanied by spasms of the colon muscles. Light massage on the abdomen may be beneficial between flare-ups.

13. *Prolapsed bowel* is a collapse of the transverse colon caused by the buildup of feces. The increased weight pulls the colon downward, resulting in pressure on the bladder, which may cause urine retention.[4] In women there may also be pressure on the fallopian tubes or the ovaries; in men, there may be pressure on the prostate gland.

14. *Pot belly.* Excess weight in the abdominal region has many negative effects. The displacement of weight puts excessive pressure on the low back and moves the abdominal organs out of position, inhibiting their proper function. Increased intra-abdominal pressure pushes the diaphragm upward, inhibiting full breathing and putting pressure on the heart. A distended, bloated belly is often the result of a build-up of feces and the resultant stagnant gases. Maintaining strong abdominal muscles contributes to proper alignment of the torso and helps to reduce pot belly conditions.

THE MIND/BODY CONNECTION

The pelvis is the body's structural center. All parts of the body come into equilibrium when balanced around the pelvis. Muscles function with their maximum efficiency in this alignment, and neuromuscular patterns generate smooth, flowing, stress-free movement. The pelvis acts as the focal point of the body, much like the hub does for a wheel. Feeling and acting from this centered place means that we operate freely from an instinctual level, not having to control movements and impulses but surrendering to the natural grace of the body and consciousness.

However, few of us function at this level of balance. For the most part, we feel our identity and initiate our actions from a place farther up in the body. The emphasis placed on intellectual processes draws most people's awareness up toward the head. Muscular initiation of movement tends to occur more from the chest and thoracic region of the spine. This not only strains the muscles responsible for breathing, but disconnects us from the more powerful and effective muscles of motion originating in the hips and thighs.

These core muscles correspond with our more instinctive nature. When living out of our core, we are more prone to incorporate feeling and intuition into our bodily experience. A more complete integration of all the modes of cognition becomes available to us. We begin to reclaim our full stature as human beings.

The pelvis houses the organs of reproduction and elimination. Culturally, we are not comfortable with these functions. Many societal constraints and restrictions are placed on both. Children are often trained to control defecation at too young of an age, before the muscles of the pelvis have developed sufficiently to operate fully in this capacity. As a result, a young child, in a vain attempt to stop elimination, will squeeze the sphincters and the muscles around them with a great deal of effort, creating a high degree of constriction in the pelvic floor and inner thighs.[5] This forms the basis of a potentially lifelong pattern of associating maintaining control with tightening the pelvic floor and inner thighs. In adults, this pattern can also be seen in rigidly contracted gluteal muscles.

Sexual issues are another area in which conflict between natural impulses and societal dictates creates inhibition in the pelvic structures. The sexual drive is a potent force that has many moral codes attached to it, defining how and where it is to be expressed. Many people withdraw from or suppress this energy by clamping down on the muscles of the pelvis, inner thigh, and/or the low back. The psychiatrist Wilhelm Reich theorized that most conditions of neurosis are created by the conflict imposed by the suppression of the sexual urge along with other expressions of the primary life force.[6]

The pelvis is designed to swing freely between the hip joints and lumbar spine. This capability can be severely limited by chronic muscular contractions in and around the pelvic region. Voluntary muscle action is controlled by the nervous system, which is ultimately under the jurisdiction of the mind. Therefore, our mental attitudes and beliefs play an important part in determining our body posture. Because of the extent of muscular interaction in determining pelvic positioning, we have a tremendous capacity to distort pelvic placement and movement through our responses to the issues associated with this body segment. Observation of a person's core may reveal much about their beliefs about control and surrender as well as attitudes about sex.[7] Some typical examples of pelvic misalignment contributed to by sexual suppression are the anterior tilt of the pelvic bowl, a tucking under of the hips, and constriction across the lumbar muscles. All of these denote some form of muscular imbalance inhibiting complete mobility of the pelvis. Clients who are interested in pursuing this subject further may be referred to a psychologist who has studied a Reichian-based approach to psychotherapy, such as bioenergetics.

The abdomen is a cylinder of soft tissue covering the viscera. Having no bony protection, this area is commonly perceived as vulnerable and weak. A feeling of apprehension is often associated with touching this body segment, partly because of a common revulsion with anything associated with the "guts."

Energetically speaking, the pelvis and abdomen are associated with the lower portion of the spine, which contains the first three chakras. The first chakra, at the base of the spine, deals with survival and security issues. The second chakra, located at the sacrum, relates to our emotional nature and ability to experience pleasure. Both of these chakras are intertwined with feelings and experiences processed through the pelvis. The third chakra, in the navel/solar plexus region, is concerned with the intellect and our sense of personal power. This chakra is physically manifested through the condition of the abdomen.

The image of the tight, washboard abdomen is considered a desirable one by most people. We are enticed by TV commercials and videos extolling the virtues of a trim, tight mid-section. By overly tightening the abdominal muscles, we effectively restrict our feelings, creating a shield of armor around our perceived vulnerabilities in an attempt to protect ourselves from our emotions.

A truly balanced abdomen has a slightly rounded contour to it. It is supple and toned, not cinched in tight. Neither is it flaccid and weak, allowing the abdomen to protrude and disorganizing the alignment of the lumbar spine and ribcage.

The abdomen and pelvis are closely related to our emotional nature. Generally, we are not encouraged to follow our emotions and allow them to thrive. We are more often directed toward rationality and the use of logic as our major mode of operation. Giving into emotions is often viewed as a form of indulgence. Again, balance is the key. When the muscles of the pelvis and abdomen are working in conjunction with each other to maintain the integrity of the trunk, the ability to experience emotions, process them, and take appropriate action or not, according to the dictates of the moment, is enhanced. Balance in the mid-section is reflective of a quality of poise and integrity that allows one to fully experience the kinesthetic unity of the body without getting caught up in distorted perceptions that manifest as chronic tightness and postural aberrations.

POSTURAL EVALUATION (TABLE 9-2)

THE PELVIS: FRONT VIEW

1. Check the level of the iliac crests. Are they on the same horizontal line?
2. Look for rotation of the pelvis. If one anterior superior iliac spine (ASIS) is more prominent than the other one, it indicates that side of the pelvis is rotated forward.
3. Is there space between the ribcage and the iliac crests, or does the waist area seem compressed, forming bulges at the sides (love handles)?
4. When the client's knees are flexed do they align over the feet properly? Incorrect tracking of the knees over the feet will affect psoas function.
5. Does the pelvis seem too large or too small for the rest of the body?

THE PELVIS: SIDE VIEW

1. Observe the direction and degree of pelvic tilt, if any.
2. From a standing position, can the pelvis swing forward and backward freely? In which motion is it restricted?

THE ABDOMINAL REGION (TABLE 9-3)

1. Check the position of the lower ribs.
   - Squeezed together, pulling downward.
   - Spread apart, lifted, protruding.
2. General shape of the abdomen.
   - Tight, withdrawn, held in.
   - Distended.
   - Lower belly larger—may indicate a constipated condition.
   - Upper belly larger—may indicate build-up of gases from the intestines.

TABLE 9–2	Body Reading for the Pelvis	
Conditions	**Muscles that May Be Shortened**
Anterior tilt—the iliac crests are tipped forward	Iliopsoas Rectus femoris Erector spinae Quadratus lumborum
Posterior tilt—the iliac crests are tipped backward	Rectus abdominus Gluteus maximus Lateral rotators Hamstrings
Lateral tilt—one iliac crest is higher than the other	Gluteus medius Quadratus lumborum Abductors on high side Adductors on low side

3. Describe the distribution of fat content.
4. Does the belly move with the breath?

EXERCISES AND SELF-TREATMENT

PELVIS

Pelvic Opening (Integrates Muscular Action in the Pelvis and Low Back Regions)

Preparation
Sit on the edge of a chair with both feet flat on the floor, or sit in a cross-legged position on the floor. Do each movement slowly and consciously. The purpose of the exercise is to increase awareness of the pelvic region.

Execution
- Roll the pelvis posteriorly, rounding the low back and taking your weight off the ischial tuberosities (Fig. 9-21A). Let your chin drop forward naturally. Return the pelvis to the vertical position. Repeat a few more times.
- Roll the pelvis anteriorly, arching the low back slightly (Fig. 9-21B). Return to the upright position and repeat several more times.
- Combine the two movements above, creating a fluid forward-and-back rocking motion of the pelvis. Rest briefly afterward, noting any changes in your level of awareness in the pelvic region.

TABLE 9–3	Body Reading for the Abdomen	
Conditions	**Muscles that May Be Shortened**
Distended belly—overall bloating accompanied by anterior tilt of the pelvis	Quadratus lumborum Iliopsoas group Rectus femoris Erector spinae
Tight midsection—rectus abdominus is overly defined, lower ribs are pulled in and down; rigid abdominal wall	Rectus abdominus Transverse abdominus Hamstrings
"Bladder belt"—upper abdominal area is distended; lower area is pulled in, as if wearing a tight belt	Obliques Pelvic floor muscles

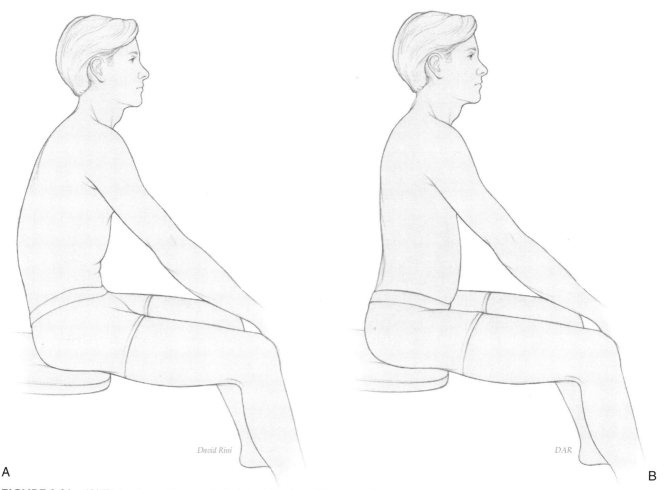

A

B

FIGURE 9-21 (**A**) Tilting the pelvis posteriorly. (**B**) Tilting the pelvis anteriorly.

■ Beginning with your weight evenly distributed over the base of the pelvis, shift slightly to the right, increasing the weight on the right ischial tuberosity. Keep the left hip on the chair or floor. Return to the center position and repeat the shift to the right several more times.

■ Beginning with your weight evenly distributed over the base of the pelvis, shift slightly to the left, increasing the weight on the left ischial tuberosity. Keep the right hip on the chair or floor. Return to the center position and repeat the shift to the left several more times.

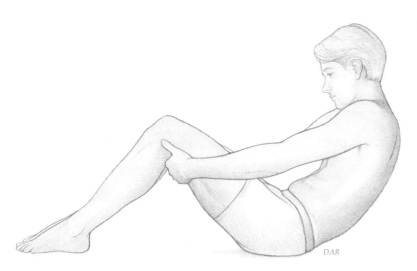

FIGURE 9-22 Sit-down exercise to strengthen rectus abdominus.

■ Combine the previous two movements, rocking your weight from side to side several times. Rest briefly afterward, noting any changes in your level of awareness in the pelvic region.

ABDOMEN

2. Sit-Downs (Strengthens Rectus Abdominus, External and Internal Obliques, Transverse Abdominus)

Preparation
Sitting on the floor, bring your knees to your chest with both feet remaining on the floor. Place your hands under the thighs just above the knees.

Execution
Exhaling, pull your abdomen in and tuck your pelvis under as you roll down the back slightly (Fig. 9-22). Hold for a few seconds as you breathe normally, then exhale strongly and roll down the back a little farther. Continue to roll toward the floor in small increments. If your back begins to hurt or the abdominal muscles cannot support the rolling motion any further, lie down on your back and rest.

3. Abdominal Stretch (Stretches Rectus Abdominus, External and Internal Obliques, Transverse Abdominus)

Lying on your back on the floor, extend your arms overhead. Exhaling, press the low back to the floor as you reach the arms behind you, until you feel a stretch in the abdominal muscles (Fig. 9-23). Hold for 20 seconds. Slightly arching the back increases the stretch. Laterally flex the trunk to the right by reaching both arms slightly to the right. Hold for 20 seconds. Laterally flex the trunk to the left by reaching both arms slightly to the left. Hold for 20 seconds.

ABDOMINAL MUSCLES ROUTINE

OBJECTIVES
■ To elongate the portion of the trunk that connects the thorax and pelvis.
■ To release the attachments of the trunk muscles along the pelvis and the lower ribs.
■ To separate the abdominal muscles so that each may function optimally.
■ To release shortness in the quadratus lumborum muscle, which can contribute to low back pain and misalignment of the pelvis.

ENERGY

Position
The client is lying supine on the table, with a bolster under the knees.

The therapist is standing at the side of the table next to the client's waist.

Polarity
Place the left palm (negative pole) on the abdomen (positive pole). Slide the right palm (positive pole) underneath the client's back to contact the lumbar spine (negative pole). Your palms should be aligned to each other vertically through the client's trunk. Keep your hands relaxed, allowing them to mold to the contours of the client's body and to be moved by the motions generated by the client's breathing action. During this polarity hold you should project feelings of trust and nurturing, allowing the client to become accustomed to being touched in the abdominal region. Hold for at least 1 minute.

Shiatsu
Slide the fingers of both hands under the client's back, palpating the lateral edge of the erector spinae in the lum-

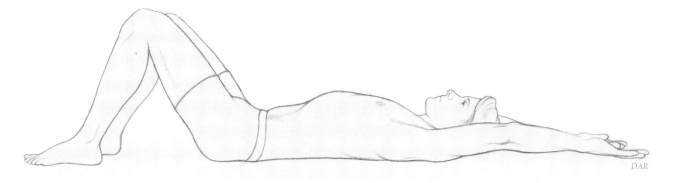

FIGURE 9-23 Stretch for rectus abdominus.

bar region with your fingertips. Straighten the fingers, allowing the weight of the client's trunk to rest on your fingertips. Repeat on the other side of the back. The outer branch of the bladder channel runs along the lateral border of the erector spinae. This move helps to relax tightness in the muscles of the low back, allowing the lumbar spine to decompress.

SWEDISH/CROSS FIBER

1. Perform circular effleurage on the abdomen.
2. Perform two-handed pétrissage on both sides of the torso between the ribcage and pelvis.
3. Perform circular friction around the abdomen in a clockwise direction.
4. Perform fingertip raking across the abdominal muscles.

CONNECTIVE TISSUE

Place your right palm on the abdomen, over the navel area. Place your left palm on top of your right hand. Begin to make a slow clockwise spiraling motion, moving the skin over the underlying tissues. Do not glide over the skin. Gradually increase the size of the spiral, stretching the skin and fascia to their maximum degree.

DEEP TISSUE/NMT

Sequence

1. Abdominal muscle attachments on the iliac crest
2. Inferior border of the costal cartilage of the ribs
3. Abdominal muscle attachments on the ribs
4. Rectus abdominus
5. Obliques—external and internal
6. Transverse abdominus
7. Quadratus lumborum
   12th rib attachment—tendon
   Iliac crest attachment—tendon
   Belly—muscle fibers

Commonly Found Trigger Points

Trigger point patterns in the abdominal muscles are not as predictable as those found in other muscle groups. Characteristically, the referred pain from these trigger points is mistaken for visceral pain. Trigger points in these muscles often cause pain bilaterally.

Check all muscle attachments thoroughly, feeling for strings and lumps that are frequently found around trigger points. The origin of the rectus abdominus at the pubic symphysis often harbors trigger points, as does its insertion along the inferior border of the ribcage just lateral to the xiphoid process.

1. Abdominal Muscle Attachments on the Iliac Crest (External and Internal Obliques, Transverse Abdominus) (Fig. 9-24)
Stand at the side of the table, facing the upper border of the client's iliac crest. Placing one or both thumbs on the upper border of the iliac crest, apply short side-to-side strokes against the inner edge of the bone. Continue around the pelvis as far as your hand can reach.

2. Inferior Border of the Costal Cartilage of Ribs 7–10 (Transverse Abdominus)
Placing the thumbs just lateral to the xiphoid process, apply short side-to-side strokes along the inferior border of the ribcage, to the tip of rib 11.

3. Abdominal Muscle Attachments on the Ribs

Rectus Abdominus
Place your fingers on the costal cartilages of ribs 5, 6, and 7 next to the xiphoid process. Using short up-and-down and side-to-side strokes with your fingertips, release the muscular attachments.

External Obliques
The attachments for this muscle are on the lower eight ribs, interweaving with the serratus anterior. Place your fingers on rib 5, near the sternum. Perform short up-and-down and side-to-side strokes on the rib. Continue to work the attachments on each rib, in succession, each time sliding your fingers a little further laterally to make contact with the muscle insertion. Use the border of the serratus anterior for a guideline.

Internal Obliques
The muscle attaches on the costal cartilages of ribs 8, 9, and 10. Place your fingers or thumbs along the lower portion of rib 8, just lateral to the rectus abdominus. Apply short side-to-side and up-and-down strokes on the attachment. Moving slightly lateral, slide down to rib 9. Repeat the same strokes on the attachment, then repeat once more on the rib 10 attachment.

4. Rectus Abdominus
Origin: Medial tendon from pubic symphysis, lateral tendon from crest of pubis.
Insertion: Costal cartilages of ribs 5, 6, and 7; xiphoid process.
Action: Flexion of spine, posterior tilt of pelvis; compresses abdominal contents.

■ Place your fingers next to the midline of the upper abdomen, just below the ribcage.
■ Slide your fingers across the fibers of the muscle, using a spreading technique (Fig. 9-25). Pause and work on abnormalities in the muscle tissue with side-to-side strokes. Release trigger points as they are found.

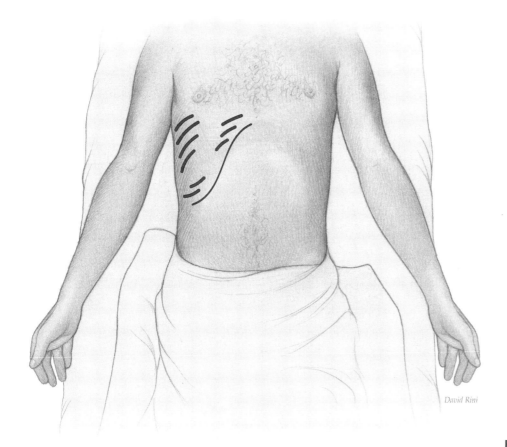

FIGURE 9-24 Abdominal muscle attachments on the ribs.

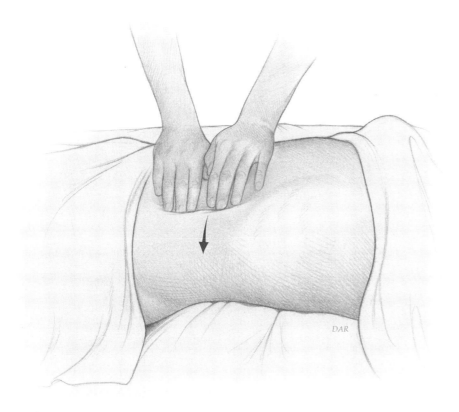

FIGURE 9-25 Cross fiber technique on rectus abdominus.

Continue, in strips, down the rectus abdominus. Be sure to palpate the tendinous sheath between each section of the muscle.

 Avoid pressure on the linea alba, which is the fascial sheath running down the midline of the rectus abdominus that joins its right and left halves. The aorta runs down the center of the trunk directly beneath this area. If you feel a strong pulse under your fingers when massaging the rectus abdominus, immediately move off it.

■ Place your thumb or fingers along the upper border of the pubic symphysis. Using short side-to-side strokes, contact the attachment of the rectus abdominus.

Note—be sure that the client is comfortable with this procedure before attempting it. Describe the move to the client first and get his or her permission to perform it.

5. External and Internal Obliques

Obliquus Externus Abdominis
Origin: Ribs 4–12, interdigitating with serratus anterior.
Insertion: Anterior part of iliac crest, abdominal aponeurosis.
Action: Flexion of trunk (bilaterally), lateral flexion of trunk and rotation of trunk (unilaterally), support and compression of abdominal viscera; assists in forced exhalation.

Obliquus Internus Abdominus
Origin: Thoracolumbar fascia, lateral two-thirds of inguinal ligament, anterior two-thirds of iliac crest.
Insertion: Cartilages of ribs 9–12, abdominal aponeurosis to linea alba.
Action: Flexion of trunk (bilaterally), lateral flexion of trunk and rotation of trunk (unilaterally), support and compression of abdominal viscera; assists in exhalation.

Begin lateral to the border of the rectus abdominus. Do a spreading stroke with your fingers across the direction of the fibers, as above. Remember that the fibers of the external obliquus angle on a lateral diagonal, so cross fiber strokes on the muscle are performed on a medial diagonal perpendicular to the fibers (Fig. 9-26A). The fibers of the internal obliquus angle on a medial diagonal, so cross fiber strokes on the muscle are performed on a lateral diagonal perpendicular to the fibers (Fig. 9-26B).

Continue outward to the lateral border of the latissimus dorsi on the side of the body. Cover the muscles thoroughly, pausing at tender areas and working in detail on tissues that feel aberrant. It is important to visualize the muscle you are working on under your fingers to be able to palpate it effectively, as the abdominal muscles overlap each other.

6. Transverse Abdominus
Origin: Lateral one-third of inguinal ligament, anterior two-thirds of lip of iliac crest, thoracolumbar fascia, costal cartilages of ribs 7–12.
Insertion: Abdominal aponeurosis to linea alba.
Action: Compresses the abdomen, assists in forced exhalation.

Place your fingers next to the lateral border of the rectus abdominus, facing in a superior direction. Apply short up-and-down strokes across the muscle fibers, covering the area between the base of the ribcage and the iliac crest thoroughly (Fig. 9-27).

7. Quadratus Lumborum
Origin: Inner lip of iliac crest, iliolumbar ligament.
Insertion: Lower border of 12th rib, transverse process of vertebrae L1–L4.
Action: Extension of lumbar spine (bilaterally), lateral flexion of spine (unilaterally), fixation and depression of 12th rib.

Trigger points in the superficial layer of the muscle are located in the lateral section, one near the attachment on the 12th rib and the other near the attachment on the iliac crest. Pain from the 12th rib attachment point is referred along the iliac crest and gluteus medius region. The referral zone for the iliac crest attachment point is to the greater trochanter and outer thigh area.

Two trigger points located in the deeper layer are found near the transverse process of L3 and between the transverse processes of L4 and L5. The trigger point at L3 refers pain to the sacroiliac joints and across the upper sacral region. The second trigger point lower down refers pain to the lower gluteal area.

Position
Place the client in side posture. Place a bolster between the knees and a small support under the side of the head. A bolster may also be placed between the side of the client's waist and the table. Have the client stretch the topmost arm overhead.

The therapist stands behind the client.

■ Place your front hand on the client's hip for support. Using the heel of your back hand, do deep circular friction on the muscles from the 12th rib to the iliac crest.
■ Slide your thumbs upward along the lateral border of the erector spinae until the 12th rib is felt. Using thumbs or a knuckle, do short side-to-side strokes across the underside of the rib to the spine. It is likely that knotted areas and trigger points will be found here.

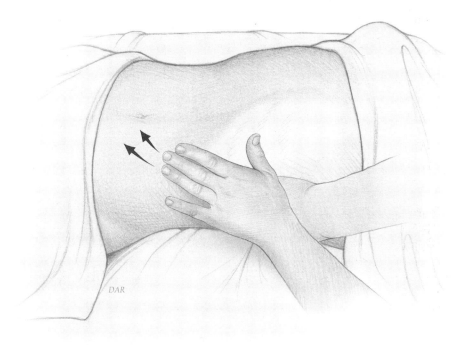

A

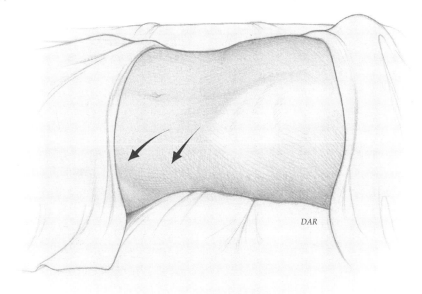

B

FIGURE 9-26   (A) Cross fiber technique on external obliques.
(B) Direction of strokes on internal obliques.

■ Turn to face the iliac crest. Apply short side-to-side strokes along the superior border of the iliac crest with knuckle or thumbs, pausing at tender points.

■ Standing behind the client's waist, place both palms on the side of the torso with the thumbs pointed downward toward the spine. Finding the edge of the erector spinae, slide the thumbs slightly anterior and press downward toward the transverse processes of the spine (Fig. 9-28). Be careful not to push into the tips of the bones. Perform short up-and-down and side-to-side strokes along the quadratus lumborum. Work between the 12th rib and the iliac crest.

Stretch

1. *Quadratus lumborum and obliques*—the client is lying in side posture. The client slides to the edge of the table near the therapist. The bottom leg is flexed at

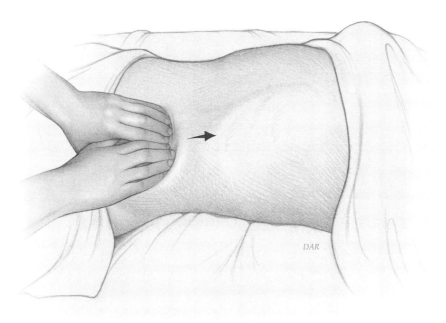

FIGURE 9-27 Cross fiber technique on transverse abdominus.

the knee, the top leg is straight, and the uppermost arm is stretched overhead, grasping the end of the table. Place one hand on the client's uppermost arm, the other hand on the client's top leg.

The straightened top leg is positioned behind the bottom leg so that it can hang off the side of the table.

Press the leg toward the floor as you push down on the top arm, until a stretch is felt in the quadratus lumborum (Fig. 9-29).

2. *Rectus abdominus*—the client is lying supine. The client slides the heels toward the hips, keeping the feet flat on the table with both knees flexed. The arms are

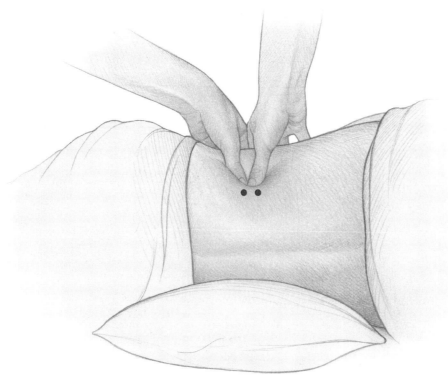

FIGURE 9-28 Contacting the lateral border of quadratus lumborum.

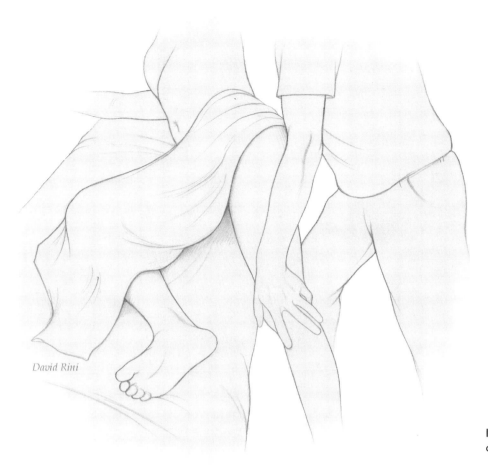

David Rini

FIGURE 9-29 Stretch for quadratus lumborum and obliques.

stretched overhead, reaching toward the head of the table (Fig. 9-30). If further stretch is required, a bolster may be slid under the client's back.

Accessory Work

1. This work should be done in conjunction with the pelvic session.

2. The solar plexus reflex point is located on the sole of the left foot slightly inferior to the bases of the metatarsal bones of the first through third toes (Fig. 9-31). Pressing this point will bring relaxation to the upper abdominal region.
3. The reflex zone for the lumbar spine is along the medial side of the instep on both feet, in the space between the first cuneiform bone and the calcaneus.

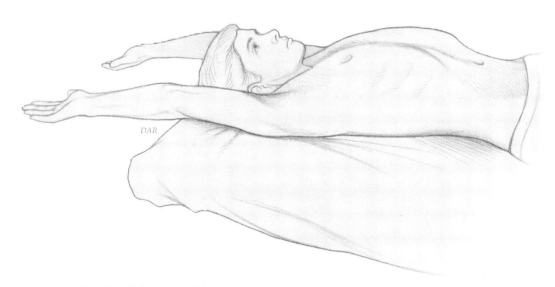

DAR

FIGURE 9-30 Stretch for rectus abdominus.

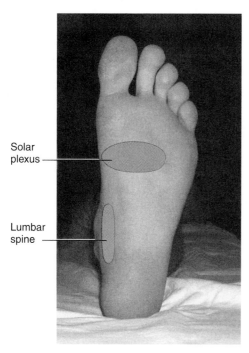

Solar plexus

Lumbar spine

FIGURE 9-31 Reflex zones on foot to accompany pelvis session.

Press this point to help relieve low back stress and pain.

Closing

Sitting at the foot of the table, lightly hold the heels of the client's feet in your hands for 30 to 60 seconds. Remove your hands slowly to complete the session.

LATERAL THIGH/INNER THIGH/INTESTINES ROUTINE

OBJECTIVES

- To balance the muscular action of the inner and outer thighs.
- To release uneven pulls on the pelvis coming from thigh muscles that attach on it.
- To improve the function of the intestines.
- To further open the abdominal cavity.

ENERGY

Position

The client is in side posture with a small pillow under the head. The leg lying against the table is slightly flexed; the top leg is flexed 90°, with a bolster placed under the knee.

The therapist is standing behind the client's hip.

Polarity

Place the palm of your top hand on the client's hip, and your bottom hand on the side of the knee. Breathe deeply and rhythmically, envisioning the client's thigh area relaxing between your two hands. Hold for at least 30 seconds.

Shiatsu

1. Top leg—using your forearm, perform Shiatsu compression movements along the side of the hip, from the iliac crest to the greater trochanter (Fig. 9-32). Both you and the client should exhale each time you lean your forearm into the hip. Continue the compression movements down the side of the leg to the knee. The gallbladder channel traverses this area.
2. Bottom leg—using your palm or the Tiger's mouth position of the hand (the webbing between the thumb and index finger), perform Shiatsu compression movements on the inner thigh from the pelvis to the knee (Fig. 9-33).

DEEP TISSUE/NMT

Sequence

Lateral Thigh
1. Vastus lateralis
2. Iliotibial tract
3. Tensor fascia latae

Inner Thigh
1. Pes anserinus
2. Adductor muscles—adductor magnus, brevis and longus; pectineus, gracilis.

Intestines
1. Large intestine
2. Small intestine

LATERAL THIGH

SWEDISH/CROSS FIBER

Position

The therapist moves to the front side of the table, facing the client's top leg.

1. Perform effleurage strokes on the top leg from the knee to the iliac crest.
2. Perform circular friction with the heel of your hand from the knee to the iliac crest.

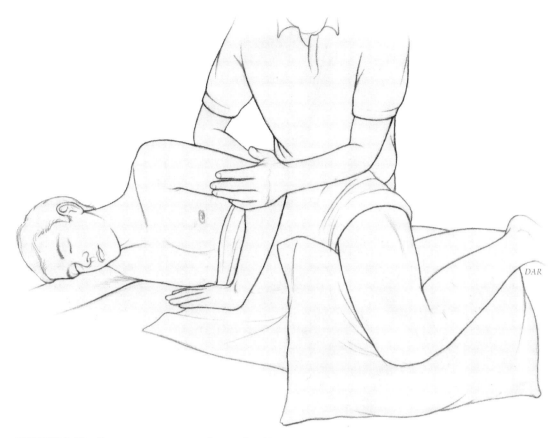

FIGURE 9-32 Forearm compression down side of hip.

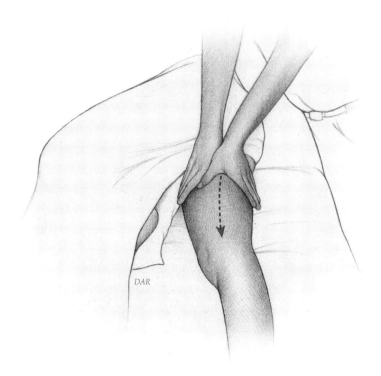

FIGURE 9-33 Tiger's mouth position on the inner thigh.

CONNECTIVE TISSUE

Myofascial Spreading

Place the heels of your hands on the midline of the thigh, at the knee. Stroke outward with both hands, spreading the tissues in opposite directions. Continue, in strips, to the iliac crest.

DEEP TISSUE/NMT

Position

The client remains in side posture.

The therapist stands at the front side of the table facing the client's flexed thigh.

1. Vastus Lateralis

Origin: Intertrochanteric line, greater trochanter, gluteal tuberosity, lateral lip of linea aspera, lateral intermuscular septum.
Insertion: Lateral border of patella, patellar ligament to tibial tuberosity.
Action: Extension of leg at knee joint.

Along the anterior portion, a group of trigger points may be found at mid-thigh level which refer pain long the length of the muscle. The majority of trigger points form along the lateral aspect of the muscle. They may be spaced just above the knee, in the middle of the thigh, and at the attachment on the upper femur.

Trigger points in the superficial fibers will fire more locally, whereas trigger points in the deeper layers shoot pain throughout the muscle and down to the side of the knee.

- Perform elongation strokes with the forearm or knuckles along the lateral thigh in the space between the rectus femoris and iliotibial tract. Pause to treat trigger points (A in Fig. 9-34).
- Perform elongation strokes with an elbow or thumbs along the distal half of the lateral thigh in the space between the iliotibial tract and biceps femoris (B in Fig. 9-34).
- Pause to treat trigger points.

2. Iliotibial Tract

With your thumbs or elbow, press a line of points along the iliotibial tract from the knee to the greater trochanter (Fig. 9-34).

3. Tensor Fascia Latae

Origin: Anterior part of outer lip of iliac crest, ASIS.
Insertion: Iliotibial tract.
Action: Flexion, abduction, medial rotation of hip.

Trigger points in this muscle usually refer pain along the iliotibial tract.

Standing behind the client at the level of the hip, place your elbow on the anterior surface of the hip. Apply short up-and-down and side-to-side strokes along the fibers of the muscle, between the iliac crest and greater trochanter (Fig. 9-35). Pause to treat trigger points.

INNER THIGH

SWEDISH/CROSS FIBER

Position

The client remains in the same position as above.

The therapist works on the inner thigh muscles of the leg that is against the table.

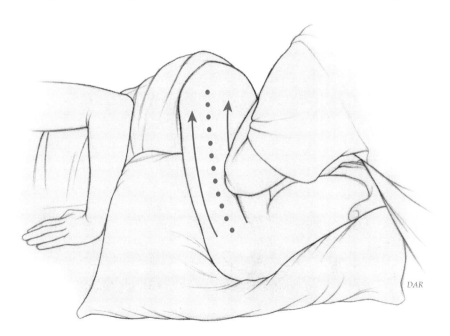

FIGURE 9-34 Deep tissue strokes on vastus lateralis and iliotibial tract.

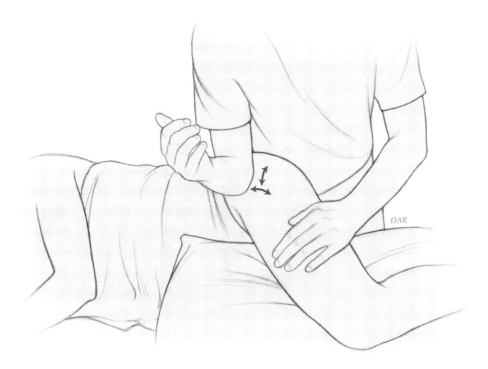

FIGURE 9-35 Position for contacting tensor fascia latae.

1. Perform effleurage strokes from the knee to the pelvis.
2. Perform circular friction on the muscle attachments at the knee.
3. Perform cross fiber fingertip raking on the adductor muscles.

CONNECTIVE TISSUE

Myofascial Spreading

Standing at the front side of the table facing the client's bottom leg, place the fingertips of both hands along the fibers of the adductor muscles, slightly above knee level. Using the spreading technique, slowly glide the fingers in a posterior direction, perpendicular to the direction of the fibers. Continue, in strips, to the pelvis.

DEEP TISSUE/NMT

Position

The client remains in side posture.

The therapist stands at the front of the table facing the inner thigh of the client's leg lying against the table.

1. Pes Anserinus (Attachment Points of Sartorius, Gracilis, and Semitendinosus)
Location—on the medial side of the proximal end of the tibia.

Press down on the insertion points on the bone with your thumbs or fingers. Move slowly up-and-down and side-to-side. Hold tender points.

2. Adductor Muscles

Adductor Magnus
Origin: Inferior ramus of pubis, inferior ramus of ischium, and inferior and lateral part of ischial tuberosity.
Insertion: Linea aspera of femur.
Action: Hip adduction, assists in hip extension and lateral rotation.

The trigger points in this muscle will probably be found in the middle portion. They project pain deep into the groin and pelvic region.

Adductor Brevis
Origin: Inferior ramus of pubis.
Insertion: Proximal third of medial lip of linea aspera, distal pectineal line.
Action: Hip adduction.

Adductor Longus
Origin: Anterior part of pubis.
Insertion: Middle third of medial lip of linea aspera.
Action: Hip adduction, assists in lateral rotation when hip is in extension.

Trigger points in these muscles are frequently located near their attachment on the pubis. Pain is referred to the upper medial thigh and into the groin region. Trigger points in the section of the muscles closer to the femur attachment will shoot pain down to the knee and perhaps over the upper tibia.

Gracilis

Origin: Inferior ramus of pubis near symphysis.
Insertion: Medial surface of shaft of tibia below tibial condyle.
Action: Hip adduction, knee flexion, assists in medial rotation of knee when leg is flexed.

There may be a trigger point found halfway up the length of the muscle and another three-quarters of the way up to the pubis. Pain from these trigger points can be intense and burning, traveling along the entire muscle.

Pectineus

Origin: Pectineal line on superior ramus of pubis.
Insertion: Femur from lesser trochanter to linea aspera.
Action: Hip adduction, assists in hip flexion.

The common trigger point is palpated on the attachment of the muscle on the pubis. It sends pain deep into the groin.

- Place the fingertips of both hands along the fibers of the adductor muscles, as in the connective tissue technique above. Use short up-and-down and side-to-side strokes on the muscle bellies to release adherent fibers and locate trigger points (Fig. 9-36).
- Find the borders of the muscles with your fingers. Slide in between the muscles and move the fingers up and

down along the borders to separate the muscles from each other. Work from the knee to the pelvis.

 Avoid any pressure in the femoral triangle, which is located in the upper third of the medial thigh. It is bounded medially by the sartorius, laterally by adductor longus, and superiorly by the inguinal ligament. The femoral nerve, artery, and vein pass through this area.

- Place your fingers or the broad side of the thumb against the pubis and move slowly side-to-side across the bone to contact the adductor muscle attachments on the pelvis (Fig. 9-37).
- Note—obtain the client's permission before performing this stroke.

Stretch

1. Tensor Fascia Latae

Position

The client is lying in side posture, with the leg to be stretched positioned on top.

Standing behind the client, take hold of the ankle of his or her top leg. Abduct the leg, medially rotate the thigh by letting the knee drop somewhat toward the bottom leg, and extend the thigh until a stretch is felt on the front of the hip at the location of the tensor fascia latae (Fig. 9-38).

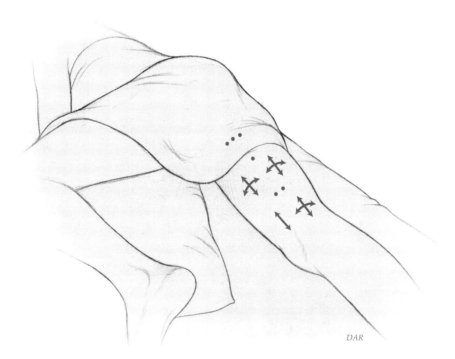

DAR

FIGURE 9-36 Direction of strokes on adductor muscles.

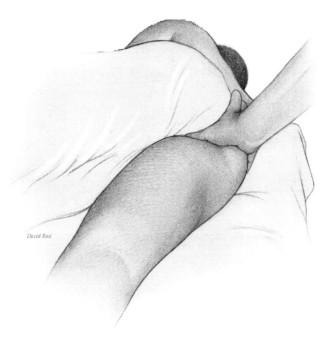

FIGURE 9-37   Contacting the adductor muscle attachments on the pubis.

2. Adductors

Position

The client is lying supine on the table, with both legs extended. The therapist stands at the foot of the table.

Holding the client's ankle, laterally rotate the leg slightly and move the leg into abduction, keeping it straight, until the client feels a stretch in the adductor muscles (Fig. 9-39).

INTESTINES

SWEDISH/CROSS FIBER

Position

The client is lying supine on the table with a bolster under the knees. Female clients are covered with a separate chest drape.

The therapist is standing at the side of the table at the level of the client's waist.

1. Perform circular effleurage on the abdomen.
2. Perform cross fiber fingertip raking on the abdominal muscles (Fig. 9-40).

CONNECTIVE TISSUE

Placing the right palm on the abdomen over the navel, left palm over the right, begin an outward spiraling, clockwise motion, stretching the fascia of the abdomen.

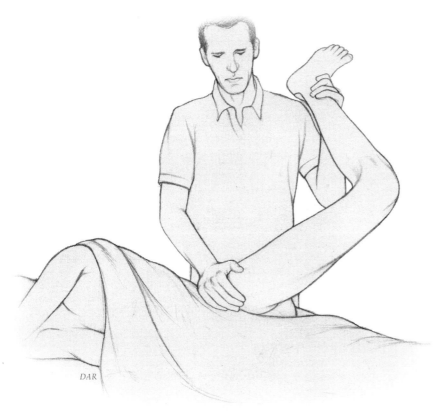

FIGURE 9-38   Stretch for tensor fascia latae.

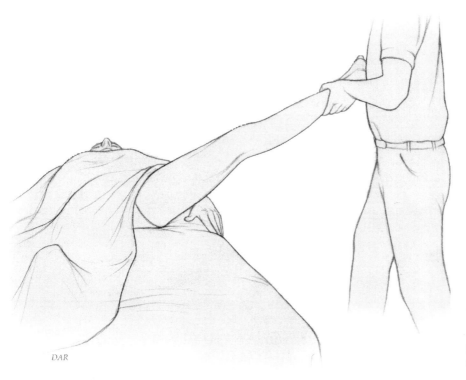

DAR

FIGURE 9-39 Stretch for adductor muscles.

Position

The client remains supine with a bolster under the knees.

The therapist is standing at the side of the table on the left side of the client's abdomen.

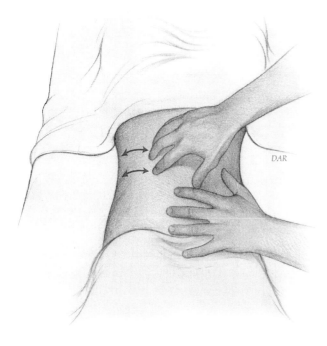

FIGURE 9-40 Cross fiber fingertip raking on rectus abdominus.

1. Large Intestine

- Reach across the table and place your fingers lateral to the ascending colon, on the right side of the client's abdomen (Fig. 9-41). Gently draw the fingers inward against the edge of the large intestine, without gliding over the skin. Continue tracing the border of the colon with your fingers, pulling it away from the outer edge of the abdomen until you reach the midline of the body. Walk around to the right side of the table and continue pulling the fingers inward along the border of the large intestine until you reach the left ASIS.
- Beginning at the ileocecal valve, do slow circular fingertip friction over the large intestine, tracing its entire length around the abdominal cavity (Fig. 9-42).
- Repeat the same path as above, doing short up-and-down and side-to-side strokes with your fingers over the large intestine. Spend extra time on impacted areas.

 Pay close attention when applying pressure over the intestines. Never push against resistance. Elicit client feedback often. Move very slowly.

2. Small Intestine

Cupping your palm, curve and spread the fingers. Place your fingertips on the abdomen, over the small intestine. Press down and circle the fingers, palpating the small intestine (Fig. 9-43). Work thoroughly, spending time on impacted areas.

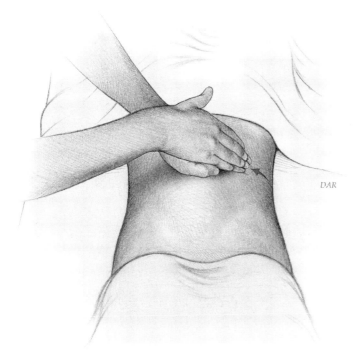

FIGURE 9-41   Contacting the lateral border of the large intestine.

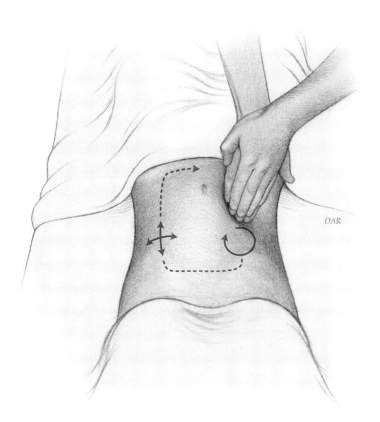

FIGURE 9-42   Sequence of deep tissue strokes on large intestine.

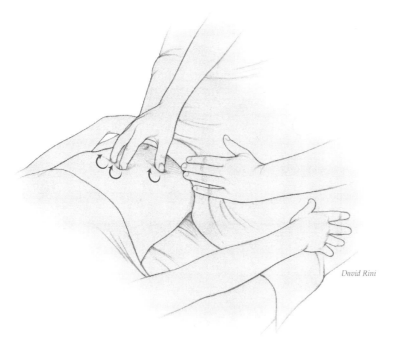

David Rini

FIGURE 9-43   Massaging the small intestine.

Accessory Work, Intestines

Reflex Points on the Feet (Fig. 9-44):
1. *Ileocecal valve point.* This point is located on the heel line on the lateral side of the right foot. Support the heel of the client's right foot with your right hand as you press the ileocecal valve point with your left thumb.
2. *Intestinal reflex zone.* To locate this zone, divide the

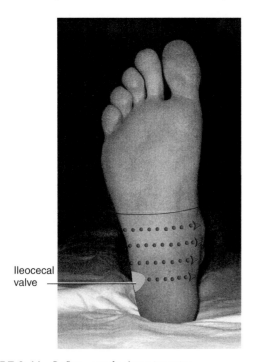

Ileocecal
valve

FIGURE 9-44   Reflex zone for large intestine.

sole of the foot into quarters, excluding the toes. The intestinal zone is located in the third quadrant, just above the heel line. To cover the area thoroughly, begin at the ileocecal point on the right foot. Press on the point with the pad of your left thumb. Move the thumb slightly forward and press on the next point (approximately one-sixteenth of an inch in front of the first point.) The thumb hinges slightly from the joint of the first phalanx.

Continue to move with the thumb tip across the foot in a horizontal direction toward the medial side, covering all points. To access the next strip of points, begin again on the lateral edge of the foot, above the first horizontal line. Repeat the sequence until the entire zone is covered. Switch hands and repeat the entire sequence, with the exception of the ileocecal point, on the left foot.

Closing

Sitting at the foot of the table, lightly hold the heels of the client's feet in your hands for 30 to 60 seconds. Remove your hands slowly to complete the session.

ANTERIOR THIGH/ILIOPSOAS ROUTINE

OBJECTIVES

- To release and lengthen the quadriceps muscles.
- To help correct anterior tilt of the pelvis.

- To complete the opening and balancing of the pelvic region.
- To achieve more efficient movement patterns, originating from the core muscles.

ENERGY

Position

The client is lying supine with the leg to be worked on fully extended. A bolster may be placed under the knee of the other leg, if desired.

The therapist is standing at the side of the table facing the client's pelvis.

Polarity

The palm of the superior hand contacts the ASIS. The palm of the inferior hand rests on the knee. Envision the thigh lengthening and the tissues reorganizing themselves along the vertical axis running along the center of the thigh. Be sensitive to any subtle movements occurring in the thigh. Let your hands softly follow them. Hold from 30 to 60 seconds.

Shiatsu

With the palms or fists, compress the thigh from the hip to the knee. These compression movements stimulate the stomach and spleen channels running approximately along the lateral and medial borders of the rectus femoris muscle.

SWEDISH/CROSS FIBER

1. Perform effleurage strokes on the anterior thigh and knee.
2. Perform kneading strokes on the anterior thigh muscles.
3. Perform friction strokes on the anterior thigh and knee.
4. Apply cross fiber strokes to the quadriceps muscles using the broad side of the thumb and/or the heel of the hand.

CONNECTIVE TISSUE

Myofascial Spreading

Place the heels of the hand on the midline of the thigh, just above the patella. Slowly draw the hands apart, spreading the tissues. Continue, in horizontal strips, to the hip.

DEEP TISSUE/NMT

Sequence

1. Patellar ligament
2. Quadriceps (vastus lateralis, rectus femoris, vastus intermedius, and vastus medialis)
3. Abdominal warm-up
4. Iliacus
5. Psoas

1. Patellar Ligament
Place your thumbs on the tibial tuberosity below the patella. Do short up-and-down and side-to-side strokes on the ligament (Fig. 9-45).

2. Quadriceps (Vastus Lateralis, Rectus Femoris, Vastus Intermedius, and Vastus Medialis)

Vastus Lateralis
Origin: Intertrochanteric line, greater trochanter, gluteal tuberosity, lateral lip of linea aspera, lateral intermuscular septum.

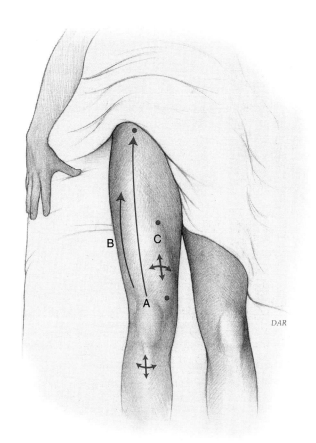

FIGURE 9-45   (A–C) Sequence of deep tissue strokes on the quadriceps.

Insertion: Lateral border of patella, patellar ligament to tibial tuberosity.

Action: Extension of leg at knee joint.

Along the anterior portion, a group of trigger points may be found at mid-thigh level which refers pain along the length of the muscle. The majority of trigger points form along the lateral aspect of the muscle. They may be spaced just above the knee, in the middle of the thigh, and at the attachment on the upper femur.

Trigger points in the superficial fibers will fire more locally, whereas trigger points in the deeper layers shoot pain throughout the muscle and down to the side of the knee.

Rectus Femoris

Origin: Anterior head—anterior inferior iliac spine.
Posterior head—groove of ilium above acetabulum.
Insertion: Patella and tibial tuberosity via patellar ligament.
Action: Extension of leg at knee joint, flexion of thigh at hip joint.

The most commonly occurring trigger point in this muscle is found just below its attachment on the AIIS. It refers pain to the knee area.

Vastus Intermedius

Origin: Anterior and lateral surfaces of upper two-thirds of shaft of femur, lower part of lateral intermuscular septum.
Insertion: Deep aspect of quadriceps tendon, patella, and tibial tuberosity via patellar ligament.
Action: Extension of leg at knee.

Trigger points in this muscle are difficult to palpate because of its position deep to the rectus femoris. They tend to develop in clusters rather than singly. The pain referral zone is most concentrated at mid-thigh level, but may extend down over the knee or to the upper thigh, depending on the location of the trigger point.

Vastus Medialis

Origin: Lower half of intertrochanteric line, medial lip of linea aspera, medial intermuscular septum, medial supracondylar line.
Insertion: Medial border of patella, tibial tuberosity via patellar ligament.
Action: Extension of the leg at the knee.

The most frequently occurring trigger point is located in the lower, thick fibers on the medial thigh slightly above the knee. Pain may be exhibited along the medial side of the muscle. A second trigger point may form about halfway up the thigh. Left untreated, these trigger points may cause a weakening in the quadriceps and bouts of buckling of the knee when the person is walking.

- Perform elongation strokes with forearm or knuckles, from the knee to the AIIS. Cover the area thoroughly

between the sartorius muscle and the iliotibial tract (A in Fig. 9-45).

- With thumbs or elbow, trace the lateral and medial borders of the rectus femoris muscle from the patella to the AIIS (B in Fig. 9-45).
- Thoroughly work small sections of the muscles with up-and-down and side-to-side strokes, using thumbs or elbow (C in Fig. 9-45).

3. Abdominal Warm-up

Position
The client is lying supine, with a bolster placed under both knees.

The therapist is standing at the side of the table next to the client's waist.

1. Perform circular effleurage on the abdomen.
2. Wave stroke—place the heels of both hands against the border of the rectus abdominus muscle on the side of the body you are standing next to, with your fingers curled around the opposite edge of the muscle (Fig. 9-46). Gently push against the abdomen with the heels of the hands, creating a bulge in front of your palms. With your fingers, reach across to the opposite side of the wave and pull the abdominal tissue back toward you. Repeat several times, creating a fluid, continuous motion.
3. Apply circular friction around the abdomen in a clockwise direction, using the heel of the hand.

4. Iliacus

Origin: Superior two-thirds of iliac fossa, inner lip of iliac crest, anterior sacroiliac and iliolumbar ligaments.
Insertion: Lesser trochanter of femur.

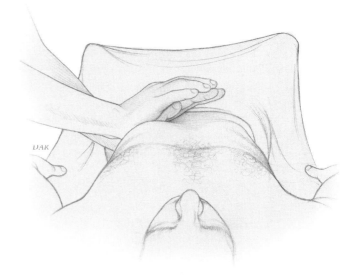

FIGURE 9-46 Beginning hand position for the wave stroke.

Action: Hip flexion, trunk flexion, hip external rotation (in conjunction with psoas).

A trigger point in the iliacus is frequently found in the upper portion of the muscle slightly superior to the ASIS.

- Place your fingers against the inner border of the iliac crest, just above the ASIS (Fig. 9-47). Allow your fingers to melt into the tissues, as if being drawn into quicksand.
- Apply short side-to-side strokes with your fingers, sinking further into the muscle. Pause at areas of resistance and/or tenderness.

5. Psoas Major

Origin: Inferior borders of transverse processes of L1–L5 vertebrae, bodies and intervertebral discs of T12–L5 vertebrae.

Insertion: Lesser trochanter of femur.

Action: Hip flexion with origin fixed, trunk flexion with insertion fixed (in conjunction with iliacus), external hip rotation, flexion of lumbar spine (bilaterally), lateral flexion of lumbar spine to same side (unilaterally).

The psoas major may manifest an active trigger point at the level of L3. The pain pattern for the iliopsoas complex is along the side of the lumbar spine and into the sacral and buttock region. Pain may also be felt in the groin and down the front of the thigh.

When pressed, these trigger points usually refer pain to the back of the body. If the trigger points are on one side only, the pain zone is more vertical along the lumbar spine. If the trigger points are bilateral, then pain may shoot in a horizontal pattern across the low back.

- Place the fingers of both hands against the border of the rectus abdominus muscle. Point your fingers slightly inward, toward the spine, reaching under the edge of the rectus abdominus (Fig. 9-48). Allow your fingers to sink into the tissues. Pause at resistance and/or tenderness, waiting for the musculature to soften.
- Perform short side-to-side strokes with your fingers, sinking further toward the psoas.
- Note—Check to be sure that you are on the psoas by having the client lift the knee a few inches to contract the muscle. You should be able to feel the muscle contracting under your fingers.
- While maintaining pressure on the psoas, have the client flex the knee and straighten the leg, aiming the foot toward the ceiling, and then lower the straight leg to the table, to alternately shorten and lengthen the muscle. Repeat a few times, moving your fingers along the length of the psoas.

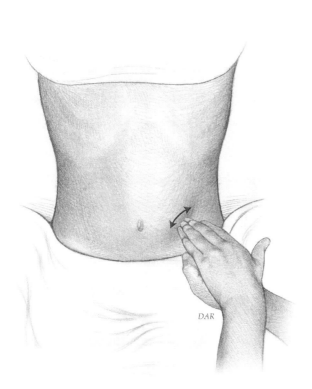

FIGURE 9-47 Contacting the iliacus on the inner rim of the tubercle of the iliac crest..

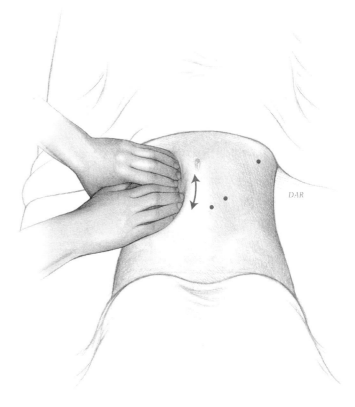

FIGURE 9-48 Contacting the psoas starting with fingertips along the border of the rectus abdominus.

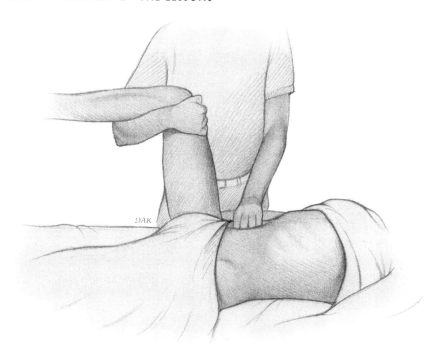

FIGURE 9-49   Position for releasing the psoas with the client's leg flexed.

■ With the client's leg flexed, slide your arm under the client's knee and lift the leg off the table. The fingers of your other hand remain in contact with the psoas. Adduct the client's thigh to access the lateral portion of the psoas. Abduct the thigh to reach the medial fibers of the muscle next to the spine (Fig. 9-49).

Stretch

The client slides toward the end of the table, so that the hips are against the edge of the table. The client then lies back on the table and holds the flexed knee of the non-stretched leg to the chest. The leg to be stretched is hanging off the end of the table, with the knee flexed.

Place one hand over the client's hands that are holding the flexed knee and assist in pressing the client's thigh toward his or her chest, as your other hand holds the thigh on the stretched side slightly above the knee. Press the thigh toward the floor (Fig. 9-50). This stretches the psoas muscle.

To stretch the rectus femoris, the client remains in the same position as above. Kneel down and hold the ankle of

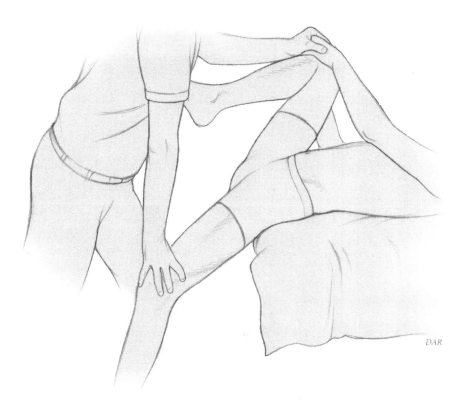

FIGURE 9-50   Stretch for psoas.

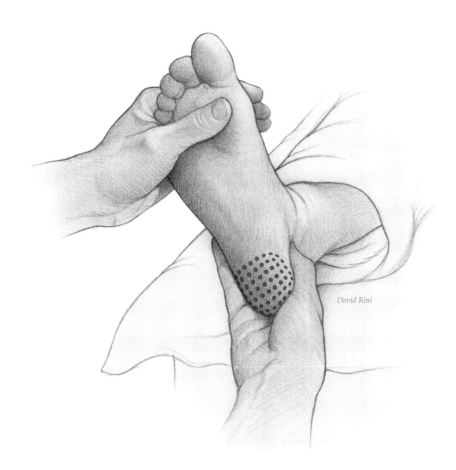

FIGURE 9-51   Reflex zone for the pelvis on the heel.

the leg to be stretched. Slowly bring the heel in the direction of the table as the client tucks the hips under. A stretch should be felt in the belly of the rectus femoris muscle.

Accessory Work

1. This session may be balanced with deep tissue work on the erector spinae, quadratus lumborum, gluteals, and hamstrings.
2. The muscles around the temporomandibular joint reflex to the pelvis and psoas. They should also be contacted to balance the upper pole of the body with the pelvis.
3. The heel is the reflex area on the foot corresponding to the pelvis. Points in the heel region on the sole of the foot may be pressed with the thumb tip. The therapist may then hold the foot around the metatarsal region with one hand while the other hand cups the heel (Fig. 9-51). With the fingers of the hand supporting the heel, the therapist may reach around to the side of the foot to press points below the malleolus. Switching hand positions allows the therapist to work on the other side of the heel.

Closing

Sitting at the foot of the table, lightly hold the heels of the client's feet in your hands for 30 to 60 seconds. Remove your hands slowly to complete the session.

REFERENCES

1. Hernandez-Reif M, Martinez A, Field T, Quintino O, Hart S, Burman I. Premenstrual syndrome symptoms are relieved by massage therapy. J Psychosom Obstet Gynaecol 2000; ZS21: 9–15.
2. Jensen B. Constipation. In: Tissue cleansing through bowel management. 6th ed. Escondido, CA; Bernard Jenson, 1981.
3. Williams DG. The ileocecal valve syndrome. In: Weinberger S. Healing within: the complete colon health guide. Larkspur, CA: Colon Health Center, 1988.
4. Jensen B. Prolapse of the transverse colon. In: Tissue cleansing through bowel management. 6th ed. Escondido, CA; Bernard Jenson, 1981: ZS48.
5. Heller J, Henkin WA. Bodywise: regaining your natural flexibility and vitality for maximum well-being. Los Angeles: Jeremy P. Tarcher, 1986; ZS156.
6. Reich W. The function of the orgasm. Volume 1 of the discovery of orgone. New York: Noonday Press, 1973.
7. The pelvis. In: Dychtwald K. Bodymind. Los Angeles: Jeremy Tarcher, 1977.

10

Balancing the Upper Pole

THE NECK AND HEAD

INTRODUCTION

The neck defines the area around the cervical vertebrae. Although it is often considered a separate body unit, the neck is actually the upper portion of the spine. Posturally, it serves the important function of balancing the head over the shoulders. The neck serves as a transitional segment, creating both space and integration between these two body parts. The adult head usually weighs between 13 and 15 pounds. Strong muscles and ligaments, anchored to the neck and shoulder girdle, are required to support it.

Releasing contracted neck muscles and repositioning the head are important elements of deep tissue release work. The neck serves as a barometer of tension throughout the body. Imbalances in lower portions of the body will be reflected in compensating displacements of the head, neck, and shoulders. In this series, neck and head

work comes after the abdomen and pelvis sessions because these two body segments counter-balance each other. If one of these segments is off-center, the other must adjust its position to maintain full-body integrity and balance.

Correct positioning of the head on the neck is crucial to proper alignment throughout the body. When the bones are stacked evenly over each other, weight transfer from the head to the feet occurs efficiently. If the head is properly poised over the atlas, the body carries a feeling of vertical lift. This sensation is the consequence of muscle balance and the body's proper relationship to gravity. The head should not tilt to either side or forward or backward.

The cranium and spine protect the brain and spinal cord. Misalignment of these bones can induce pressure and restriction on the nerves passing through the spinal cord, thus inhibiting the function of the nervous system.

Proper alignment of the head can occur only if the condyles of the atlas, on which the head sits, are on the horizontal plane. The cervical vertebrae will be displaced to the degree that the head deviates from this position, and muscles will be called into action to hold the head to prevent it from sliding further off center. Balance of the head can be checked by noting if the two ears are on the horizontal plane. From a side view, a vertical line from the center of the ear should pass through the center of the shoulder.

The deepest layer of neck muscles, the intervertebral muscles, serve as scaffolding for the vertebrae. They are responsible for stabilizing and moving the cervical vertebrae. More superficial muscles, notably the sternocleidomastoid (SCM), levator scapulae, and trapezius, serve to connect the head to the shoulder girdle. When the head-neck relationship is off, the more superficial muscles that connect the head to the shoulder girdle tend to take over the job of stabilizing the head and cervical spine. This situation occurs because the deeper, intrinsic muscles have become more or less frozen in their effort to constantly brace the vertebrae against further misalignment. This muscle action imbalance results in diminished movement in the neck and a sensation of tension. When the superficial muscles are overworked, they appear ropy, with their tendons prominent.

Patterns of chronic muscular contraction diminish the flow of fluids to the neck muscles and into the brain. Muscle tissues that receive inadequate nutrition through the blood and lymph become very dysfunctional. As the tissues atrophy, the neck area shortens further, compressing vertebrae and restricting nerves. Some types of headache are the result of this lack of circulation to the neck and head. Over time, reduction of fluid flow can lead to deposits in the arteries and diminished oxygen to the brain. It is possible that some signs of senility may be a result of lack of oxygen to brain cells.[1]

MUSCULOSKELETAL ANATOMY AND FUNCTION (ESSENTIAL ANATOMY BOX 10-1 AND FIG. 10-1A TO C)

The cervical spine consists of seven vertebrae. The first two vertebrae (C1 and C2) are uniquely designed to allow support and movement of the head. The other five vertebrae (C3–C7) are similar to those of the thoracic and lumbar spine, except that their bodies are smaller, with thinner discs between them. This design favors greater mobility in the cervical spine. However, later bending of the vertebrae is limited by the rectangular shape of the bodies and short, broad transverse processes that block further lateral movement after they make contact with each other.

As a group, the posterior neck muscles are responsible for extension when acting bilaterally and lateral flexion and rotation when acting unilaterally. Muscles acting on the head alternate with those acting on the cervical spine throughout the muscle layers of the posterior neck.

The most superficial muscle, the **trapezius**, extends the head, as does **splenius capitis** in the intermediate layer.

ESSENTIAL ANATOMY BOX 10-1

The Neck Routines

Muscles

Upper trapezius

Splenius capitis, splenius cervicis, levator scapula,

Longissimus capitis, semispinalis capitis

The transversospinal muscles—semispinalis, multifidus, rotatores

The suboccipital muscles

Platysma

Sternocleidomastoid

Scalenes

Suprahyoid muscles—digastric, stylohyoid, mylohyoid

Infrahyoid muscles—omohyoid, sternohyoid, sternothyroid

Prevertebral muscles—longus capitis, longus colli

Bones and Landmarks

Cervical vertebrae

Occipital ridge

Clavicle

Sternum

Mastoid process

Styloid process

Mandible

Digastric fossa

Hyoid

Greater horns of hyoid

Lesser horn of hyoid

Trachea

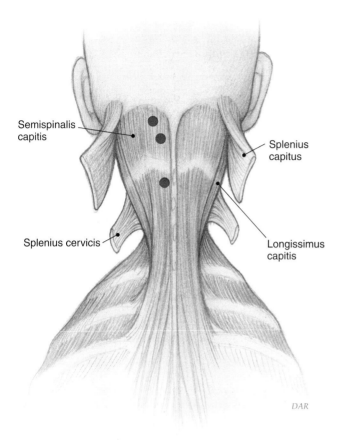

A

Semispinalis capitis

Splenius capitus

Splenius cervicis

Longissimus capitis

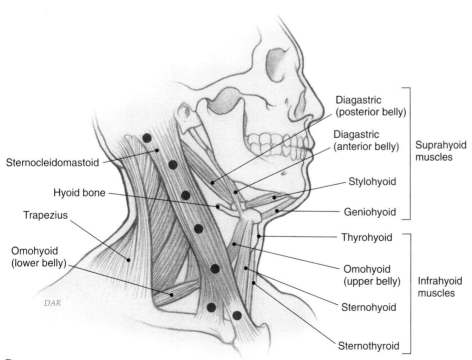

B

Sternocleidomastoid

Hyoid bone

Trapezius

Omohyoid (lower belly)

Diagastric (posterior belly)

Diagastric (anterior belly)

Suprahyoid muscles

Stylohyoid

Geniohyoid

Thyrohyoid

Omohyoid (upper belly)

Infrahyoid muscles

Sternohyoid

Sternothyroid

FIGURE 10-1 (**A**) Posterior neck muscles—deep layer. (**B**) Hyoid muscles with sternocleidomastoid and trapezius. *(continued)*

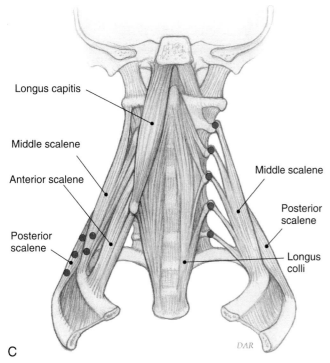

C

DAR

FIGURE 10-1   *Continued.* (**C**) Prevertebral muscles.

Longus capitis

Middle scalene

Anterior scalene

Posterior scalene

Middle scalene

Posterior scalene

Longus colli

The two other muscles in the intermediate later, **splenius cervicis** and **levator scapula**, extend the cervical spine (Fig. 10-1A). In the first layer of deep muscles, the **longissimus capitis** and **semispinalis capitis** are capital (head) extensors. The transversospinalis muscles, which link the vertebrae, are cervical extensors. They are **semispinalis, multifidus,** and **rotatores.** The deepest-lying muscles, the **suboccipitals,** extend the head. This alternating of actions throughout the layers provides additional strength and support to neck and head movements.

All the posterior neck muscles are subject to strain to varying degrees. Trauma to the neck and head occurs easily due to their rather fragile design. Trigger points that develop in these muscles often refer into the head or shoulders and can be a major contributing factor in certain headache pain.

The **sternocleidomastoid (SCM)** is the largest neck flexor. It has two branches, both originating on the mastoid process and inserting separately on the sternum and clavicle (Fig. 10-1B). This muscle serves several functions. When contracted bilaterally, the SCM flexes the neck and draws the head forward and downward toward the chin. Unilateral contraction produces lateral flexion of the head to the same side and rotation of the head to the opposite side. When the neck is in a straight-up or extended position and the head is still, the SCM elevates the sternum and clavicle, assisting inspiration.

The SCM provides an important stabilizing function. It prevents hyperextension of the neck when the head is turned upward and resists strong backward movement of the head during sudden body shifts, such as a backward fall. It aids the trapezius in maintaining a stable head position when the mandible is moving, as in talking and chewing. Active trigger points in the SCM are mostly commonly felt in the head rather than in the neck. They can also be responsible for feelings of disequilibrium when standing or moving.

The **scalenes** have three divisions: anterior, medial, and posterior (Fig. 10-1C). They all originate on the transverse processes of the cervical vertebrae. The anterior and middle scalenes insert on the first rib. The posterior scalene muscle inserts on the second rib.

When contracting unilaterally, all three scalenes contribute to lateral flexion of the cervical spine, particularly the posterior scalene, due to its almost vertical position along the side of the neck. The anterior and middle scalenes are positioned at a forward oblique angle to the cervical spine. When they contract bilaterally, they increase the curve in the neck. They are opposed in this action by the **longus colli** and **longus capitis,** which straighten the cervical spine. All three scalenes aid in respiration by lifting the first two ribs during forced inspiration.

The space formed between the anterior and middle scalenes is known as the thoracic outlet. The brachial plexus (composed of spinal nerves C5–8 and T1) and the subclavian artery emerge from this opening and then pass through the space between the clavicle and first rib. The spinal nerves merge into cords to become the median, radial, and ulnar nerves, which continue down the arm to the hand and fingers.

The hyoid bone is a horseshoe-shaped bone located on the front of the neck, between the mandible and larynx. It does not articulate with any other bone, but rather is suspended in place by a series of muscles and a ligament. The main purpose of the hyoid is to provide an attachment for muscles that control movements of the tongue. It also assists in cervical flexion.

The muscles that attach above the hyoid are called the suprahyoid muscles (Fig.10-1B). They are the **digastric, hyoglossus, geniohyoid, mylohyoid,** and **stylohyoid.** The muscles that originate below the hyoid, on the sternum, clavicle, and scapula, are called the infrahyoid muscles. They are the **sternohyoid, thyrohyoid,** and **omohyoid.** Restrictions in the hyoid muscles can interfere with the mechanics of sound articulation in speech and with the function of swallowing. Trigger points in these muscles have led to chronic sore throats and to diminished thyroid activity.

The longus colli and longus capitis are both located on the anterior side of the spinal column, deep to the trachea (Fig. 10-1C). Longus colli extends from the atlas to the body of the third thoracic vertebra. Longus capitis runs from the transverse processes of C3–C6 vertebrae to the base of the occiput. Longus colli flexes the cervical spine while longus capitis flexes and stabilizes the head. Both muscles contribute to side-bending of the cervical spine.

There are several structures located in the anterior neck that need to be taken into consideration when performing massage in this area. The thyroid gland is located on the anterior surface of the trachea from the level of C5–T1 vertebrae. It is deep to the sternothyroid and sternohyoid muscles. The vertebral artery passes through the foramen of the transverse processes of the cervical vertebrae. The common carotid artery runs along the anterior border and posterior to the SCM muscle. Its pulse can be palpated by pressing lightly near the tips of the transverse processes of the cervical vertebrae. The internal jugular vein is located lateral to the common carotid artery. The vagus nerve lies posteriorly between the two.

The first cervical vertebra is called the atlas. It rests on the second cervical vertebra, called the axis. A small, peg-like projection on the axis, called the odontoid process (or dens), fits into the inside of the anterior arch of the atlas above it. It is held in place by a transverse ligament. The head and atlas can pivot around the dens, allowing for rotational movements. The atlas is the only vertebra capable of independent movement. All the other vertebrae move as a unit. This limits the range of motion at each joint of the spine, protecting the spinal cord from damage caused by excessive bending in one place.

The cranium consists of eight bones: the frontal, sphenoid, ethmoid, two temporal, two parietal, and the occipital. The head shares a design feature with the pelvis in that it is not a massive singular structure, but rather a series of bones connected together to form a bowl, or basin. The cranium is filled with air spaces, called sinuses, to decrease its weight. The bones of the head are joined by sutures that are saw-toothed shaped and fit together like jigsaw puzzle pieces. They are supported by fascial tissues and require little muscular reinforcement. These sutures are pliable, allowing the cranium to subtly shift and absorb trauma that might otherwise injure the brain. (The perspective of moveable cranial joints is advocated by craniosacral practitioners. The classic anatomy view is that these sutures are immobile. For a complete explanation of craniosacral theory refer to Upledger and Vredevoogd J.[2]) Easing tension in the scalp helps to mobilize the sutures and retains their springiness. Reducing pressure between the cranial bones has been known to ease sinus congestion brought about by blockage in the small sinus drainage ducts.

The occipital bone is located at the posterior and inferior portion of the skull. The spinal cord passes through a hole in its base, called the foramen magnum, and into the tunnel formed by the cervical vertebrae below. On either side of the foramen magnum are two oval, convex condyles. They fit into two corresponding concave articular facets on the first cervical vertebra, or atlas. The atlas is ring-shaped; it does not have a central body, like the other vertebrae. This design allows the spinal cord to pass through it freely.

The rounded surfaces of the articulations form an enarthrosis, which is a ball-and-socket type joint that can perform movements in all three planes.[3] However, the oval shape of the condyles, which are longer than they are wide, favor forward and backward motions, like those of a rocking chair. Due to its weight, the head tends to slide forward on the condyles. Many daily activities, such as reading, writing, and working at a computer, can lead to a forward tilting of the head. The posterior muscles of the neck have to work to prevent the head from sliding further forward in this position, leading to strain and possible trigger point formation. Attaining proper alignment of the head is a primary goal in reducing tension in the neck.

Several muscles play an important role in stabilizing the head on the atlas. They are the multifidus, interspinalis, semispinalis capitis, and semispinalis cervicis. It is essential that these muscles do not become chronically contracted for the head to subtly adjust its position as needed to maintain equilibrium in the body and to prevent restriction of the arteries, veins, and nerves that pass into the head from the neck.

Maintaining the head in a horizontal balance over the atlas is important for many reasons. Chronically holding the head in altered positions affects the flow of blood, lymph, and spinal fluid and changes internal pressures. According to craniosacral theory, the cranium and spine form a hydraulic pump whose uninhibited operation forms the basic rhythm on which many of the metabolic processes of the body rely.[4] Any alterations in internal pressures affect this pumping system, which can potentially damage brain and nervous system functions.

CONDITIONS (INDICATIONS/ CONTRAINDICATIONS BOX 10-1)

1. *"Forward head"* is a commonly seen postural deviation, where the head is held forward of proper alignment. It can be easily observed by having the subject stand in profile next to a plumb line. The ear lobe will be forward of the plumb. Holding the head forward of the center of gravity proportionally increases its weight. As stated previously, the head normally weighs about 15 pounds. A head held 3 inches forward of the vertical line of gravity weighs approximately 30 pounds.[5] In this position the cervical spine is compressed, setting the stage for disc problems. The thoracic curve is often exaggerated.

   This postural deviation can be caused by poor postural habits, like slumping while reading or watching a computer screen. Spinal conditions such as osteoporosis, kyphosis, and degenerative arthritis can also cause the head to be projected forward. If the cause is

INDICATIONS/
CONTRAINDICATIONS
BOX 10-1

Conditions
Affecting
Neck Massage

Indications	Contraindications
Stiff neck	Severe trauma
Pain in neck/shoulders	Fever
Pain/numbness in arm	Skin disorders
Whiplash	Recent injury/surgery
Tension in throat	Severe hypertension
Postural deviations	

poor postural habits, a simple exercise can help to re-establish proper head position. The person should spend some time each day performing common activities with a small weight, like a bean bag, balanced on top of the head. Proper head positioning becomes mandatory to prevent the object from sliding off the head. Additional weight on top of the head also contributes to the feeling of heaviness when the head is held forward, thus reminding a person to maintain proper vertical alignment.

2. *"Military neck"* is the opposite deviation of forward head. In this posture, the cervical curve is diminished or absent. The back of the neck appears elongated. The chin may be drawn downward, and a noticeable strain can often be seen in the tendons of the SCM muscles. The SCM's assist in capital and cervical flexion and are involved in maintaining this position along with longus colli and longus capitis.

3. *Torticollis* is a condition commonly referred to as "stiff neck." It is a twisting or tilt of the head caused by spasms in the neck muscles. Torticollis can be brought about by some disease conditions, trauma to the neck area, or tension. When the cause is neck tension, some precipitating factors are sleeping in an awkward position, allowing the neck to become chilled, watching a sporting event that requires moving the head back and forth, leaning over a desk, and reading. The muscles most often involved are the levator scapula, the trapezius, and the posterior cervical muscles.

4. *Whiplash* is a general term referring to injuries to the tissues of the neck caused by rapid front-to-back or side-to-side movements of the head. These movements cause the neck muscles to be hypercontracted and hyperstretched. Damage to the neck can consist of microscopic tears to the muscles and ligaments, as well as damage to the other structures of the cervical region. A massage therapist should always be sure that

a medical doctor has examined the client before he or she attempts any massage work.

5. *Bulging discs* in the cervical region can manifest in a number of problems. Irritated nerves can produce tingling down the arm all the way to the hand. Weakness may be present in the affected arm and hand. To check for disc involvement, have the client perform range-of-motion movements for the neck. If severe pain occurs in one direction of movement but not the other, it is a good indicator of a disc problem. Clients exhibiting signs of disc problems should be referred to a medical doctor for evaluation.

6. *Ligament tears*. Damage to neck ligaments can occur from injury or chronic misuse and poor alignment of the head and neck, causing a weakening of the ligamentous tissue. This injury is characterized by pain, particularly during resisted head movements.

7. *Thoracic outlet syndrome* is caused by entrapment of the neurovascular bundle that passes through the space between the anterior and middle scalenes, and the space between the clavicle and first rib. Symptoms of nerve compression include pain and paresthesia (tingling) in the neck, shoulder, arm, hand, and fingers. Vascular compression may produce numbness, pain, cold, and fatigue in the shoulder and arm. The syndrome can be diagnosed by electromyographic (EMG) measurements.

Causes of thoracic outlet syndrome include build-up of the fascial tissue around the scalenes, which decreases the size of the spaces that the nerves and blood vessels pass through. Rounded shoulders accompanied by kyphosis and an increased cervical curve lead to chronic shortness and fascial thickening in the scalenes. Restrictions in the breathing muscles, resulting in shallow upper chest breathing, also strain the scalenes. Treatment includes deep tissue massage to the scalenes, correction of faulty postural and breathing habits, and regular, slow stretching of the scalenes.

THE MIND/BODY CONNECTION

The neck serves as a channel linking the head with the rest of the body. Passageways in the neck function in the transfer of food, air, and nerve impulses. The neck is also responsible for balancing the head. The constant activity occurring through the neck makes it an area of transition. For having so many duties, it is a small, weak region, making it vulnerable to overuse and stress conditions.

Integration is a quality associated with the neck. It acts as a bridge between the intellect and the heart, or emotions. In this role, the neck serves as a mediator. We often have a choice whether to process an internal impulse as a thought or a feeling. The neck helps to determine the route the expression will take—to the thinking center in the head or the emotional center in the chest.

Constantly rerouting emotional experiences to the thinking facility diminishes their power and can serve as a form of repression or avoidance. This may be reflected in tension in the neck muscles. The opposite case can also be problematic, in which we indulge emotions rather than seeking rational alternatives. Exercising choice over how and when to express ourselves is a desirable state and will help to maintain an open, healthy condition of the neck and throat.

The neck is a vulnerable area that may lodge much repressed fear. It is very likely that someone who has been attacked or raped was grabbed and held at the neck. Having that area touched, particularly the anterior neck region, may elicit feelings of fear, rage, or panic. The therapist should always check with a client before touching the anterior neck to ensure that the client is comfortable receiving massage there.

If a client has experienced neck trauma and decides to proceed with the work, the therapist should move slowly and deliberately, allowing the client time to relax and verbalize any feelings of discomfort. The client must always feel in control and know that he or she can have the massage stopped at any time, if desired.

POSTURAL EVALUATION (TABLES 10-1 AND 10-2)

FRONTAL VIEW

1. Does the head appear to be resting on a horizontal base?
2. Are the two sides of the neck of equal length?
3. Does the head tilt or rotate to one side or the other?
4. Assess the musculature of the neck.
   - Are one or both of the SCM muscles prominent?
   - Are the tendons of the SCM muscles at the manubrium prominent?
   - Are there hollows above the clavicles? (Hollows denote shortness of the scalenes.)

SIDE VIEW

1. Are the centers of the earlobe, shoulder, hip, knee, and ankle aligned in a straight line?
2. Check the tilt of the head.
   - Forward
   - Backward
   - Neutral
3. Is there the appearance of vertical lift in the body, a sense of being led upward by the head?
4. Does the body appear to be compressed, with the head pushing down into the neck?

TABLE 10-1	*Body Reading for the Neck*
Conditions	**Muscles that May by Shortened**
Lateral tilt of the head	Sternocleidomastoid
	Scalenes
	Upper trapezius
	Levator scapula
Military neck	Sternocleidomastoid
	Longus capitis
	Longus colli
Forward head	Scalenes
	Splenius capitis
	Upper trapezius
	Semispinalis capitis

TABLE 10-2	**Range of Motion (ROM) for the Neck**

Action	Muscles
Flexion (ROM 45°)	Longus capitis
	Longus colli
	Scalenes
	Sternocleidomastoid
Extension (ROM 55°)	Splenius cervicis
	Splenius capitis
	Upper trapezius
	Semispinalis capitis
	Semispinalis cervicis
Lateral flexion (ROM 40°)	Longus colli
	Scalenes
	Sternocleidomastoid
	Splenius capitis
	Splenius cervicis
	Upper trapezius
Rotation same side (ROM 70°)	Longus colli
	Longus capitis
	Splenius cervicis
	Splenius capitis
Rotation opposite side (ROM 70°)	Scalenes
	Sternocleidomastoid
	Trapezius
	Semispinalis

EXERCISES AND SELF-TREATMENT

1. *Forward flexion* (stretches the neck extensor muscles—splenius cervicis, splenius capitis, upper trapezius, semispinalis capitis, semispinalis cervicis). Tilt your head forward, bringing your chin toward the chest. Place your hands on the back of the head, gently pressing down until you feel a mild stretch in the back of the neck.
2. *Extension* (stretches the neck flexor muscles—longus capitis, longus colli, scalenes, SCM). Slowly raise your head to look up toward the ceiling. Reach up from the back of the neck and the front to prevent compression of the cervical vertebrae. Draw your lower teeth up over the upper teeth to further stretch the anterior neck muscles.
3. *Lateral flexion* (stretches scalenes, SCM, splenius capitis, splenius cervicis, upper trapezius).
   - Looking straight ahead with your head upright, place your right hand on the left side of your head above the left ear. Slowly move your right ear toward the right shoulder. Press against the left side of your head gently to increase the feeling of stretch. Relax and imagine breathing into the tight muscles on the left side of your neck.
   - Place your left hand on the right side of your head above the right ear. Slowly move your left ear toward the left shoulder. Press against the right side of your head gently to increase the stretch. Relax and imagine breathing into the tight muscles on the right side of your neck.
4. *Relaxation of the neck and head*. Lie on your back on the floor with the knees flexed and both feet on the floor. As you breathe deeply imagine that your head is a heavy bag filled with sand. Visualize the sand slowly flowing out of the bag from a small hole located just below the external occipital protuberance (EOP), emptying the interior of the head and neck of all stress and tightness. Rest in this position for several minutes.

NECK AND HEAD EXTENSORS ROUTINE

OBJECTIVES

- To lengthen the posterior neck.
- To begin the process of repositioning the head on the cervical spine.

- To relieve tightness in neck muscles which may be contributing to neck or head pain.
- To reduce muscular pulls on cervical vertebrae.
- To assist the client in acquiring more effective neck and head alignment in everyday activities to help reduce stress factors.

ENERGY

Position

The client is in side posture. A small pad is placed under the side of the head; a bolster is positioned between the knees.

The therapist is standing behind the table at the client's neck and head region.

Polarity

The palm of one hand is lightly placed across the occipital ridge. The palm of the other hand contacts C7. Envision the neck lengthening as the cervical vertebrae decompress and the musculature of the neck relaxes. Maintain contact for at least 1 minute.

Shiatsu

Place one hand on the client's shoulder. Wrap your other hand around the posterior neck, just below the occipital ridge, with the thumb on one side of the trapezius and the fingers on the other side. Slowly squeeze the neck and hold for a few seconds (Fig. 10-2). Release, slide your hand to the middle of the neck, and repeat. Then, putting your hand at the base of the neck, squeeze again. This move helps to stimulate the points on the portion of

the bladder channel that passes through the posterior neck

SWEDISH/CROSS FIBER

1. Perform effleurage strokes from the acromion to the occipital ridge.
2. Perform one-handed pétrissage:
   - From the shoulder to the base of the neck.
   - From the base of the neck to the occiput.
3. Perform fingertip raking across the posterior neck, in horizontal strips, from C7 to the occiput.

CONNECTIVE TISSUE

Reaching across the posterior neck, place the fingers of one hand just posterior to the transverse processes of the cervical spine on the opposite side from where you are standing. Allow your fingers to sink into the tissues. As the tissues melt under your touch, let your fingers glide toward you to the sides of the spinous processes of the cervical spine (Fig. 10-3).

DEEP TISSUE/NMT

Sequence

1. Superficial layer—upper trapezius
2. Intermediate layer—splenius capitis, splenius cervicis, levator scapula
3. Deep layer—longissimus capitis, semispinalis capitis
   Transversospinal muscles—semispinalis, multifidus, rotatores
   Suboccipital muscles—obliquus capitis superior, obliquus capitis inferior, rectus capitis posterior major, rectus capitis posterior minor

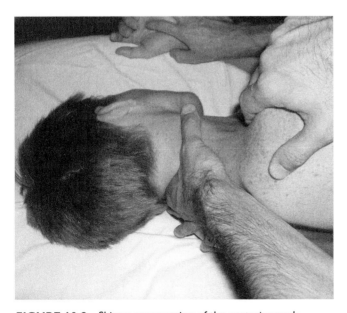

FIGURE 10-2   Shiatsu compression of the posterior neck.

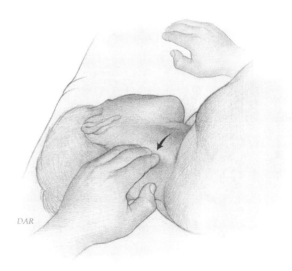

FIGURE 10-3   Connective tissue release of the posterior neck.

1. Superficial Layer

Upper Trapezius
Origin: Medial third of the superior nuchal line and EOP, ligamentum nuchae and the spinal processes of C1–C5 vertebrae.
Insertion: Lateral third of the clavicle.
Action: Elevation and upward rotation of scapula, capital extension.

Trigger points in this muscle are frequently responsible for tension headaches that may be felt at the temple, behind the eye, and sometimes at the mastoid process and down the posterior neck. Trigger points are located in the fibers slightly behind the border of the muscle, near where it attaches on the lateral portion of the clavicle. They are best palpated by squeezing the edge of the muscle between the thumb and fingers.

■ Wrap your hand around the base of the neck, as in the Shiatsu procedure above, with the thumb pad at the border of the trapezius. Using the thumb pad, stroke posteriorly, from the border of the trapezius to the spinous process of C7 (Fig. 10-4).
■ Sliding your thumb half an inch superior, repeat the stroke. Continue, in strips, to the occipital ridge.
■ Apply up-and-down and side-to-side strokes, with the thumbs, to the attachment of the upper trapezius on the superior nuchal line on the occiput.

2. Intermediate Layer

Splenius Capitis
Origin: Ligamentum nuchae from C3–C7, spinous processes of C7–T4 vertebrae.

Insertion: Mastoid process of temporal bone, lateral third of superior nuchal line of occiput.
Action: Extension of head, lateral flexion of head to same side.

A trigger point may be found in the upper portion of the muscle, on the occiput, in the space between the trapezius and SCM. It refers pain to the highest point on the head on the same side as the trigger point.

■ Using your thumb pad, stroke at an oblique angle from the spinous processes of C3 and C4 to the mastoid process. Repeat the stroke, beginning at C5. Continue, in strips, to T3 (Fig. 10-5).
■ Roll your thumb across the fibers of the muscle, feeling for taut bands. Check for trigger points.

Splenius Cervicis
Origin: Spinous processes of T3–T6 vertebrae.
Insertion: Transverse processes of C1–C3 (varies).
Action: Extension of cervical spine, rotation of cervical spine to same side, flexion of cervical spine to same side.

A commonly experienced trigger point can be palpated near the transverse process of C3. It refers pain to the eye on the same side. In some cases, treatment of this trigger point may relieve blurred vision in that eye.

With your fingertips, find the posterior aspects of the transverse processes of C2–C4. Do short up-and-down strokes (Fig. 10-6). Pause at tender points and hold.

3. Deep Layer
There are three areas of trigger point activity that form in the line of the lamina groove:

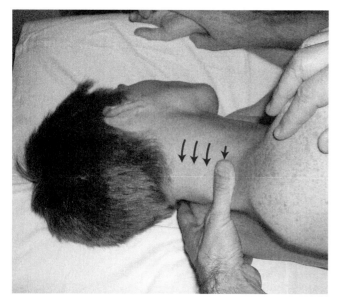

FIGURE 10-4 Deep tissue stroking on the upper trapezius from C7 to the occiput.

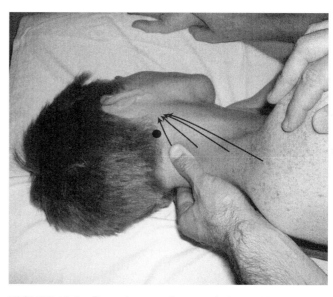

FIGURE 10-5 Deep tissue strokes on splenius capitis.

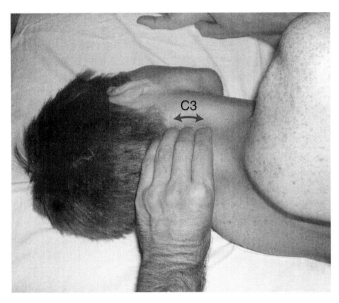

FIGURE 10-6 Working the attachments of splenius cervicis and levator scapula from C2–C4.

■ *The first one is found at the level of C4 and C5. Pain can be referred up to the suboccipital area and also down to the upper vertebral border of the scapula.*
■ *The second area of trigger point activity is located at the level of C2. The pain referral zone is around the occiput and upward toward the top of the head.*
■ *The third location of trigger points is right below the occipital ridge at the attachment point of semispinalis capitis. The pain pattern forms a band around the head with the most severe sensation felt at the temple and forehead over the eye.*

Longissimus Capitis and Semispinalis Capitis

Longissimus Capitis
Origin: Transverse processes of T1–T5 vertebrae, articular processes of C4–C7 vertebrae.
Insertion: Posterior margin of mastoid process of temporal bone.
Action: Extension of head, lateral flexion and rotation of head to same side.

Semispinalis capitis
Origin: Transverse processes of T1–T7 vertebrae (varies), articular processes of C4–C6.
Insertion: Occiput between superior and inferior nuchal lines.
Action: Extension and lateral flexion of head.

■ With your thumb, do combination stroking (up-and-down and side-to-side) in small sections at a time in the space between the spinous processes and the transverse processes of the cervical vertebrae. Begin at the level of

C7; continue to the occiput (Fig. 10-7). Treat trigger points when you find them.
■ Work on the attachments of the muscles on the occiput using the combination strokes:
  ■ Longissimus capitis—posterior margin of the mastoid process.
  ■ Semispinalis capitis—the space between the superior and inferior nuchal lines.

Transversospinal Muscles (Semispinalis, Multifidus, Rotatores)

Locations on Cervical Spine
Semispinalis cervicis—spinous processes of C2–C5. Multifidi—spinous process of two to four vertebrae above origin. Rotatores—base of spinous process of next highest vertebra.
Action: Extension of cervical spine.

With your thumb, perform the combination stroke in the lamina groove of the cervical spine, from C7 to the occiput (Fig. 10-8). Work in small sections, paying attention to soft tissue dysfunction at the deepest level, next to the bone. Treat trigger points as you find them.

Suboccipital Muscles (Obliquus Capitis Superior, Obliquus Capitis Inferior, Rectus Capitis Posterior Major, Rectus Capitis Posterior Minor)

Obliquus Capitis Superior
Origin: Transverse process and superior surface of atlas.
Insertion: Occiput between superior and inferior nuchal lines (lateral to semispinalis capitis).
Action: Extension of head on atlas, lateral flexion to same side.

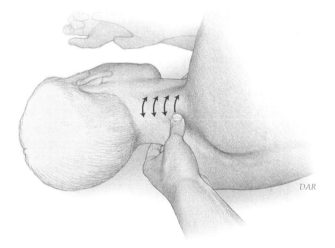

FIGURE 10-7 Deep tissue strokes on longissimus capitis and semispinalis capitis from C7 to the occiput.

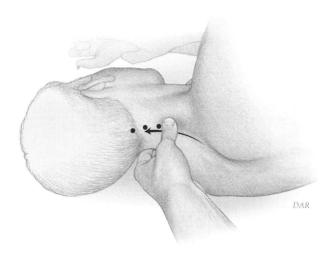

FIGURE 10-8 Deep tissue strokes on the transversospinalis muscles.

Obliquus Capitis Inferior
Origin: Apex of spinous process of atlas.
Insertion: Inferior and dorsal part of transverse process of atlas.
Action: Extension of head, lateral flexion to same side.

Rectus Capitis Posterior Major
Origin: Spinous process of axis.
Insertion: Lateral part of inferior nuchal line of occiput.
Action: Extension of head, rotation of head to same side, lateral flexion of head to same side.

Rectus Capitis Posterior Minor
Origin: Tubercle on posterior arch of atlas.
Insertion: Medial part of inferior nuchal line of occiput.
Action: Extension of head, lateral flexion of head to same side.

- Standing at the head of the table, cup your palm over the back of the cranium, hooking your fingers under the occipital ridge. Allow them to sink in as far as the client's tissues will allow without discomfort (Fig. 10-9A). Do slow up-and-down and side-to-side strokes.
- Standing at the side of the table facing the client's head, place the thumbs on the occipital ridge, next to the EOP. The thumbs are in a horizontal position, one above the other (Fig. 10-9B). Alternately, roll the thumbs upward along the base of the cranium and slightly below, on the neck, at the level of C1 and C2.

Stretch

The client sits upright on the edge of the table. Sitting or standing behind the client, place one palm on the shoulder and the other palm on the same side of the head, above the ear. Laterally flex the head while stabilizing the shoulder (Fig. 10-10). Have the client slowly rotate the head to bring the chin toward the chest. Pause and maintain the stretch where tightness and/or tenderness are experienced. Be careful not to overstretch the neck in this position. Direct the client to imagine breathing into the muscles being stretched as they relax and lengthen.

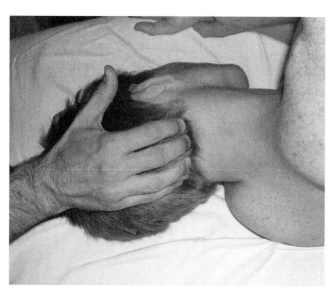

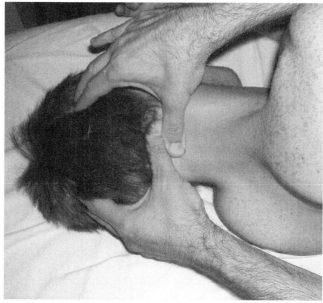

A   B

FIGURE 10-9 (**A**) Using fingertips to release the suboccipital muscles. (**B**) Deep tissue thumb strokes to release the suboccipital muscles.

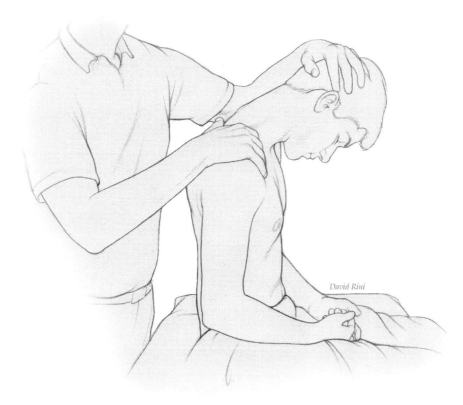

FIGURE 10-10   Stretch for posterior neck muscles.

David Rini

Accessory Work

1. Neck and head extensors should be worked on in conjunction with the neck and head flexors to balance the musculature of the cervical region.
2. Jaw work should accompany the neck session as imbalance is almost always reflected in both segments simultaneously.
3. Work on the feet synchronizes the upper and lower poles of the body and grounds the client after neck and head massage.

Closing

Sitting at the foot of the table, lightly hold the heels of the client's feet in your hands for 30 to 60 seconds. Remove your hands slowly to complete the session.

NECK AND HEAD FLEXORS ROUTINE

OBJECTIVES

- To elongate the muscles of the anterior neck.
- To balance the anterior neck muscles with the posterior neck muscles.
- To continue the process of balancing the head on the cervical spine.

- To relieve painful conditions due to shortened flexor muscles.
- To reduce uneven pulls on the hyoid bone.

ENERGY

Position

The client is lying supine on the table.

The therapist is sitting at the head of the table

Polarity

The therapist holds the client's head by placing his or her right palm (positive pole) across the client's occipital ridge (negative pole), and his or her left palm (positive pole) across the forehead (negative pole) (Fig. 10-11). This head hold is very relaxing. It is sometimes referred to as the " brain drain" because of its effectiveness in easing excessive mental activity. The position is held for at least 1 minute.

Shiatsu

Press the **conception vessel** (CV) 22 point, located in the notch at the base of the throat, just above the sternum (Fig. 10-12). This point helps open the throat passage and relieve sore throat and other inflammatory conditions of the throat and chest.

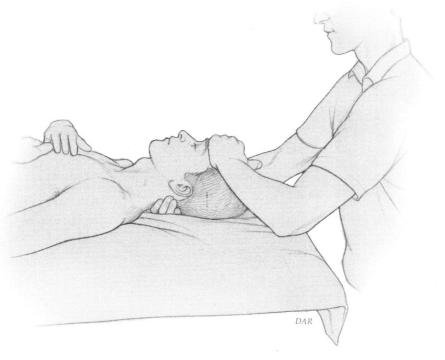

FIGURE 10-11   Polarity balancing head hold.

 Keep your finger on the superior edge of the manubrium. Do not press into the soft tissues above it, as nerves and blood vessels are close to the surface here.

SWEDISH/CROSS FIBER

1. Perform effleurage strokes down the sides of the neck.
2. Apply circular fingertip friction along both sides of the neck.

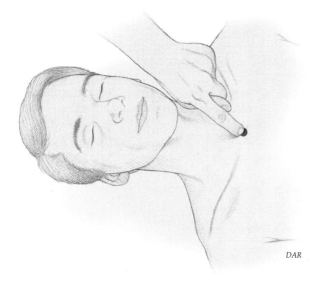

FIGURE 10-12   Contacting conception vessel 22 point.

3. Perform thumb sweeping on the side of the neck. Stroke each side individually.

CONNECTIVE TISSUE

Holding the client's head in one hand, slightly rotate it to the side. Place the fingers of your other hand along the anterior border of the SCM. Allow your finger pads to sink into the muscle. As the tissues yield, let your fingers slowly glide in a posterior direction. Repeat along the length of the neck.

DEEP TISSUE/NMT

Sequence

1. Platysma
2. SCM
3. Scalenes
4. Suprahyoid muscles—digastric, stylohyoid, mylohyoid
5. Infrahyoid muscles—omohyoid, sternohyoid, sternothyroid
6. Prevertebral muscles—longus capitis, longus colli

1. Platysma

Origin: Fascia covering upper portion of the chest.
Insertion: Mandible, subcutaneous fascia, and muscles of the chin and jaw.
Action: Depresses lower lip and draws it backward, lifts skin of chest.

Active trigger points in this muscle are usually found where it covers the SCM. They may best be palpated by sifting the platysma between the thumb and fingers. The trigger points refer to the area of the mandible. The sensation of pain is superficial, as if originating in the skin over the jaw.

Place the fingers of one hand on the mandible, just below the corner of the mouth. Do a slow elongation stroke, following the fibers of the muscle, down the neck, over the clavicle, and onto the upper chest (Fig. 10-13).

2. Sternocleidomastoid

Origin: Sternal head—sternum, ventral surface of manubrium. Clavicular head—superior and anterior surface of medial third of clavicle.

Insertion: Mastoid process of temporal bone, lateral half of superior nuchal line of occiput.

Action: Flexion of cervical spine (both muscles), lateral flexion of cervical spine to same side, rotation of head to opposite side, capital extension (posterior fibers), lifts sternum in forced inhalation.

Trigger points may be found almost anywhere along the length of the sternal and clavicular branches of the muscle.

Sternal Division

A trigger point in the lower portion of the muscle refers pain downward over the upper part of the sternum.

Trigger points in the middle section tend to shoot pain across the cheek area, around the eye orbit and into the eye, and sometimes into the external part of the ear canal. Trigger points along the medial border of the middle SCM refer pain into the throat and back of the tongue, creating the sensation of a sore throat. Trigger points in the upper

section refer pain to the occipital ridge and to the top of the head.

An associated autonomic response to trigger points in the sternal division of the SCM can be eye problems such as blurred vision and an inability to control eye muscles fully.

Clavicular Division

Trigger points in the middle section refer pain to the forehead.

An associated autonomic response to trigger points in the clavicular division can be dizziness, particularly after the SCM muscle has been stretched.

- Holding the client's head in one hand, rotate the head slightly. Place your thumb pad on the mastoid process. Using the broad side of the thumb, do an elongation stroke along the fibers of the SCM, ending at the sternum.
- With the thumb or index finger, apply cross fiber strokes to the SCM attachment on the sternum. Glide your thumb along the top edge of the clavicle to the clavicular attachment of the SCM and apply cross fiber strokes to it.
- Grasp the SCM muscle between your fingers and thumbs and sift the muscle fibers thoroughly, searching for trigger point activity (Fig. 10-14). Begin near the insertion on the mastoid process and continue down to the origins on the sternum and clavicle.

3. Scalenes

Scalenus Anterior

Origin: Transverse processes of C3–C6 vertebrae.

Insertion: Scalene tubercle on inner border of 1st rib.

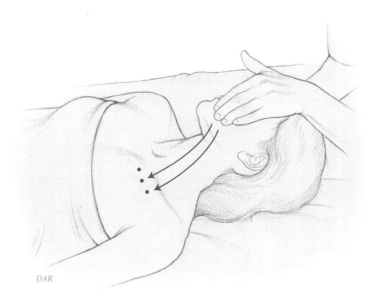

DAR

FIGURE 10-13   Direction of deep tissue stroking on the platysma.

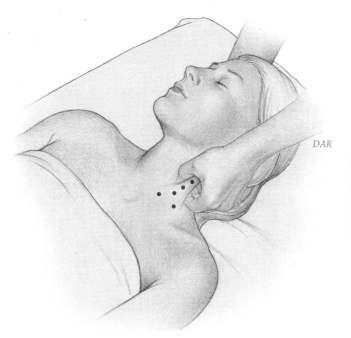

DAR

FIGURE 10-14   Sifting the sternocleidomastoid.

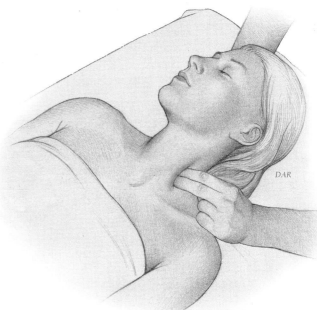

DAR

FIGURE 10-15   Contacting the scalene attachments on the transverse processes of C3–C6.

Action: Flexion of cervical spine, elevation of 1st rib on inhalation, rotation of cervical spine to opposite side, lateral flexion of cervical spine to same side.

Scalenus Medius

Origin: Transverse processes of C2–C7 vertebrae.
Insertion: Superior surface of 1st rib.
Action: Flexion of cervical spine (weak), elevation of 1st rib on inhalation, lateral flexion of cervical spine to same side, cervical spine rotation to opposite side.

Scalenus Posterior

Origin: Transverse processes of C4–C6 (variable).
Insertion: Outer surface of 2nd rib.
Action: Cervical flexion (weak), elevation of 2nd rib on inhalation, lateral flexion of cervical spine (assists), cervical spine rotation to opposite side.

The order of frequency of trigger point activity in the scalene muscles is from anterior to medial to posterior. Trigger points in the three scalenes may refer pain to the chest, the upper arm and shoulder, and in the back of the body to the medial border of the scapula. Trigger points in these muscles often form secondarily to trigger points in the SCM, so it is important to check both muscles together.

■ Find the posterior border of the SCM with your fingers. Moving it slightly anterior and avoiding the jugular vein, press your fingers down gently on the front portion of the transverse processes of the cervical vertebrae (Fig. 10-15). Hold tender points.
■ Using the broad side of your thumb, do an elongation stroke in the triangle formed by the posterior border of

the SCM and the anterior border of the upper trapezius (Fig. 10-16). Move in an inferior direction, to the clavicle (A in Fig. 10-16). Then, with your fingers, stroke across the direction of the muscle fibers of the medial scalene, seeking taut bands of tissue (B in Fig. 10-16). Pause to treat trigger points.

 Do not apply deep pressure in the posterior triangle area because the subclavian artery and vein are located here. Light cross fiber strokes are sufficient to relax the scalene muscles.

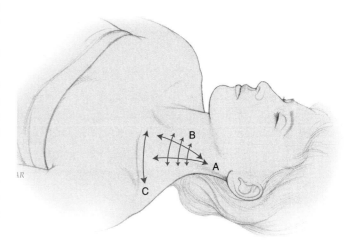

AR

FIGURE 10-16   Sequence of deep tissue strokes on the scalenes.

- With your index finger, reach under the superior edge of the clavicle toward the scalene attachments on the first and second ribs (C in Fig. 10-16). Apply cross fiber strokes to the attachments. Keep your finger against the inside surface of the clavicle to avoid pressing on nerves.

4. Suprahyoid Muscles (Digastric, Mylohyoid, Stylohyoid)

Digastric

Origin: Posterior belly—mastoid notch on temporal bone. Anterior belly—inner side of inferior border of mandible near symphysis.
Insertion: Intermediate tendon and to hyoid bone via a fibrous sling.
Action: Mandibular depression, elevation of hyoid bone during swallowing, anterior belly draws hyoid forward, posterior belly draws hyoid backward.

A trigger point may be found in the digastric muscle near its attachment on the mandible, just under the chin. It refers to the lower front teeth and the alveolar ridge below them.

- Digastric and mylohyoid attachments on the mandible. Place the pad of your index finger on the underside of the mandible near the center, at the digastric fossa. Slowly stroke across the inside border of the bone, to the angle of the mandible (Fig. 10-17).
- Belly of digastric. Beginning with your index finger at the digastric fossa of the mandible, stroke along the fibers of the muscle on the underside of the chin, to the fibrous loop on the superior border of the hyoid (Fig. 10-18).

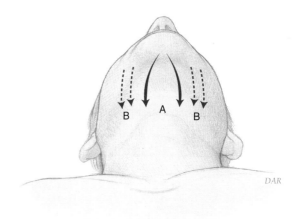

FIGURE 10-18 Direction of deep tissue strokes on the bellies of digastric (A) and mylohyoid and stylohyoid (B).

Mylohyoid

Origin: Mylohyoid line (from symphysis to molars) on inside surface of mandible.
Insertion: Hyoid bone.
Action: Raises hyoid bone and tongue for swallowing.

Stylohyoid

Origin: Styloid process of temporal bone.
Insertion: Hyoid bone.
Action: Hyoid bone drawn upward and backward, assists in opening mouth, possible participation in mastication and speech.

- Belly of mylohyoid and stylohyoid. Place your fingers at the inferior border of the mandible. Stroke in an inferior direction from the mandible to the hyoid bone (Fig. 10-18).
  - Note—The mylohyoid muscle forms the floor of the mouth.
  - Repeat the stroke, starting more laterally on the mandible, covering the entire surface area of the muscles. Feel for taut bands; hold at tender points. This stroke moves across the fibers of the muscles, rather than parallel to them.

 Be careful to not move off the mylohyoid muscle fibers on the lateral side because the submandibular gland is located here.

- Attachments on the hyoid bone:
  - To locate the hyoid bone, slide the fingers of one hand downward from the inferior border of the mandible until they touch the superior border of the hyoid bone (Fig. 10-19).
  - To stabilize the hyoid, keep the index finger on the

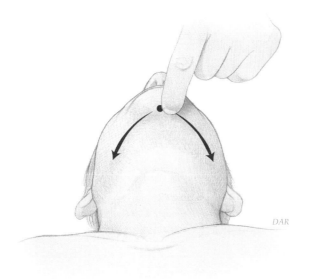

FIGURE 10-17 Working the digastric and mylohyoid attachments on the inside border of the mandible.

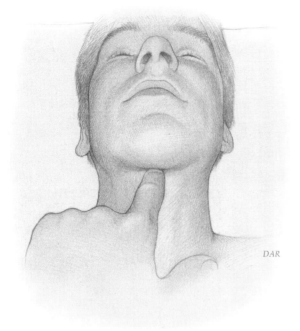

FIGURE 10-19   Palpating the superior border of the hyoid bone.

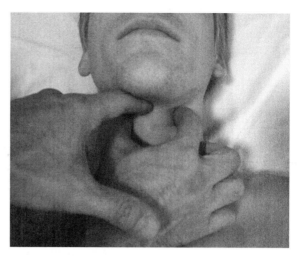

FIGURE 10-20   Hand position for contacting muscle attachments on the hyoid bone.

superior border of the bone while you place the thumb on the tip of the greater horn of the hyoid on one side and your middle finger on the tip of the greater horn on the other side.

■ To relax the muscles that attach to the hyoid bone, remove your index finger from the superior border. Maintaining the hold on the ends of the bone, slowly shift the hyoid from side to side.

 The hyoid bone is fragile. Do not squeeze it tightly or apply strong pressure to it.

■ To work the suprahyoid muscle attachments, place the index finger of your other hand on the superior border of the hyoid while you continue to hold on to the ends of the bone (Fig. 10-20). Move your finger across the edge of the bone, getting client feedback about tenderness. Pay special attention to the fibrous loop on the lesser horn of the hyoid that connects the digastric muscle to the bone.

5. Infrahyoid Muscles

■ Still stabilizing the hyoid with one hand, place the index finger of your other hand on the body of the hyoid and slowly stroke side-to-side. Hold sensitive points.
■ Slide your finger down slightly and stroke side-to-side on the inferior border of the hyoid.
■ Slide the pad of your index finger onto the inner surface of the clavicle and stroke side-to-side on the medial end to contact the attachment of the sternohyoid.

6. Prevertebral Muscles (Longus Capitis, Longus Colli)

Longus Capitis
Origin: Transverse processes of C3–C6 vertebrae.
Insertion: Inferior basilar part of occiput (anterior to foramen magnum).
Action: Capital flexion, rotation of head to same side.

Longus Colli

Superior Oblique Part
Origin: Transverse processes of C3–C5 vertebrae.
Insertion: Tubercle of anterior arch of atlas.

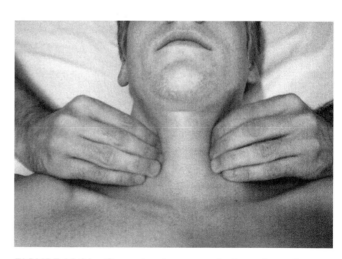

FIGURE 10-21   Contacting the prevertebral muscles underneath the trachea.

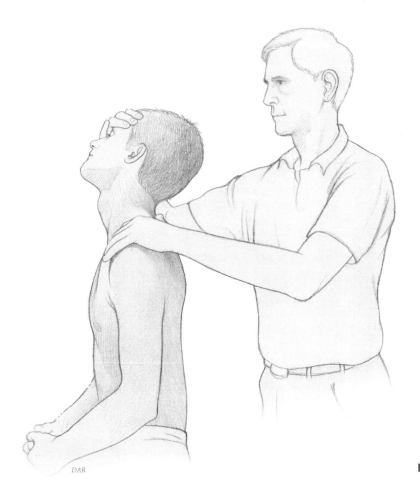

FIGURE 10-22 Stretch for the anterior neck.

Inferior Oblique Part
Origin: Anterior bodies of T1–T3 vertebrae (variable).
Insertion: Transverse processes of C5–C6 vertebrae.

Vertical Portion
Origin: Anterior bodies of C5–C7, T1–T3 vertebrae.
Insertion: Anterior bodies of C2–C4. **Action of all three parts: Cervical flexion (weak), cervical rotation to opposite side (inferior oblique), lateral flexion (superior and inferior oblique).**
■ Place the fingers of both hands lengthwise along the borders of the trachea. Slowly and lightly slide the fingers medial under the trachea toward the anterior bodies of the cervical vertebrae (Fig. 10-21).

 Do not press on the top of the trachea, so that the thyroid gland can be avoided. Move slowly and sensitively in this area as the vertebral artery runs parallel to the trachea. If you feel a pulse as you slide under the trachea, lift your fingers slightly and move them more medial to take pressure off the artery.

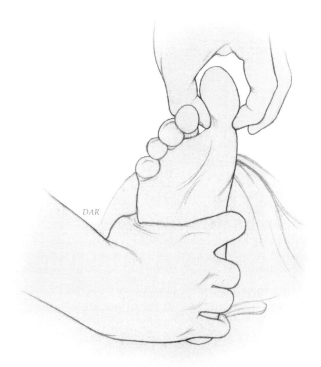

FIGURE 10-23 Contacting the neck reflex zone on the big toe.

- Slowly move the fingers of one hand at a time up-and-down and side-to-side along the prevertebral muscles, feeling for knots and taut bands. Work each side individually. Get client feedback about tenderness. Hold trigger points.
- Note—A cough reflex may be encountered at the base of the neck near the sternal attachment of the SCM.

Stretch

The client sits upright on the edge of the table. Sitting or standing behind the client, place one palm on the shoulder and the other palm on the same side of the head, above the ear.

Laterally flex the head while stabilizing the shoulder. Slowly turn the client's head toward extension (Fig. 10-22). Move in small increments, pausing to hold as the various muscle groups just worked on are stretched.

Accessory Work

1. Occipital release. Sitting at the head of the table, slide your fingers under the client's occipital ridge. Let them sink into the tissues under the base of the cranium. Hold for 1 or 2 minutes.
2. The reflex zone on the foot that corresponds to the neck is the shaft of the big toe. Hold the sides of the big toe, near the base, with your thumb and index finger (Fig. 10-23). Glide the fingers up and down in small movements. Repeat on the other foot. Press and hold tender points.

Closing

Sitting at the foot of the table, lightly hold the heels of the client's feet in your hands for 30 to 60 seconds. Remove your hands slowly to complete the session.

THE FACIAL MUSCLES AND TEMPOROMANDIBULAR JOINT

INTRODUCTION

Probably more than any other part of the body, the head and face tend to define a person's identity. Many people have the image of themselves as a head carrying around the body like baggage. When asked the question, "Where do you feel yourself to reside in your body?" the majority of people will answer, "In my head." One of the greatest benefits of deep tissue bodywork is the reconnection of the head with the rest of the body.

In our society, the values most appreciated are those associated with the head. In the workplace, people are generally judged and valued more for their mental abilities than for physical prowess. Most occupations rely on mental and sensory acuity for success and advancement. In part because of these factors, the head and face readily accumulate stress. Headaches related to tension are common and often debilitating. Massage to the scalp and facial muscles has a relaxing, rejuvenating quality that does much to counteract the effects of strain on the face.

The temporomandibular joint (TMJ) of the jaw is one of the most frequently used joints in the body. Its movement accompanies talking and eating, two of the most commonly occurring functions in which we engage. Therefore, the muscles that control the TMJ need to be strong and have quite a bit of stamina. These muscles are subject to stress and dysfunction due to overuse and emotional factors. Tightening the jaw by clenching the teeth is a frequent response to tension. It is often done unconsciously, even while a person is asleep. Chronically shortened jaw muscles can generate painful trigger points and misalign the TMJ.

TMJ dysfunction is becoming recognized as a major problem that is often misdiagnosed and untreated. In addition to muscle overuse and fatigue, other causes of TMJ disorder include trauma to the jaw, keeping the mouth open for long periods (as during a dental examination), and loss of teeth.

TMJ disorder causes many possible symptoms. Pain may occur around the joint itself, in the jaw muscles, and in or above the ears. Dizziness is also common. Referred pain patterns may be perceived as toothache or neck pain. It may be difficult to open or close the mouth, and a clicking sound may be heard. TMJ dysfunction may affect the position of the facial and cranial bones. They can become compressed, resulting in ringing in the ears, vision disorders, headaches, and/or chronic sinus inflammation.

There is often a correspondence between tension areas in the jaw and the pelvis. The two are connected by a polarity relationship, being at both ends of the spinal cord. The head and jaw represent the positive pole, and the pelvis acts as the negative pole. There is even a similarity in shape between the mandible and the pelvis. The balance of both poles helps to integrate the entire body.

Muscles	Bones and Landmarks	ESSENTIAL ANATOMY BOX 10–2
Temporalis	Occipital	
Occipitalis	Temporal	
Galea aponeurotica	Parietal	
Auricularis	Frontal	*The Cranium and Facial Routines*
Frontalis	Orbital ridge	
Procerus	Maxilla	
Orbicularis oculi	Mandible	
Masseter	Zygomatic arch	
Buccinator		

MUSCULOSKELETAL ANATOMY AND FUNCTION (ESSENTIAL ANATOMY BOXES 10-2 AND 10-3 AND FIG. 10-24A AND B)

The TMJ is the articulation of the mandible with the temporal bone of the cranium. This joint is unique in the body in that the lower portion hangs from the upper portion, requiring muscular action to keep the jaw shut. The joint consists of the convex-shaped mandibular condyle, the concave articular eminence of the temporal bone, and a disc between these bony surfaces. There are actually two joints, an upper and a lower portion. The articulation of the temporal bone and disc form the upper joint, while the mandible and disc form the lower joint. Complete opening and closing of the mouth is dependent on coordinated action of these two joints.

The disc is irregularly shaped, being narrower in the center than at the two ends, causing its center to be concave at both the top and bottom surfaces. This allows for a greater adaptability of fit against differently shaped bony surfaces. The disc is attached to the medial and lateral sides of the condyle of the mandible, allowing it to rotate around it without sliding off. The anterior end of the disc is attached to both the joint capsule and the **lateral pterygoid** muscle. At the posterior end, the disc is attached to two bands of fibers, called the bilaminar retrodiscal pad. The other end of the upper band attaches to the tympanic plate. It is composed of elastic fibers that stretch when the disc slides anteriorly and help pull the disc back into position posteriorly when the jaw closes. The lower band is composed of inelastic fibers attached to the neck of the condyle. The function of this band is to prevent the disc from sliding too far forward.

The mandible is a U-shaped bone that articulates with the temporal bone on both ends. It is capable of depression and elevation (opening and closing the mouth), protrusion and retrusion (jutting the jaw forward and back), and lateral deviation or sliding from side to side. The

Muscles	Bones and Landmarks	ESSENTIAL ANATOMY BOX 10–3
Temporalis	Temporal	
Tendon of temporalis	Sphenoid	
Masseter	Lateral pterygoid plate	
Lateral pterygoid	Mandible	*The TMJ Routine*
Medial pterygoid	Ramus of mandible	
Digastric	Condyle of mandible	
	Coronoid process	

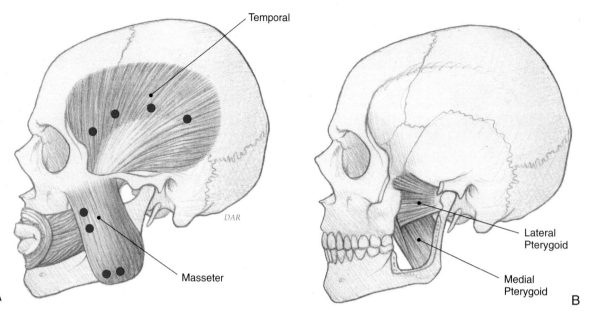

FIGURE 10-24 (**A** and **B**) Muscles acting on the temporomandibular joint.

mandible can also move asymmetrically around its condyles, a motion that is used in chewing. The TMJ is frequently called into action during chewing, talking, and swallowing.

When the jaw first opens, the mandibular condyle rotates on the inferior surface of the disc, allowing between 11 and 25 mm of opening. To open the mouth further, the disc and condyle unit glide anteriorly along the articular eminence of the temporal bone. The normal vertical span of a fully open mouth is between 40 and 50 mm. To close the mouth, these actions occur in reversed order.

The muscles of the jaw are very strong, particularly the masseter, and at the same time able to control small, precise movements. The articular surfaces of the joint are covered with fibrocartilage, which is resistant to damage and capable of quick healing.

Mandibular depression is accomplished primarily by the digastric muscle. The lower portion of the lateral pterygoid also assists in this action. Elevation of the mandible is performed by the **masseter, temporalis,** and **medial pterygoid** as well as the upper portion of the lateral pterygoid muscle.

Because of its prominent role in closing the jaw and chewing, the masseter is prone to dysfunction, including trigger point formation. Eating hard, chewy foods, such as gristly meat and bagels, causes the masseter to overwork. Biting down hard on ice or trying to hold things between the teeth can also be aggravating to this muscle. Emotional distress is often reflected in chronic contraction of the masseter, accompanied by gritting the teeth. Shortness in the masseter can be assessed by a person's inability to fully open the mouth vertically.

The temporalis assists the masseter in mandibular ele-

vation. The posterior section of the muscle assists in retraction of the jaw and lateral deviation of the mandible to the same side. Dysfunction in this muscle due to trigger points may manifest as hypersensitivity in the muscle and tension headaches caused by referred pain patterns. Sometimes pain in the upper incisor teeth originates from trigger points in the temporalis muscle.

The lateral pterygoid consists of two segments that work in opposition to each other. The upper portion, which is attached to the anterior end of the disc and to the condyle of the mandible, acts in unison with the temporalis and masseter to elevate the mandible. It also maintains traction on the disc when the jaw closes. When the upper lateral pterygoid becomes chronically short, it pulls the disc forward of the condyle as the jaw closes, causing a clicking sound and making closing the mouth difficult.

The lower portion of the lateral pterygoid acts to open the jaw, to protract the jaw when both sides of the muscle are contracting, and when contracting unilaterally, to pull the jaw to the opposite side. Pain felt in the TMJ frequently comes from a shortened lateral pterygoid muscle.

CONDITIONS (INDICATIONS/ CONTRAINDICATIONS BOXES 10-2 AND 10-3)

1. *Bell's palsy* is a partial facial paralysis involving cranial nerve VII, also known as the facial nerve. Symptoms may include a drooping mouth or eye and in some cases severe one-sided facial distortion. There are several factors that can cause the nerve to swell

Indications	Contraindications	
Sinusitis	Recent trauma	**INDICATIONS/ CONTRAINDICATIONS BOX 10-2**
Earache	Broken facial bones	
Headache	Cranial fractures	*Conditions Affecting Cranial and Facial Massage*
Facial pain	Black eye or bruising	
Fatigue	Sunburn	
Tension	Recent dental surgery	
Eye strain		

and become impinged, including viral diseases. In some cases, onset of Bell's palsy is precipitated by an emotionally upsetting circumstance. Recovery usually takes several months. Massage treatments may help to relieve some of the stress accompanying the condition.

2. *Headaches.* There are many types and causes of headaches. Listed below are some of the more common types, but there are many others.

   a. *Tension.* Tension headaches are caused by chronic contraction or spasm of the muscles of the neck, causing a restriction of blood flow to the cranial region. Massage to the tight muscles will frequently bring relief.

   b. *Allergic.* Allergic headaches are brought on by the body's reaction to foods or environmental factors. They are usually characterized by a dull, aching sensation over the forehead and cheeks. Monosodium glutamate (MSG), caffeine, nitrites, and other additives frequently trigger allergic headaches. Some foods that contain common allergens include wines, cheeses, processed foods, pickled foods, chocolate, and many others. The most effective treatment is to trace the allergy-producing food or foods and remove them from the diet.

   c. *Migraine.* This form of headache is brought about by dilation of the extracranial blood vessels. It is characterized by sharp and debilitating pain on one side of the head, sometimes behind the eye. It may be accompanied by visual disturbances, such as seeing lights or ropes floating in front of the eyes, and possibly vomiting. The headache may last from several hours to several days. There are many precipitating factors, including stress, exposure to bright light, and allergic reactions. Treatment consists of reversing blood flow out of the head by applying ice compresses to the forehead and/or occiput and immersing the hands and feet in warm water.

3. *Some types of hair loss.* In some cases, a person loses hair due to tightness of the scalp muscles strangling hair follicles, which prevents them from receiving adequate nutrition. Deep tissue massage will increase circulation to the area and may restimulate hair growth.

4. *Sinus congestion* may be relieved through a combination of heat, massage, and acupressure treatment to the appropriate areas of the face.

THE MIND/BODY CONNECTION

The face projects our persona, or the part of us that we present to the world. A person's face is often the primary criterion used to assess his or her quality of character. We

Indications	Contraindications	
Headaches	Abscesses	**INDICATIONS/ CONTRAINDICATIONS BOX 10-3**
Pain in teeth	Recent trauma	
Facial pain	Broken facial bones	*Conditions Affecting TMJ Massage*
Earaches	Gum surgery	
Sore throat	Serious illness	
Bruxism (teeth grinding)	Fever	

can frequently deduce a person's emotional state by interpreting facial features.

The face can be thought of as the mask we take off or put on to either reveal ourselves or hide what we are thinking or feeling. When the face is open and relaxed it can reflect our inner state. It has been said that a person's soul can be seen through the eyes. In the same way, we can block or limit what we reveal about ourselves by holding the face frozen or in a fixed expression.

The conflict between the outer facade and inner sensation is often a source of tension. It can be frightening and confrontational to have the face scrutinized and the muscles relaxed if a person is blocking access to his or her inner feelings through a fixed facial expression. Make-up and glasses are sometimes used as a means to shield the face in an attempt to hide or protect the person inside.

It is fairly common to encounter people who do not want their faces massaged or even touched. The therapist should therefore ask permission before massaging a client's face to avoid a possible adverse reaction

The jaw is used in eating and speaking. The jaw and teeth are strong and capable of tearing and grinding. Animals frequently use the jaw and teeth as weapons. We assert ourselves through the use of the jaw, claiming what we want through speech.

Tightness in the jaw muscles usually accompanies clamping down of the teeth and denotes a withholding of feeling or expression. A person who is contracting the jaw muscles might be blocking the communication of strong emotion. It is a common experience for many of us to "swallow my feelings" or "hold my tongue." This bottling up of expression can become chronic.

Bruxism, or grinding down the teeth by contracting the jaw muscles, is a condition that dentists deal with frequently. The release of tension in the jaw might be accompanied by a desire to speak out loud what one has been holding inside. Sometimes just making sounds of different varieties can be very liberating. We tend to limit our vocal expression to words. Sounds like grunting, hissing, or screaming can release the more primal parts of our nature and are very therapeutic, when expressed in an appropriate setting.

EVALUATION OF THE FACIAL AREA (TABLE 10-3)

1. Observe the overall shape and contours of the head.
2. Check for symmetry in the face.
   - Imagine a vertical line dividing the face into right and left segments.
   - Compare the two sides.

3. Observe the eyes.
   - Are they the same size?
   - Are they on the same horizontal plane?
   - Where are they looking?

4. Make note of any lines of stress on the face.
   - Across the forehead.
   - Between the eyebrows.
   - Outside corners of eyes and mouth.

5. Observe any muscular tension in the face and neck region.

EVALUATION OF THE TEMPOROMANDIBULAR JOINT

1. Have the client open and close the mouth a few times.
   - Observe the motion of the jaw. It should move symmetrically on both sides.
   - The bone at the TMJ junction should not jut out on either side when the mouth opens and closes.
   - Observe the alignment of the upper and lower teeth. There should not be a lateral shift of the teeth as the mouth opens and closes.

TABLE 10-3	Body Reading for the Face	
Conditions	**Muscles that May be Shortened**	
Furrowed brow—lines on the forehead and/or between the eyebrows	Frontalis Temporalis Procerus	
Constant frown—the corners of the lips are turned down	Platysma Digastric	
Facial misalignment—asymmetry of the features and/or bone structure of the face	Treat the tight muscles that seem to be distorting the face Some imbalances may be permanent	

2. Place your fingers on both sides of the client's jaw, at the TMJ. Have the client slowly open and close the mouth a few times.
   - Feel for a smooth, gliding motion on both sides. Note any deviations.
   - Listen for any clicking or popping sounds.

   Note—A number of injuries can displace the TMJ. These include blows to the jaw and whiplash injuries that cause the cervical spine and jaw to hyperextend. Biting down on hard food and overindulgence in chewing gum may also be culprits.

EXERCISES AND SELF-TREATMENT

1. Eye exercises
   - Slowly look straight upward toward the eyebrows, then downward toward the cheeks. Perform the movement three times. Close the eyelids and rest for a few moments.
   - Slowly look across a horizontal path to the right corners of the eyes. Look across a horizontal path to the left corners of the eyes. Perform the movement three times. Close the eyelids and rest for a few moments.
   - Look around the eye sockets in a clockwise direction, making a full circle. Begin by looking upward toward the eyebrows and then continue around the eye orbit to the left. Perform the movement three times. Rest for a few moments, then trace three slow circles in a counterclockwise direction.
   - Lie down on your back. Rub both palms together vigorously to generate heat, then rest the palms over your closed eyes. Allow the warmth and energy to penetrate into the eyes and cheeks, feeling the entire area around the eyes relaxing. Rest, with the eyes closed, for several minutes.

2. Facial tension release
   This exercise may be performed sitting or lying down. As you inhale, expand the face by slowly making a look of surprise. Open the eyes very wide, open the mouth as far as you can, flare the nostrils. Hold for a few moments. Exhaling, pull all the features of the face toward the center by closing the eyes tight, draw the cheeks in, and pucker the mouth. Squeeze and hold for a few moments. Repeat both facial expressions two more times, then rest, allowing all the tension to flow out of the facial muscles.

3. Jaw and tongue tension release
   - Place the pads of both thumbs on the underside of your chin. Slowly begin to yawn as you press against the underside of the chin with the thumbs, creating a resistance to the opening of the mouth. Repeat a couple of times and then rest the jaw muscles.
   - With the mouth closed, circle your tongue in a clockwise direction over the upper and lower teeth. Repeat 9 more times. Reverse the direction of the tongue circling, completing 10 repetitions counterclockwise.

HEAD/FACE/JAW ROUTINE

OBJECTIVES

- To release tightness in the cranial muscles, which can be a major stress reliever.
- To help alleviate aggravating factors in headaches and facial pain.
- To reduce tension in muscles affecting the jaw and TMJ.
- To reduce muscular stresses in the facial muscles.

ENERGY

Position

The client is lying supine on the table. A bolster may be placed under the knees for comfort.

The therapist is sitting at the head of the table.

Polarity

Place your right palm (positive pole) under the client's occipital ridge (negative pole), and your left palm (negative pole) across the forehead (positive pole). Imagine your hands drawing all the tension out of the head. Breathe deeply and relax fully as you maintain the contact. Hold for 1 to 2 minutes.

Shiatsu

Place your fingers on the sides of the client's head, above the ears. With your fingers curved and separated, press in against the cranium. Move your fingers to several different places on the sides of the head and repeat. This move stimulates points on the gallbladder and triple heater channels.

SWEDISH/CROSS FIBER

1. Perform circular friction with the fingertips on the scalp. Start from the back of the head and work forward to the forehead.
2. Perform effleurage strokes with the fingertips across the forehead, cheeks, and chin.
3. Perform circular friction with the fingertips under the cheekbones and down the sides of the jaw.

DEEP TISSUE/NMT

Sequence

1. Cranium—temporalis, occipitalis, galea aponeurotica
2. Facial muscles—frontalis, procerus, orbicularis oculi
3. Jaw—tendon of temporalis, masseter, lateral pterygoid

1. Cranium

Temporalis

Origin: Temporal fossa, temporal fascia.
Insertion: Coronoid process and anterior border of ramus of mandible.
Action: Elevates mandible, clenches teeth, posterior fibers retract mandible, assists in lateral grinding motion.

Several trigger points may form in this muscle. They usually occur in an arc around the section where the muscle fibers join the tendon. These trigger points often account for headache pain in the temple region and pain around the eyes into the upper teeth.

The first trigger point, in the lower anterior portion of the muscle, refers pain along the supraorbital ridge and inferiorly into the upper front teeth. The second and third trigger point regions are located in the middle lower portion of the muscle and send pain to the temple and into the maxillary teeth. The fourth section of trigger point formation, in the posterior aspect of the muscle, has a referral zone located behind and above the trigger point

- Place your fingertips or thumb on the side of the client's head, slightly above the ear (Fig. 10-25). Put the palm of your other hand against the temporalis muscle on the other side, to stabilize the head.
- Move up-and-down and side-to-side, on small sections of the muscle, feeling for stringy fibers and points of tenderness. Cover the entire muscle. Treat trigger points as you find them. Repeat on the other side.

Occipitalis

Origin: Lateral two-thirds of superior nuchal line on occipital bone, mastoid process on temporal bone.
Insertion: Galea aponeurotica.
Action: Draws back scalp, helps frontalis to raise the eyebrows and wrinkle the forehead.

Trigger points in this muscle are common culprits in the formation of headaches that shoot pain over the top of the head and into the eye.

- From the EOP, slide your fingers laterally along the superior nuchal line to the mastoid process part of the temporal bone.
- Move your fingers up and down and side to side, on small sections of the muscle (Fig. 10-26). Feel for taut bands and points of tenderness. Treat trigger points as you find them. Both sides may be worked simultaneously, or each side separately.

Galea Aponeurotica (Tendinous Sheet Connecting the Occipitalis and Frontalis)

- Positioning the fingers of both hands above the occipitalis muscles, move the scalp up and down, in small sections, sliding it over the cranium. Pay attention to sections of tissue that are immobile. Hold tender points until they become less sensitive.
- Continue, moving up over the top of the head to the frontalis. Be thorough, covering the galea aponeurotica completely.

2. Facial Muscles

Frontalis

Origin: Fascia of facial muscles above nose and eyes and the skin.
Insertion: Galea aponeurotica.
Action: Along with occipitalis draws scalp back, raises eyebrows, wrinkles forehead. Working alone, raises eyebrow on same side.

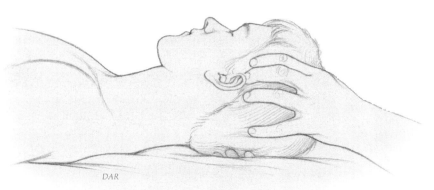

DAR

FIGURE 10-25   Hand position for releasing the temporalis.

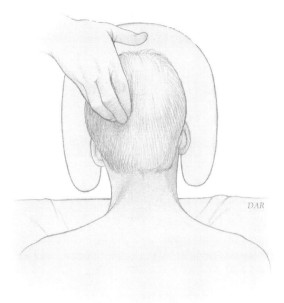

FIGURE 10-26   Palpating the occipitalis above the superior nuchal line.

A trigger point may be found about halfway between the eyebrow and the hairline, toward the mid-line of the forehead. It refers pain over the forehead on the same side that the trigger point is located.

■ Place the fingers of both hands on the front portion of the scalp, above the hairline. Move the fingers up and down and side to side, in small sections, over the fibers of the muscle (Fig. 10-27). Feel for taut, stringy fibers, and painful, stuck areas.
■ Continue the stroke in an inferior direction, covering the entire forehead to the eyebrows.

Procerus
Origin: Nasal bone and nasal cartilage.
Insertion: Skin of forehead between eyebrows.
Action: Wrinkles skin between eyebrows, draws medial part of eyebrows downward.

■ Place your thumbs horizontally and parallel to each other on the bridge of the nose, in the space between the eyebrows (Fig. 10-28).
■ Alternately roll the thumbs over each other, in the direction of the forehead, in a small, continuous motion without moving them off the space between the eyebrows.

Orbicularis Oculi
Origin: Nasal part of frontal bone, frontal process in front of lacrimal groove of maxilla.
Insertion: All around orbit of the eye, blends with occipitofrontalis and corrugator, skin of eyelid.

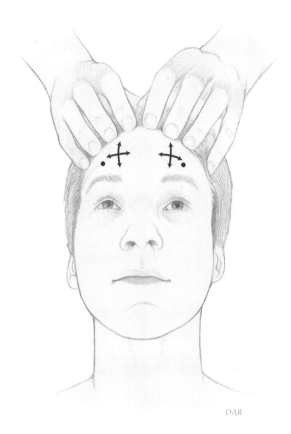

FIGURE 10-27   Releasing the frontalis muscle.

Action: Closes eyelids gently or forcibly, draws eyelids and lacrimal canals medially.
   Trigger points along the upper ridge of the eye socket may refer pain to the nose.

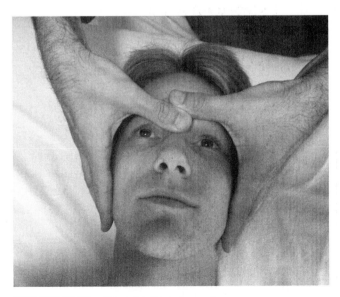

FIGURE 10-28   Deep tissue stroke on the procerus.

- Place the pads of your index fingers against the medial side of the upper portion of the eye sockets (supraorbital ridge). Both sides may be worked simultaneously.
- Slowly trace the border of the bone with your finger to the lateral side of the upper part of the eye socket, pausing at areas of tenderness (Fig. 10-29). Repeat several times.

3. Jaw (Tendon of Temporalis, Masseter, Lateral Pterygoid)

Tendon of Temporalis

- Place your fingers or thumb slightly above the lateral portion of the superior border of the zygomatic process of the temporal bone.
- Pressing your fingers against the tendon, move side to side slowly, feeling for taut bands and tender points. Having the client open the mouth stretches the tendinous fibers, making them easier to palpate.
- The client's mouth is open. Place your index finger in the space between the zygomatic bone and the coronoid process. Stroke side to side across the tendon.
- Stroke side to side on the top edge of the coronoid process. Pause and hold on points of tenderness (Fig. 10-30).

Procedures and Precautions for Performing Intraoral Techniques

1. Check the local ordinances to ascertain that performing intraoral procedures is legal in the area where you practice massage therapy.
2. Obtain the client's permission before attempting this work. Although every precaution is taken to maintain the client's comfort and prevent pain, the act of con-

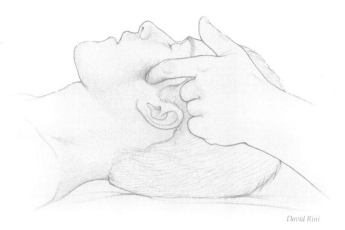

David Rini

FIGURE 10-30   Contacting the insertion of temporalis on the superior edge of the coronoid process.

tacting interior jaw muscles can be intense and may generate an emotional response. The client should be informed of this possibility before giving consent to receive the work.

3. Always describe the procedure to your client beforehand. Explain how releasing the masseter and especially the lateral pterygoid muscles can alleviate many of the symptoms of TMJ syndrome and relax the jaw area in general. To ease any feelings of apprehension, explain where your fingers will be placed inside of the mouth and which muscles will be addressed. Showing clients an illustration of the jaw muscles may be helpful in furthering their understanding of the procedure.
4. Do the necessary preparatory work before performing intraoral techniques. These procedures are the final ones described in the book. All the sessions learned beforehand have led to this culmination point. It is not necessary to have completed all the deep tissue sessions on a client to perform these procedures, but the client's body should be in a fairly relaxed and healthy state before attempting this work. Intraoral massage procedures are always preceded by massage of the neck, cranial, and facial muscles.
5. The therapist always wears a latex glove or finger cot when performing intraoral techniques. These items may be purchased at massage or medical supply stores. Rinse off any powder on the latex surface with water before putting your finger in the client's mouth. The latex should always be moistened before placing your finger against the tissues inside the mouth. This can be accomplished by dabbing your finger on the client's tongue to coat the working surface of the glove with a layer of saliva. Dry latex can stick to the delicate tissues inside the mouth and cause minor abrasions.
6. Communication with the client is extremely important throughout the procedure. However, it may be difficult for the client to speak with your finger in his or

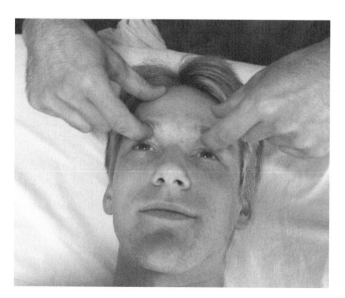

FIGURE 10-29   Pressing against the supraorbital ridge to release the orbicularis oculi muscles.

her mouth. A system of finger signals may be incorporated to allow the client to communicate reactions to the work. Explain to the client that raising the thumb means more pressure can be applied. Lifting the index finger means the pressure is adequate and comfortable. Raising the middle finger means the pressure is too intense and needs to be reduced. Raising the entire hand signals that the client needs to have the work halted immediately and the therapist's finger removed from the mouth. The therapist should remind the client of the meaning of each signal while performing the procedure, so that the client does not forget or become confused.

7. The approach to treating the internal jaw muscles is very gentle. The tissues are contacted only to the point of mild resistance and held without applying any further pressure until a softening of the muscles is sensed. Proceed slowly, maintaining your full attention on where your finger is placed, the response of the tissues, and the client's reaction to what is occurring.

Masseter

Origin: Superficial part—zygomatic process of maxilla, maxillary process, and inferior border of arch of zygomatic bone. Intermediate part—inner surface of anterior two-thirds of zygomatic arch. Deep part—posterior one-third of zygomatic arch.

Insertion: Superficial part—angle and lower half of lateral surface of ramus of mandible. Intermediate part—central part of ramus of mandible. Deep part—superior half of ramus and coronoid process of mandible.

Action: Elevates the mandible.

Trigger points in the superficial and deeper layers of this muscle have different referral zones. The layers are best distinguished using the sifting technique.

Trigger points in the superficial layer send pain to the lower jaw, maxilla, and molars and gums. Trigger points along the anterior border, in the upper portion, refer to the maxilla, upper molars, and the gums around them. Pain coming from these trigger points is often misinterpreted by the client as inflammation of the sinus cavities.

Trigger points along the base of the mandible send pain in an arc across the temple and eyebrow.

The deeper layer trigger points can send pain into the cheek, around the lateral pterygoid, and sometimes into the ear, which is perceived as a ringing sensation.

■ Place your fingers or thumbs on the anterior fibers of the muscle at the inferior border of the zygomatic arch (Fig. 10-31). Do an elongation stroke downward, to the base of the mandible. Press both sides simultaneously.

 Avoid pressing on the most posterior fibers of the muscle, as the parotid gland covers them.

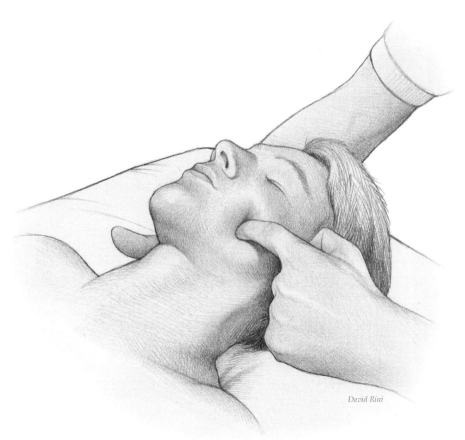

David Rini

FIGURE 10-31   Palpating the anterior border of the masseter muscle.

- Have the client open the mouth to stretch the masseter. Place your thumbs or index fingers on the anterior borders of the masseter, at the origin. Press in and up toward the zygomatic bone and hold for a minimum of 10 seconds. This is an excellent tension release point. Continue to stroke along the border, inferiorly, to the base of the mandible.

    Note—The next two moves are performed inside the client's mouth and require the therapist to wear a latex glove or finger cot.

- Sift the muscle by squeezing the fibers between your thumb and index finger, one of which is placed on the cheek, the other inside the mouth (Fig. 10-32). As you roll the fibers, check for trigger points.

Lateral Pterygoid

Origin: Superior head—lateral surface of greater wing of sphenoid. Inferior head—lateral surface of lateral pterygoid plate of mandible.

Insertion: Condylar neck of mandible, anterior margin of articular capsule and disc of the TMJ.

Action: Aids opening the mouth by protracting mandibular condyle and disc of TMJ joint forward while the mandibular head rotates on disc. Protracts jaw, bringing lower teeth forward of upper teeth. Acting on same side with medial pterygoid—causes the mandible and jaw to rotate to the opposite side (chewing motion).

Trigger points in this muscle are a major source of TMJ pain. They can also refer to the maxillary sinus.

- Have the client open the mouth slightly. Slide the pad of your index finger along the upper gum, fitting it into the pocket formed between the inside surface of the mandible and the lateral pterygoid plate on the sphenoid bone, behind the back upper molars.

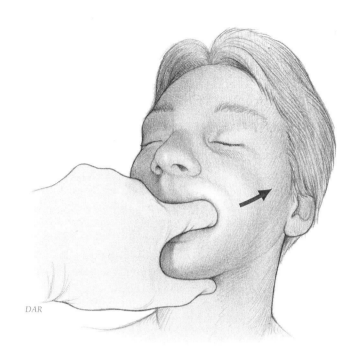

FIGURE 10-33 Palpating the lateral pterygoid.

- Press inward and upward, along the roof of the cheek, aiming the finger toward the condylar neck of the mandible, where the lateral pterygoid inserts (Fig. 10-33). Move slowly, as extremely painful trigger points may be encountered.

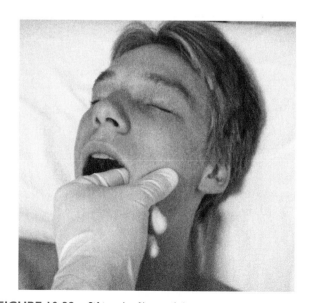

FIGURE 10-32 Sifting the fibers of the masseter.

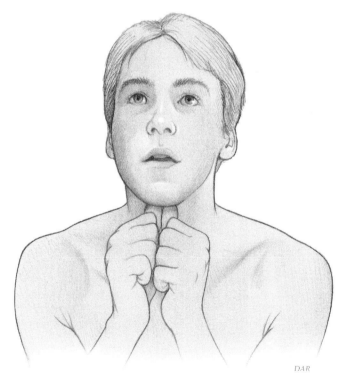

FIGURE 10-34 Tension release exercise for the temporomandibular joint muscles.

Stretch

The client places both thumbs under the center of the chin. The client then yawns, pressing up against the base of the chin to apply resistance to the downward movement of the mandible (Fig. 10-34). This stretch helps to relieve tension in the muscles of the jaw.

Accessory Work

1. Posterior and anterior neck work should accompany any work done on the jaw.
2. The pelvis is a reflex zone for the jaw. Simultaneously contacting tender points in both areas often brings relief of pain and balance to the body.
3. Working on the feet completes a session done on the cranium.

Closing

Sitting at the foot of the table, lightly hold the heels of the client's feet in your hands for 30 to 60 seconds. Remove your hands slowly to complete the session.

REFERENCES

1. Rolf IP. Rolfing: the integration of human structures. New York, NY: Harper and Row, 1977: 238.
2. Upledger J, Vredevoogd J. Craniosacral theory. Seattle, WA: Eastland Press, 1983.
3. Kapandji IA. The physiology of the joints. 2nd ed. New York, NY: Churchill Livingstone, 1974; ZS3: 180.
4. Upledger JD. Your inner physician and you: craniosacral therapy and somatoemotional release. 2nd ed. Berkeley, CA: North Atlantic Books, 1997.
5. Cailliet R. Soft tissue pain and disability. 2nd ed. Philadelphia, PA: FA Davis, 1988: 154.

CASE STUDIES

CASE STUDY 1 (EMOTIONAL RELEASE WORK)

The subject is a 28-year-old man named Brian, who works as a medical technician. He received a series of massage sessions several years ago and enjoyed them. He wants to experience massage therapy again because he is feeling out of touch with his body and thinks that receiving bodywork will help to bring him more physical awareness. Another reason he would like to achieve greater physical presence is that Brian has been experiencing problems with low self-esteem. He contends that a lack of assertiveness is causing problems at work and with his relationships. As a result, he feels weak and ineffective. As well as beginning massage therapy sessions, Brian bought a health club membership and has started a weight-training program to build himself up, as part of his program to increase self-confidence.

Physically, there is a lack of symmetry between Brian's upper and lower body. His torso is rather well developed, with good muscular definition in the chest and arms. The abdominal region appears to be overly contracted. The lower ribs are drawn inward toward the midline, creating compression in the solar plexus region. This restriction is partially due to tightness in the rectus abdominus.

Viewing Brian from the side, his back appears to be overly straight. Shortness in the abdominal wall has caused the pelvis to be drawn into a posterior tilt, causing a reduction in the lordotic curve. There is a band of tension wrapping around the mid-section. The cervical curve is also reduced. Brian's jaw is slightly retracted. The sternocleidomastoid muscles are clearly visible, with both tendons prominent at the base of the anterior neck. His lower body lacks the definition of his upper body. His hips are broad. The quadriceps muscles lack tone. His ankles are thick and both feet are turned out. The piriformis and hamstring muscles appear to be contracted.

One of the initial goals in working with this client is to help him to feel more supported by his legs and feet. He seems to control his body from the waist up, creating areas of tension in the torso and neck. When he walks he throws each leg forward rather than swinging the thigh freely from the hip. Each step lands flat on the entire plantar surface of the foot rather than rolling smoothly from heel to toe to cushion the impact. In addition to receiving deep tissue therapy, Brian is encouraged to engage in exercise activities in which he must use his legs and feet actively and with awareness. Tai chi classes and walking daily are recommended.

The plan for the first session was to begin the process of balancing the musculature of the legs. The initial contact was a polarity head hold followed by Swedish massage on the neck with deep tissue strokes performed along the lamina groove in the cervical region. Next the feet were addressed. Some time will be spent on the feet in each session to increase their mobility so that they will become more active during walking actions. Freeing restrictions in the feet will also enhance Brian's feeling of being grounded and help build awareness through the lower body.

After the work on the feet was completed, focus was shifted to the tibialis anterior and peroneal muscles. These muscles were found to be quite tense, contributing to a lack of fluidity throughout the feet. The quadriceps muscles were then massaged. This sequence was repeated on the left leg.

As the quadriceps were reached on the left side, the client began to complain of an uneasy feeling in his abdomen, almost a feeling of light spasm. With Brian's permission, the therapist moved on to the abdominal area to explore the feelings being generated there. The therapist lightly placed his right hand on Brian's abdomen while the left hand cradled the back of Brian's head. Brian was encouraged to breathe deeply into his abdomen, trying to push up the therapist's hand by expanding his abdomen as he inhaled and allowing the therapist's hand to sink toward his spine as he exhaled.

After a few rounds of deep breathing, Brian's breathing rhythm became choppy, especially on exhalation. He began to complain of tightness rising into his upper chest. The therapist asked him if he wished to continue to investigate these sensations. Brian responded that he would, so the therapist removed his left hand from behind Brian's head and placed it on the upper chest, just below the clavicles. Brian took a few breaths and began to clench his jaw. His neck and face were becoming flushed. The therapist asked if he was aware that he had begun to grit his teeth. He said no, he had not realized it, he was only aware that it was a little difficult to take a deep breath, but he wanted to continue. The therapist asked him to open his mouth slightly and allow his lower jaw to drop. He did so, and at that point began to cry. The therapist removed his hand from Brian's chest, reached for a tissue, put the tissue in Brian's hand, and asked if Brian wanted to describe what he was experiencing. He said he wasn't sure what was happening but felt comfortable staying with the feelings. He closed his eyes and continued to breathe slowly and deeply. The therapist's right hand remained on his abdomen while the left hand lightly touched his shoulder in a reassuring manner. Soon his body started shaking as waves of movement began to ripple through his trunk and legs. The crying became deeper.

After several minutes, the movement in his body calmed and the crying subsided. He lay there for a while continuing to breathe rhythmically but more slowly. The therapist gradually removed his hands from Brian's abdomen and shoulder and asked him how he felt. He began to smile and said he could sense a buzzing, tingling sensation across his forehead and in his hands. He then related that his breathing felt much easier and the tension in his abdomen was totally gone. He was very aware of the sensations in his body as he lay on the table. He said it felt as if a tight, heavy belt had been removed from around his waist, allowing him to sense his legs and feet much more fully. The therapist asked Brian if he would like to try to sit up on the table, and he answered that he would. The therapist helped lift him to a sitting position with his legs hanging off the side of the table and then brought him a glass of water, which he slowly sipped. When the therapist was sure that he was all right, he left the room to allow Brian to get dressed.

Upon entering the room again, the therapist encouraged Brian to walk around a little and relate what he was experiencing. He said his legs felt much freer and easy to move and he could sense himself land lightly on each foot as he took a step. When he walked, he was also more aware of the movement of his arms coordinated with the swinging of his legs. He said he felt as if a huge amount of bottled-up tension had been released during this session. Brian is now looking forward to continuing to become better acquainted with his body through deep tissue therapy.

CASE STUDY 2 (CONNECTIVE TISSUE)

The client is a 36-year-old woman named Margaret, who works in sales. She views her job as fairly high stress. She is constantly dealing with people, either in person or on the telephone. Although she exercises regularly, doing stretching and aerobics at least three times a week, she feels unable to relax fully. At times it is difficult to take a deep breath because her chest cavity feels muscularly tight and constricted. Her blood pressure is borderline high. Her goal in seeking massage therapy is to be able to relax and reduce the feelings of muscular tension that build up on a daily basis.

On observation, her muscles appear to be well toned. She was athletic in high school, having been on the swimming team, and her body still has an athletic quality. The musculature in her upper trunk and shoulders appears constricted. Her shoulders are medially rotated, with a slight degree of kyphosis in the upper back. Her sternum is depressed, causing her chest to appear somewhat sunken. Her head projects forward, causing the T1 vertebra to be prominent. There is a build-up of connective tissue around the upper thoracic vertebrae. Her pelvis is posteriorly rotated. She stands with her knees slightly flexed. This postural stance points to short hamstring muscles. Overall, she appears to be vertically compressed when standing, as if she was carrying a heavy load on her shoulders.

The plan for the initial session was to help relieve the feelings of muscular constriction due to built-up stress and to open the chest and shoulder region so that the client can experience fuller breathing. Future sessions will deal with lengthening the spinal column and bringing the head and pelvis into a better relationship to each other.

Soon after the session began, it became apparent that the client was unable to accept deep direct pressure to the muscles. The muscles were held tightly, in a seemingly protective mode. When moderate pressure was applied, the client reported feeling uncomfortable pain and her upper body retreated further into its medially rotated stance. The therapist decided that a connective tissue approach was the preferred treatment for this client. The fascial compartments needed to be stretched so that her muscles could lengthen and relax. She was uncomfortable with firm pressure and did not like sustained pressure to specific areas of soft tissue, even if the contact was light.

Myofascial mobilization and spreading techniques were applied to the pectoralis major and minor and to the serratus anterior to help expand the chest region and widen space across the shoulder girdle. The fanning stroke was also used in the upper thoracic region to help lift the sternum. Long Swedish strokes combined with connective tissue spreading were used on the rest of body to promote feelings of length and relaxation. Overhead stretching of the arms was used at the end of the session to stretch the chest.

The client reported feeling much lighter at the end of the session. Her breathing felt much fuller without forcing it. Her comment was, "I feel like a burden has been lifted off of me."

CASE STUDY 3 (THE CHEST)

The client is a 10-year old boy named Joey, who has asthma. His mother wants him to receive deep tissue therapy to help alleviate the condition and to possibly boost his self-esteem. He has been picked on in school because of his small stature and because he cannot participate fully in sports activities.

Postural evaluation of Joey revealed that his chest area was severely constricted. There were noticeable hollow areas under the clavicles and along the borders of the anterior deltoids, indicating that the pectoralis minor muscles were very contracted. The central sternal region of the chest was lifted but in a strained manner due to the boy's conscious attempt to make himself appear bigger. This position of the chest may also be partly a consequence of struggling to breathe during asthma attacks.

The focus of the session was to relieve tension in the chest to ease restrictions in the breathing muscles. The boy, being rather shy, was afraid to be left alone; therefore, his mother sat in on the session. Based on observation and the information gathered about his asthmatic condition, the areas chosen to focus on included pectoralis major and minor, subclavius, the scalenes, the intercostals, and the diaphragm. A connective tissue approach to these muscles was mandated due to the child's age and his sensitivity to touch in the chest area.

Joey responded very well to the front-to-back polarity contact on his sternum and upper back. He visibly relaxed and his breath deepened. Swedish massage strokes were used to warm up the muscles thoroughly before the deep tissue/connective tissue strokes were applied. The deep tissue protocol was followed but with full attention given to sensing a melting of the tissues before applying any further pressure or moving through the muscle fibers.

The chest muscles were released in layers, from superficial to deep. Many trigger points were encountered in the intercostal muscles. As a trigger point was pressed, Joey was encouraged to breathe deeply and imagine the point melting. He enjoyed participating in the process and felt a sense of accomplishment when the uncomfortable feelings generated by the trigger points dissolved. The diaphragm was contacted and massaged very carefully. It is not advised to work that area intensively on children, because much of their muscular tension is emotionally rooted, and deep, aggressive work on the diaphragm confronts that tension too strongly.[1] (See Kogan[2] for Reich's caution to therapists about approaching the diaphragm aggressively.)

The session was concluded with long Swedish strokes along the erector spinae and fingertip raking into the intercostal spaces between the ribs in the back to balance the release work performed on the front of the chest cavity. After the session, Joey's mood was much lighter. He was thrilled to be able to take fuller breaths without struggling and commented to his mother how much broader his chest and shoulders felt. He was very proud of himself. Joey was shown the door frame stretches for the chest muscles. It was suggested that he practice them every day to maintain the new-found length in his pectoralis major and minor muscles.

CASE STUDY 4 (THE BACK)

The client is a 29-year-old man named Clint. He works in real estate. He has received massage treatments from different therapists on an irregular basis over several years. His goal is to relax and relieve tension in tight neck, shoulder, and back muscles. Clint is tall and muscular. He used to lift weights but quit because he strained his low back and found that weightlifting put stress on his neck muscles. Recently, he has felt the need to return to exercising and has just begun to work out again. He is in good health. His only physical problem is residual tightness in low back muscles from the weightlifting injury 4 years ago.

Clint's upper body is more developed than his lower body. His shoulders and arms carry more bulk, relatively speaking, than his hip and thigh muscles. He exhibits a small degree of posterior pelvic tilt. His erector spinae muscles are very pronounced, particularly on the right side. He used to play baseball regularly and exhibits the right-left side muscular imbalance that one-handed sports generate. His neck appears short due to contracted trapezius muscles as well as other shortened head and neck extensors. The focus of this session will be to elongate the spinal column by releasing the erector spinae and deep paraspinal muscles.

Initial work on the back revealed that the superficial musculature was fairly relaxed. However, the deep muscles along the spine were extremely contracted. The client requested very deep pressure on these muscles. He barely felt any sensation in the deep paraspinal muscles regardless of the depth of pressure. They seemed to be numb. Deep pressure applied with the elbow did not cause the contractions in the muscles to yield. The lack of feeling and response from these muscles seemed to indicate the tension may be psychologically based. In other words, the

client may contract these muscles on a subconscious level to prevent certain feelings from arising to conscious awareness. This is known as armoring.[3]

Although the client wanted very deep pressure applied to these muscles so that he could feel something other than numbness there, the tissues were guarding against the invasion by contracting further. It was explained to the client that this deep, invasive pressure was being counter-productive, so the pressure was decreased. Although the client could not feel anything in the deep muscles, they relaxed to a small degree when the pressure was lessened.

The session continued with deep tissue strokes applied to the muscles along the entire spinal column. Then the client turned supine so that balancing work could be applied to the anterior neck and chest areas. Shiatsu compression moves were performed on the legs, and the session was completed with massage of the spinal reflex points on the feet.

After the session, the client described himself as high strung and unable to relax. This description matched the assessment of the condition of the soft tissues of the back. It was suggested that, if interested, the client should participate in a yoga class, where he could learn slow, sustained stretching movements along with coordinated deep breathing to begin to relieve some of the deep-seated stress in his intrinsic muscles. Regular yoga practice, along with deep tissue therapy sessions, would help to uncover and release the tightly held tension that has accumulated along his spinal column. The client appreciated the suggestion and added that he has wanted to start taking yoga and this session had been a good incentive for him to follow through on it.

CASE STUDY 5 (THE SHOULDERS AND ARMS)

The client is a 43-year-old massage therapist named Doris. She has been practicing massage therapy professionally for 10 years. For the past several months she has been experiencing tightness and pain in her neck, shoulders, and upper back. The tightness is exacerbated by giving a massage. During the previous 2 weeks she has begun to experience sharp pains in her right forearm muscles. It is becoming increasingly difficult for her to administer pressure with her right arm, as the pain in her forearm becomes intense when she pushes with her right hand.

Doris is a frail-looking woman. She is small-boned and does not have well-developed musculature. She is somewhat stooped over, with a slight kyphosis in her upper back. Her scapulae are protracted, with her arms medially rotated and the upper chest collapsed. She also exhibits a forward position of the head. Based on observing her posture and listening to the description of her arm complaint, the likelihood that she may be lacking in body mechanics skills is being considered. It is probable that she tries to push too much with her arm and back muscles when applying pressure during massage strokes, rather than leaning forward and distributing force throughout her entire body.

This and future deep tissue sessions will focus on releasing the muscles of the scapulae and relieving tension in the neck, around the clavicles, in the serratus anterior and pectoralis minor muscles, and throughout the muscles of the forearms and hands. She will obviously require a series of deep tissue sessions to address all the problems arising from her poor posture and lack of proper body mechanics.

Because of the protraction of the scapulae, collapse of the chest, and medial rotation of the arms, the serratus anterior, pectoralis major and minor, and anterior deltoid muscles were emphasized in the session. Numerous trigger points were encountered, particularly in the lateral section of the pectoralis minor. Working on the right forearm, the common extensor tendon was found to be very tender, perhaps inflamed. It was recommended that the client apply ice to it regularly. The borders of the forearm muscles were carefully traced and separated. The client found that the degree of mobility in both hands was greatly increased following the session. The muscles of the thenar eminence were tender on both hands, but particularly on the right side.

After the session, the likelihood that she is favoring her right arm and hand while performing massage was discussed. Doris is also overusing her arm and hand muscles to apply pressure, instead of allowing the weight of her body to flow through her arm and supply the force needed for the massage strokes. It was suggested that she diminish her massage client workload until the strain in her muscles from incorrect body mechanics is reduced. In addition to receiving deep tissue therapy treatments twice a week for the next month, she is going to engage in daily stretching of the chest, shoulder, arm, and hand muscles. She will also receive coaching in proper body mechanics. Once the initial trauma to the upper body muscles is reduced and better alignment of the shoulder girdle is achieved, she will begin a very mild weight-training program to build strength and acquire more kinesthetic awareness of her entire body.

CASE STUDY 6 (THE FOOT AND LEG)

The client is a 50-year-old man named Eugene, who is the head manager of a fast-food franchise. The duties of his job require that he stand all day. He is constantly moving around the store, ensuring the smooth operation of the business. He sought out deep tissue therapy because his feet and legs are becoming extremely sore and swollen, especially by the end of the workweek. It has become increasingly difficult for him to carry out the functions of his job because he is so uncomfortable.

Postural evaluation revealed that Eugene has flat feet. This causes the medial side of the knees to fall inward, creating stress on the medial collateral ligaments. He also exhibits a high degree of lordosis, and his scapulae are depressed. His clavicles angle downward, and his arms hang forward of his sides. Eugene also exhibits a forward head position, with his chin held abnormally high.

To deal fully with the problems in his lower body, a series of deep tissue sessions was commenced to align the entire body. Isolated massage to his feet and legs would not resolve the problems in his feet because they are reflective of postural imbalances throughout the entire body. Massage to the feet was performed in every deep session. However, the current case study details the fourth session performed, during which the muscles of the lower limb were emphasized.

Eugene's feet are very stiff and immobile. There is limited movement in the ankles and throughout the joints of the foot. After the first session, he was shown foot exercises to practice at home to begin to alleviate some of the inflexibility of the foot muscles.

The session focusing on the feet began with work on the intrinsic muscles of the foot. The deep tissue strokes revealed tiny granular-feeling lumps accumulated along the toe tendons and extreme sensitivity to pressure in many areas on the plantar surface of the foot. Sustained therapist-assisted flexion and extension of the toes was administered to stretch the muscles and fascia of the foot, along with plantar flexion, dorsiflexion, inversion, and eversion movements.

Low medial arches force both feet into eversion while the client is standing. Therefore, the peroneal muscles, which evert the foot, are extremely contracted. They felt like concrete. Slow, deep strokes with the elbow were performed on these muscles. A high degree of softening of the peroneal longus and brevis was achieved. To balance the release of the peroneals, the client was taught an exercise to strengthen the tibialis anterior muscle, which lifts the medial arch. Its action counter-balances that of the peroneal muscles. The lesson took place after the session. Eugene was taught to sit in a chair with his leg flexed at the hip, knee, and ankle. He was to hang a petite-size gift bag containing two soup cans from his flexed foot. He would then slowly invert his foot (turn the plantar surface inward) and hold for 3 seconds. This movement was to be repeated 10 times on the right and left sides.

The gastrocnemius and soleus muscles were also massaged. The heads of the gastrocnemii were sensitive to touch. Extensive Swedish pétrissage and friction strokes were used to relax the muscles. Cross fiber strokes were incorporated rather than deep tissue elongation strokes because the muscles were too sensitive to withstand sus-

tained direct pressure. All the muscle attachments around the knee were treated. The muscle attachments of the pes anserinus were particularly sensitive.

Deep tissue therapy to the legs and feet was followed by shoulder, neck, and cranial massage to complete the session. To supplement the foot exercises, additional home care suggestions (including elevation of the legs following a long day at work and regular foot soaks in warm water with epsom salts) were made.

CASE STUDY 7 (THE HIP)

This case demonstrates the pervasive effects an injury can have on the soft tissues. The client is a 31-year-old homemaker named Mia, who is a former ballet dancer. She sustained an injury to her left hip while stretching in a dance class when she was 16 years old. She was sitting in a spread open-leg position on the floor with her upper body flexed forward and her arms extended along the floor in front of her. After a few seconds in the stretch she felt a shift of the left femur in the hip socket and a sharp pain running down the inside of her left thigh.

For several months after the injury Mia experienced sharp pains extending down the inside of her left thigh. Over time the pain became less pronounced, but she still experiences a dull throbbing in that area. The most dramatic effect of the injury was a loss of full turn-out of the left leg due to restriction of the femur in the hip socket. Mia found that this lack of turn-out on the left side affected her knee, as it was difficult to plié (flex) the left leg while keeping the left knee properly aligned over the foot. She would experience pain and swelling in that knee after dancing.

The bracing of the muscles around the left hip has caused a build-up and hardening of connective tissue on the left side of the body, extending well up into the back. There is a hardened mass of connective tissue along the lateral border of the iliocostalis muscle under the 12th rib that feels like another rib. Viewing the hips from the anterior position, the left hip appears narrower and posteri-

orly rotated. There is a small but noticeable limp on the left side when Mia walks.

The plan for the session was to attempt to improve alignment of the muscles on the left side which have been strained over the years in bracing the hip. These include the adductor muscles, gluteus medius and minimus, and the erector spinae (particularly iliocostalis). Deep tissue strokes along the borders of these muscles were incorporated extensively to relieve adhering of the muscles. Connective tissue spreading techniques and deep tissue elongation strokes were also applied to the muscles where there was a build-up of connective tissue. Deep tissue techniques were used to release the lateral rotator muscles of the posterior hip. Therapist-assisted stretches for the left hip included flexion, adduction, and abduction. The client was encouraged to continue to perform these stretches regularly between sessions.

A visit to a chiropractor or osteopath was recommended to evaluate the condition of the hip. An adjustment to the left hip joint may alleviate some of the stress around the joint. Although the problem was not resolved by the deep tissue session (i.e., the left hip joint did not become unrestricted), the client felt much more range of motion in the left hip after the session and wishes to continue to receive deep tissue therapy. She feels that it will be of great benefit in halting the further build-up of connective tissue above the left hip.

CASE STUDY 8 (RECTUS FEMORIS AND ILIOPSOAS)

The subject is a 27-year-old man named Eric, who is an actor. Eric is in good physical health. He enjoys reading about and becoming involved in activities that contribute

to his health and self-improvement. He participates in yoga and dance classes regularly and tries to maintain a low-fat diet. Eric enjoys outdoor activities like bicycling and hiking. He has been receiving a series of deep tissue therapy sessions as part of his health and high-level wellness regimen. This case study describes the session focusing on his hip flexors.

Eric has a well-balanced musculature overall. However, his anterior thigh and gluteal muscles appear to be overdeveloped in relation to the rest of his body. He exhibits an anterior pelvic tilt and slight pelvic rotation, with the left iliac crest drawn forward and downward. Observing his walking pattern reveals that he initiates thigh movements primarily with the rectus femoris muscles. This is apparent on observation because instead of allowing his thighs to swing from a mobile pelvis when he walks, he lifts his knees toward his chest and remains rigid in the pelvic region.

Eric complains that his thighs become very sore after dance classes and after hiking. He also gets winded sooner than he feels he should during strenuous activities and sometimes experiences cramping (a "stitch") under his ribcage. At irregular intervals, he experiences pain in his low back, more concentrated on the left side, near the sacrum.

Eric provides an example of someone who does not move from his core. His rectus femoris muscles overwork during hip flexion movements, while the psoas muscles are underactive. He has gained fairly good control of his body, but his movements are not as fluid as they could be if initiated from the pelvic center. His poor stamina reflects the lack of coordinated action between the extrinsic and intrinsic muscles. This is the fourth session dealing with the core, with the abdominal and thigh muscles worked on previously. Getting Eric more in touch with the iliopsoas complex will likely provide the missing key for him in understanding how to control his body movements properly.

The rectus femoris muscles were fairly sore. Elongation strokes along the fibers were performed extremely slowly, giving time for the client to relax and the muscle to lengthen. At least 10 minutes were spent on each rectus femoris muscle, allowing it to soften and lengthen fully. The attachment of the rectus femoris on the anterior inferior iliac spine was particularly sensitive. Initially, the client experienced extreme ticklishness when the attachment was contacted. After being directed to focus on slowing his breathing and relax into the sensations, the ticklishness transformed into extreme pain. The pressure was adjusted to a tolerable level and maintained without any movement until the client reported a considerable diminishing of the sensation. At that point, the therapist began a cross-fiber motion on the tendon to complete the release of the rectus femoris.

After warming up the abdominal region, the border of the iliacus was contacted along the rim of the ilium. There was surprisingly little discomfort there. The muscle responded well to the strokes and softened considerably. After placing his fingers in the left lower quadrant of the abdominal cavity in the proper location to palpate the psoas, the therapist had the client flex his left thigh to contract the muscle fibers. It was difficult to locate the psoas initially. When the muscle was finally palpated, the fibers felt extremely taut, like a thin cord. This was an unusual occurrence because the psoas is a thick, cylindrically shaped muscle. It was obviously extremely contracted, appearing to be frozen in position. The therapist very gradually moved the fingers up the length of the muscle, parallel to the bodies of the lumbar vertebrae. The client was not experiencing much sensation other than awareness of the presence of the fingers deep in his abdomen. However, at the level of L3 vertebra, he experienced a sharp pain as the therapist rolled across a tight knot of fibers. The pain was radiating into his low back, near the sacrum. This was exactly the area where he reported experiencing intermittent low back pain. The point was held until he reported an almost complete disappearance of the pain in his low back.

After the psoas muscles were worked on both sides, the client expressed feeling a wonderful sense of freedom, almost euphoria. He said he felt much more of a sense of being in his body. He felt light and open in his legs and feet and was actually aware of his spinal column, an experience he had never had before. It is not uncommon for clients to have a renewed burst of self-awareness after receiving psoas work. It is often the most profound deep tissue session they experience.

CASE STUDY 9 (THE NECK)

The subject is a 20-year-old woman named Chloe, who is a college student. Chloe is not a regular massage client. She schedules appoints sporadically, usually during high stress periods in her life. Her reason for seeking deep tissue therapy at this time is that for the past week she has been experiencing severe pain in her posterior neck. It radiates down her upper back to the level of T12 and up to the occiput. She is experiencing pain in the temporal region of her head that she feels is being generated by the tight muscles in her neck. It is difficult for her to study because the act of leaning forward at a desk to read causes shooting pains to radiate to the top of her head and throughout the posterior neck and upper back.

Chloe has been involved in several car accidents over 5 years. She has never been seriously injured but has experienced whiplash to varying degrees as a result of each accident. She received medical treatment for neck injuries sustained from the accidents and currently visits a chiropractor twice a month.

Although she has a history of neck injuries, she feels that the source of the pain is as much psychological as physical. It is always much worse during times of high stress. In addition to studying for exams, she is experiencing relationship problems that have her concerned to the point that she is not sleeping well at night. She often wakes up in the morning with a stiff, painful neck. The focus of this session will be deep tissue work on the posterior and anterior neck, the muscles of the upper back (particularly the trapezius), the cranium, some work on the jaw muscles, and stimulation of spinal reflex points on the feet.

With the client lying in a prone position, the layers of posterior neck muscles were meticulously worked, from superficial to deep. As expected, the muscles were very tender. Trigger points were discovered along the borders of the upper trapezius that radiated pain to the anterior portion of the temporal muscle, where she frequently experiences headache pain. A significant softening of the region was noted following the completion of deep tissue therapy on the neck. The entire upper back was massaged with careful attention paid to the entire trapezius.

Immediately after the client turned supine, the occipital release procedure was applied. When the therapist initially placed the fingers under her occipital ridge, she reported feeling a throbbing pain near the top of her head. It was triggered by pressure to the fibers of the upper portion of splenius capitis, between the borders of the trapez-

ius and sternocleidomastoid. She was willing to stay with the sensation, however, so the therapist continued to apply the occipital release technique. During approximately the first 30 seconds of the procedure, her head was held suspended away from the palms of the therapist's hands due to constrictions in the neck muscles. After about 1 minute of holding, her head began to sink toward the therapist's palms. Within another minute of holding, the back of her head was resting in the palms and she was smiling broadly. She reported that the pain at the top of her head was completely gone, and her head felt light and free.

Massage to the cranium and facial muscles was followed by deep tissue therapy to the sternocleidomastoid, scalenes, and prevertebral muscles. All these muscles were tender and elicited much radiated pain, particularly the attachments to the scalenes on the anterior side of the transverse processes of the cervical vertebrae. Swedish and cross fiber strokes were applied to the pectoralis major to balance the work done on the upper and mid-back. The session was completed with foot massage accompanied by reflexology and polarity.

After the session, the client reported feeling "like a new person." She said it felt as if someone had lifted her head off her shoulders. Due to the extreme tenderness in some of the neck muscles and the high incidence of radiating pain that was uncovered, the client decided to schedule another massage for the following week. She was shown neck stretches to perform whenever she began to feel strain in her neck muscles. The benefits of purchasing a portable editor's desk or bookstand to use when studying so that she does not have to flex her neck and head was discussed. She was also going to consider using a smaller pillow when she sleeps so that her head is not elevated so much, causing her neck to remain flexed all night.

CASE STUDY 10 (TEMPOROMANDIBULAR JOINT)

The subject is a 29-year-old woman named Rachel, who works as a part-time secretary. She moved to the Southeast from the West Coast about 8 months ago. Her experience with massage therapy is limited. She has received several relaxation-style massages as gifts. Since moving, she has been experiencing sinus headaches on a weekly basis, which she attributes to allergic reactions to the vegetation. She is also experiencing severe jaw pain and some restriction when opening her mouth wide. The jaw pain seems to be worse when she wakes up in the morning. Rachel's dentist has informed her that she is clenching and grinding her teeth at night. She is going to

be fitted with a night guard this week. The dentist recommended that she also receive massage therapy for the cranial and jaw muscles to reduce tension in those areas.

Rachel was asked if she had a history of temporomandibular joint (TMJ) dysfunction. She said that she did not; her problems began after her move. She has never been struck in the face, nor has she suffered whiplash. However, about 5 years ago, as she was biting into an apple her jaw momentarily stuck in an open position. It scared her quite a bit, but the mandible immediately slipped back into place and the incident has not recurred.

To evaluate movement of the jaw, Rachel was asked to

slowly open and close her mouth as the therapist lightly held his fingers on her right and left TMJs. When her mouth reached about a 0.75-inch opening, the mandible slipped to the left and there was a clicking sound. When the mouth reached an opening of 1.25 inches, the client began to experience pain in the jaw muscles.

The session focused on the TMJ and related muscles. The neck area was massaged first, followed by cranial massage. The temporalis muscles were sore, but the client said that pressure on the muscles felt good. Therefore, the therapist held points on both sides simultaneously for several seconds. After the entire cranial area was relaxed, the facial muscles were addressed. Focused attention was paid to the tendon of the temporalis muscle above the zygomatic bone. It was quite tender. The masseter muscles were bulky and unyielding to pressure. Circular friction strokes helped to relax the muscles. Numerous trigger points were found in the masseters.

The lateral pterygoids were the final muscles in the facial area to be massaged. Because the mandible pulled to the left, the left lateral pterygoid was most likely more contracted. The therapist explained the intraoral procedures to the client and put on a latex glove. The right lateral pterygoid was massaged first to accustom the client to the protocol and to induce relaxation in the less involved muscle before the more problematic left side was contacted. Even though there was much tenderness in both lateral pterygoid muscles, the client handled the procedure very well.

The procedure was done slowly to allow the client to breathe and relax throughout. The therapist removed his finger from inside the client's mouth several times during the procedure to allow her to relax and assimilate the release as well as to report her feelings toward the work. She said that, amazingly, when the therapist touched the lateral pterygoids, it triggered the pain in her sinus cavities that she had been attributing to allergies. Her eyes watered a little during the work, so she was given a tissue to wipe away the tears. She said the tears were not from pain or emotions, but more of a reflexive reaction.

After the completion of the session, Rachel observed her face in a mirror. She noted that she looked like she had shed about 5 years of age in her face. She felt completely relaxed and elated at gaining some insight into her sinus pain as well as feeling pain relief in the jaw muscles. When her jaw movement was evaluated after the session, the click was minimal and the mandible barely shifted. It was agreed that she should receive more TMJ work along with deep tissue therapy to other areas of her body.

Rachel had a realization that much of her TMJ problem was a stress reaction to moving to a new part of the country and starting her life over again. She also realized that she had been holding back from saying some important things to certain people in her life and that the suppression of those feelings was contributing to her jaw pain. She greatly appreciated the support she was receiving through massage therapy and from her dentist. As part of a home care plan, she was taught deep abdominal breathing to incorporate as a stress reduction technique to help minimize nighttime teeth clenching.

REFERENCES

1. Benjamin BE. Are you tense? The Benjamin system of muscular therapy: tension relief through deep massage and body care. 1st ed. New York, NY: Pantheon Books, 1978: 10.
2. Kogan G, ed. Your body works: a guide to health energy and balance. Berkeley, CA: Transformation Press, 1981: 34.
3. Benjamin BE. Are you tense? The Benjamin system of muscular therapy: tension relief through deep massage and body care. 1st ed. New York, NY: Pantheon Books, 1978: 4.

GLOSSARY OF TERMS

Brachial plexus—the network of nerves that supply the arm, forearm, and hand. It is made up of lower cervical and upper dorsal spinal nerves.

Chakra—a Sanskrit word meaning "wheel." The chakras are seven subtle energy centers located along the spine that correspond in location to the major endocrine glands. They are responsible for governing functions on the physical, mental, and emotional levels.

Conception vessel—one of the two central meridians, along with the governing vessel. It runs up the front of the body from the perineum to the brain. It regulates all the yin channels in the body.

Enarthrosis—a ball-and-socket joint.

External occipital protuberance (EOP)—a prominence at the center of the outer surface of the squama of the occipital bone which gives attachment to the ligamentum nuchae.

Facilitated nerve pathways—routes developed within the neural structures from areas of hyperirritation to other segments of the musculoskeletal system.

Fibrils—minute fibers located in the sarcoplasm of muscle fibers.

Fingertip raking—a cross fiber stroke executed with the finger pads of one hand. The fingers stroke back and forth perpendicular to the direction the muscle fibers are running while remaining in contact with the skin.

Golgi tendon organ—a nerve receptor located in muscle tendons that senses tension, or stretching.

Hara—a Japanese word that refers to the core of the body, the abdominal-pelvic cavity, where the life force is concentrated.

Meridians—also known as channels. They are energetic pathways often associated with the organs. Meridians distribute qi throughout the body.

Muscle spindles—also called intrafusal fibers. Spindles are a specialized type of muscle fiber arranged in bundles within the larger muscle fibers. They register changes in the length of muscle fibers.

Pronation—a rotational movement. A pronated foot is rotated so that the plantar surface faces in a lateral or outward direction. In standing, the medial arch is collapsed, placing more weight on the medial side of the foot.

Qi—a Chinese word referring to the vital life force.

Qi gong—exercises design to cultivate or enhance the level of qi in the body.

Referred pain zone—a site within the myofascial tissues that registers pain, numbness, weakness, or paresthesia from a stimulus originating in another area.

Reflex arcs—nerve feedback loops operating through the spinal cord that link the sensory and motor systems. They monitor and direct muscle actions, mostly at an unconscious level.

Shingles—a Swedish massage stroke. It is a variety of effleurage that utilizes an overlapping movement of the hands where one hand replaces the other continuously.

Soft fist—a hand position used in Shiatsu. It is a modification of a fist, with the distal phalanges of the fingers held in an extended position instead of tucked in against the palm.

Sternocleidomastoid (SCM)—the largest neck flexor.

Temporomandibular joint (TMJ)—articulation of the mandible with the temporal bone of the cranium.

Thumb sweep—a cross fiber stroke done with the broad side of the thumb. The thumb rolls back and forth across the muscle to release adherent fibers and spread the fascia.

Tiger's mouth—a hand position incorporated in Shiatsu in which pressure is exerted on a limb with one or both hands using the webbing between the thumb and index finger.

Two-joint muscle—a muscle that crosses two joints, influencing the actions of both.

Yang—the primary energetic movement of expansion or dispersion. Its qualities include light, heat, action, and dryness.

Yin—the primary energetic movement of contraction or congealing. Its qualities include dark, cold, stillness, and dampness.

Yoga—an ancient self-development system from India with several branches that emphasize meditation, postures, breathing, service, devotion, and knowledge.

BIBLIOGRAPHY

Agur AMR, Lee MJ. Grant's atlas of anatomy. 10th ed. Baltimore, MD: Lippincott Williams & Wilkins, 1999.

Chaitow L. Muscle energy techniques. New York, NY: Churchill Livingstone, 1996.

Chapman CF. Medical dictionary for the non-professional. Woodbury, NY: Barron's Education Series, 1984.

Clemente CD. Anatomy: a regional atlas of the human body, Baltimore, MD: Urban and Schwarzenberg, 1987.

Dychtwald K. Bodymind. Los Angeles, CA: Jeremy Tarcher, 1977.

Fahey BW. The power of balance: a Rolfing view of health. Portland, OR: Metamorphous Press, 1989.

Finando D, Finando F. Informed touch: a clinician's guide to the evaluation and treatment of myofascial disorders. Rochester, NY: Healing Arts Press, 1999.

Fritz S. Mosby's fundamentals of therapeutic massage. St. Louis, MO: Mosby Year-Book, 1995.

Gillanders A. The joy of reflexology: healing techniques for the hands and feet to reduce stress and reclaim health. Boston, MA: Little, Brown and Co., 1995.

Heller J, Henkin WA. Bodywise: regaining your natural flexibility and vitality for maximum well-being. New York, NY: Jeremy P. Tarcher, 1986.

Kurtz R, Hector D. The body reveals: what your body says about you. New York, NY: Harper & Row, 1977.

McCellan S, Monte T. Integrative acupressure: a hands-on guide to balancing the body's structure and energy for health and healing, New York, NY: Berkeley Publishing Group, 1998.

Menkin D. Transformation through bodywork: using touch therapies for inner peace. Santa Fe, NM: Bear & Company, 1996.

Norking CC, Levangie PK. Joint structure and function: a comprehensive analysis. 2nd ed. Philadelphia, PA: FA Davis, 1992.

Olsen A, McHose C. Body stories: a guide to experiential anatomy. Barrytown, NY: Station Hill Press, 1991.

Peters LM. Manual muscle testing: a visual guide. Atlanta, GA: Susan Hunter Publishing, 1986.

Rolf IP. Rolfing: the integration of human structures. New York, NY: Harper and Row, 1977.

Scheumann DW. Deep tissue therapy student training guide. Atlanta, GA: Atlanta School of Massage Press, 1994.

Sweigard L. Human movement potential: its ideokinetic facilitation. New York, NY: Dodd, Mead, and Company, 1975.

Thomas CL, ed. Taber's cyclopedic medical dictionary. Philadelphia. PA: FA Davis, 1989.

Todd ME. The thinking body. Brooklyn, NY: Dance Horizons, 1972.

Travell JG, Simmons DG. Myofascial pain and dysfunction: the trigger point manual. Baltimore, MD: Williams & Wilkins, 1992: 1, 2.

Travis JW, Regina SR. Wellness workbook. 2nd ed. Berkeley, CA: Ten Speed Press, 1988.

Zemach-Bersin D, Zemach-Bersin K, Reese M. Relaxercise: the easy new way to health and vitality. New York, NY: Harper Collins, 1990.

Index

Page numbers in italics followed by f denote figures; those followed by t denote tables.